Health Organizations: Theory, Behavior, and Development

Edited by

James A. Johnson, PhD

JONES AND BARTLETT PUBLISHERS
Sudbury, Massachusetts
BOSTON   TORONTO   LONDON   SINGAPORE

World Headquarters
Jones and Bartlett Publishers
40 Tall Pine Drive
Sudbury, MA 01776
978-443-5000
info@jbpub.com
www.jbpub.com

Jones and Bartlett Publishers
Canada
6339 Ormindale Way
Mississauga, Ontario L5V 1J2
Canada

Jones and Bartlett Publishers
International
Barb House, Barb Mews
London W6 7PA
United Kingdom

Jones and Bartlett's books and products are available through most bookstores and online booksellers. To contact Jones and Bartlett Publishers directly, call 800-832-0034, fax 978-443-8000, or visit our website www.jbpub.com.

Substantial discounts on bulk quantities of Jones and Bartlett's publications are available to corporations, professional associations, and other qualified organizations. For details and specific discount information, contact the special sales department at Jones and Bartlett via the above contact information or send an email to specialsales@jbpub.com.

Copyright © 2009 by Jones and Bartlett Publishers, LLC

All rights reserved. No part of the material protected by this copyright may be reproduced or utilized in any form, electronic or mechanical, including photocopying, recording, or by any information storage and retrieval system, without written permission from the copyright owner.

This publication is designed to provide accurate and authoritative information in regard to the Subject Matter covered. It is sold with the understanding that the publisher is not engaged in rendering legal, accounting, or other professional service. If legal advice or other expert assistance is required, the service of a competent professional person should be sought.

Production Credits
Publisher: Michael Brown
Production Director: Amy Rose
Associate Editor: Katey Birtcher
Production Editor: Tracey Chapman
Production Assistant: Roya Millard
Marketing Manager: Sophie Fleck
Manufacturing Buyer: Therese Connell
Composition: Arlene Apone
Cover Design: Kristin E. Ohlin
Cover Image: © Andy Platt/ShutterStock, Inc.
Printing and Binding: Malloy, Inc.
Cover Printing: Malloy, Inc.

Library of Congress Cataloging-in-Publication Data
Health organizations : theory, behavior, and development / [edited by] James A. Johnson.
   p. ; cm.
Includes bibliographical references and index.
ISBN-13: 978-0-7637-5053-4 (pbk.)
ISBN-10: 0-7637-5053-0 (pbk.)
1. Health services administration. 2. Organizational behavior. 3. Organizational sociology. I. Johnson, James A., 1954-
[DNLM: 1. Health Facilities--organization & administration. 2. Models, Organizational. 3. Organizational Culture. WX 100 H4345 2008]
   RA971.H398 2008
   362.1068--dc22
                                    2007023328

6048

Printed in the United States of America
12 11 10 09 08   10 9 8 7 6 5 4 3 2

ACKNOWLEDGMENTS

Many thanks to the talented and tireless authors who contributed to this book and to the publisher, Michael Brown, for encouraging me to do it. As always, I remain grateful to my three children, Allen, Adam, and Elizabeth for the inspiration they provide me everyday, simply by being who they are.

CONTENTS

FOREWORD

During the last ten years in my work, I have had the privilege of visiting numerous healthcare organizations; some expansive healthcare organizations with unlimited resources, others, small community hospitals with limited resources; all have endured significant new demands and unexpected challenges.

The world has witnessed unprecedented events that have affected the foundation of health care. The September 11th terrorist attacks and multiple natural disasters, such as Hurricane Katrina, have impacted different healthcare organizations in ways that we never envisioned. With globalization and the push for universal care in many states, there has been a ripple effect throughout society.

Other new requirements have surfaced for healthcare organizations. Much is known about the impact of medical errors on the patient population. As an effort to develop a body of basic rules of engagement to improve the care provided to the patient population and to guarantee safety to the patients, the National Patient Safety Goals have been instituted to address some of the concern. Only the healthcare organizations with well-developed organization structures have succeeded with its implementation. Others, not so well organized, are still struggling with such tasks.

Finally, much is known about the limited human resources (ex. nurses shortage), the aging healthcare infrastructure, and the struggle organizations go through in an attempt to adjust to various regulations imposed by the agencies that govern the industry. Some organizational behaviorist has described misalignment between human resources and capital resources as the factors that have lead to a less than desirable outcome in health care. Those, with sound and sometimes adaptable organizational structures, who have integrated their human and capital resources by aligning all of their resources, have succeeded in the face of the various stressors we have seen.

Healthcare organization theory has often focused on extending the concepts of business organizations applied to the healthcare field. Much of the knowledge about healthcare organization theory has been an extrapolation of the concepts developed to explain how businesses organize. Until now, there has been no integrated view on healthcare organization theory.

This book comes as a much-needed initiative of Dr. James Allen Johnson and a group of scholars and experts in an attempt fill a void existent in health administration education. It provides an integrated view of Organization Theory; Organization Behavior; and Organization Development making it one of the first books on the integration of these three critical interconnected domains.

Integrated knowledge and understanding is needed in health care in order to prepare organizations for an uncertain future. This compendium of knowledge will attract significant attention from the healthcare administration and public health academic communities with its potential to enhance the professional development and education of our future leaders.

Lorenzo Gonzalez, MD
The Joint Commission

PREFACE

This book was written to address a significant need in health administration education. While there are many textbooks available for courses in organizational behavior, there are few that address organization theory and even fewer that discuss organization development in any significant way. Many university professors and instructors prefer to have a text that addresses all three domains. Drawing upon the expertise and experience of colleagues in various disciplines from universities, government, and corporations, I have brought these three interconnected domains together in this book. It is comprised of three sections: Part I Organization Theory; Part II Organization Behavior; and Part III Organization Development; each containing key chapters that address foundations, research, and new directions. A summary of these themes follows:

Organization Theory: Health organizations are complex human systems that have evolved over time and continue to do so. There have been many theories drawing from the fields of psychology, sociology, economics, political science, anthropology, and, lately, physics in an attempt to explain the phenomenon of organization. Each of the theories has changed as social science and behavioral research offered new findings and perspectives on human behavior in groups and larger aggregates. The classical theories of organization were primarily mechanistic and relied heavily on the knowledge advanced in the industrial age. Modern organization theory takes more of a contingency approach and accounts for human dynamics. Today, emerging theories draw upon new insights from biology and physics where organizations are seen as systems interconnected with the larger environment. Postmodern theory and our increasing understanding of complexity take us even further.

Organization Behavior and Dynamics: By virtue of their distinct care mission, health organizations have unique behavioral qualities. This book examines power, influence, conflict, motivation, group dynamics, values, communication, and leadership in the context of care giving. Additionally, organization dysfunction and stakeholder dynamics is addressed. Health organizations are comprised of highly credentialed professionals who function under considerable scrutiny within many prescribed guidelines. The challenge of managing in this environment is great. The bases of any level of effectiveness come from the understanding of individual, group, and organization behavior.

Organization Change and Development: Lastly, health organizations are not static. The one constant seems to be change. Leaders and managers are tasked to facilitate and manage the change that is inevitable in modern organizations. This can be done in a systematic planned way utilizing approaches found in organization development and team building. This section of the book helps the student and practitioner put to use theories of organization and knowledge of organization behavior in ways that foster change in productive and sustainable ways resulting in better outcomes. Team development, board development, physician development, and organization development and learning are all addressed. Likewise, current challenges such as disaster preparedness, globalization, and sustainability are discussed.

As you read the book and engage in the discussions and exercises recommended in each chapter, it is important to remember the significant responsibility you have as a current or future healthcare manger and leader. You will have a responsibility to yourself, co-workers, the organization, and the individuals and communities you serve. Part of this responsibility can be met by committing to life-long learning and continuously seeking to better understand physical and social phenomena. This includes an understanding of organizations as human created systems. As our insightful colleague, Margaret Wheatley once said, "Rather than thinking of organization as an imposed structure, plan, design, or role, it is clear that in life, organization arises from the interactions and needs of individuals who have decided to come together." It is in this coming together that purpose manifests and then demonstrates the great potential of health organizations in making the world a better place for all.

James A. Johnson, PhD

CONTRIBUTORS

Ahmed Adu-Oppong, PhD

Program in Health Services Administration
Jiann-Ping Hsu College of Public Health
Georgia Southern University

Lee W. Bewley, MHA, PhD, FACHE

US Army Medical Department
Army-Baylor Program in Health and Business Administration
Baylor University

M. Nicholas Coppola, MHA, PhD, FACHE

Health Sciences Center
Texas Tech University

Jo-Ann Costa

Hughes Corporation (Retired)

Mark A. Cwiek, MHA, JD, FACHE

Doctoral Program in Health Administration
Herbert and Grace Dow College of Health Professions
Central Michigan University

Mark L. Diana, MBA, MSIS, PhD

Department of Health Systems Management
School of Public Health and Tropical Medicine
Tulane University

Dawn Erckenbrack, MHA, EdD, FACHE

Health Program Analysis and Evaluation
Office of the Assistant Secretary for Health Affairs
US Department of Defense

Dmitry A. Erofeev, MA, PhD

Express Personnel Services

Dennis G. Erwin, MST, DHSc, CPA

E2 Consulting Group

Rupert M. Evans, Sr., MPA, DHA, FACHE

Division of Health Administration
College of Health Professions
Governors State University

Andrew N. Garman, MS, PsyD

Department of Health Systems Management
College of Health Sciences
Rush University

Sharon Glazer, MS, PhD

Department of Psychology
College of Social Sciences
San Jose State University

Lorenzo Gonzalez, MD

The Joint Commission

David R. Graber, MPH, PhD

Department of Health Administration and Policy
College of Health Professions
Medical University of South Carolina

Lana V. Ivanitskaya, MA, PhD

Doctoral Program in Health Administration
Herbert and Grace Dow College of Health Professions
Central Michigan University

James A. Johnson, MS, MPA, PhD

Doctoral Program in Health Administration
Herbert and Grace Dow College of Health Professions
Central Michigan University

Michele E. Jordan, EdD

School of Education
University of Texas at Austin

Gerald R. Ledlow, MHA, PhD, FACHE

Program in Health Services Administration
Jiann-Ping Hsu College of Public Health
Georgia Southern University

Reuben R. McDaniel, Jr., MS, EdD

Department of Information, Risk, and Operations Management
McCombs School of Business
University of Texas at Austin

Peter C. Olden, MHA, PhD

Department of Health Administration and Human Resources
Panuska College of Professional Studies
University of Scranton

Mary S. O'Shaughnessy, MS, MHSA, DHA

Department of Health Services Administration
College of Health Professions
University of Detroit Mercy

James H. Stephens, DHA, FACHE

Program in Health Administration
College of Health and Human Services
Ohio University

James Whitlock, DHA, FACHE

Healthcare Management Program
Department of Business Administration
Brenau University, Georgia

Sudha Xirasagar, MD, PhD

Department of Health Policy and Management
Arnold School of Public Health
University of South Carolina

ABOUT THE EDITOR

Dr. James Allen Johnson, Jr. is a Professor in the Herbert and Grace Dow College of Health Professions at Central Michigan University. He is also a medical social scientist working in international health development. He has published 10 books and over 100 articles on a wide range of healthcare and management issues. His most recent book is *Managing Health Education and Promotion: Leadership for the 21st Century* published by Jones and Bartlett of Sudbury, MA. Dr. Johnson is the past Editor of the *Journal of Healthcare Management* published by the American College of Healthcare Executives and was Senior Editor for the *Journal of Management Practice*. He is the founding editor of the *Carolina Health Policy and Management Review* and has been a Special Issue Editor for the *Journal of Management Development;* the *Journal of Health and Human Services Administration;* the *Organizational Ethics Journal;* and the *Journal of Health Administration Education.* Additionally, he is the Senior Editor of the Praeger series, *Community Preparedness,* and Co-Editor of the *Handbook of Health Administration and Policy.* Dr. Johnson's work and travels have taken him to 21 different countries including work with the World Health Organization and organization development consultation with numerous hospitals, government agencies, and health organizations. He has chaired and served on many non-profit boards, most recently the National Diabetes Trust Foundation. Dr. Johnson was previously on the faculty of the Medical University of South Carolina where he served as Chair of the Department of Health Administration and Policy for many years and was the founding director of the Doctor of Health Administration Program. He has also lectured at Oxford University in England; Beijing University in China; the University of Colima in Mexico; the University of Dublin in Ireland; and is an Adjunct Professor at Auburn University Montgomery. His PhD is from Florida State University.

PART

I

Organization Theory and Foundations

"Whenever a theory appears to you as the only possible one, take this as a sign that you have neither understood the theory nor the problem, which it was intended to solve."

Karl Popper

CHAPTER

1

Introduction

James A. Johnson and Peter C. Olden

As long as there have been human endeavors, there have been people engaged in organizing.[1] Perhaps even nature itself, as a system, is involved in the processes of organizing.

Probably the natural emergence of organization grew out of our instinct for survival. In the hostile world of early humankind, food, shelter, and safety needs usually required cooperative efforts, and cooperative efforts required some form of organization. Certainly, the patriarchal system vested leadership in the heads of early families. The oldest member of the family was the most experienced and presumed to be the wisest member of the family and thus was the natural leader.

Complex forms of organization were required and did evolve as families grew into tribes and tribes evolved into nations. The earliest written record, the clay tablets of the Sumerians, recorded division of labor and supervision practices. In Sumerian society, as in many others since then, the wisest and best leaders were thought to be the priests and other religious leaders.

Likewise, the ancient Babylonian cities developed very strict codes, such as the code of Hammurabi. King Nebuchadnezzar used color codes to control production of the hanging gardens and there were weekly and annual reports, norms for productivity, and rewards for piecework.

The Egyptians organized their people and their slaves to build cities and pyramids. Construction of one pyramid, around 5000 B.C., required the labor of 100,000 people working for approximately 20 years. Planning, organizing, and controlling were essential elements.

China perfected military organization based on line-and-staff principles and used these same principles in the early Chinese dynasties. Confucius wrote parables that offered practical suggestions for public administration.

The city-states of ancient Greece were commonwealths, with councils, courts, administrative officials, and boards of generals. Socrates talked about management as a skill separate from technical knowledge and experience. Plato wrote about specialization and proposed notions of a healthy republic.

Many think the Roman Empire was so successful because of the Romans' great ability to organize the military and conquer new lands. Similarly, those sent to govern the far-flung parts of the empire were effective administrators and were able to maintain relationships with the other provinces and the empire as a whole.

There are numerous other ancient examples of organization development, such as Hannibal leading a massive army across the Alps, Alexander the Great building a vast interconnected empire, and the first emperor of China building the Great Wall. Many of the practices employed today in leading, managing, and administering modern organizations have their origins in antiquity.

The Industrial Revolution created a need for new thinking and the refinement of old thinking. However, modern management theory, as discussed in this book and applied specifically to health organizations, is primarily a phenomenon of the 20th century with new theoretical constructs and practices emerging now in the early 21st century.

Today organizations have become a constant part of people's lives. Most people spend their professional lives working in an organization. Additionally, they spend their personal lives in and with organizations (e.g., churches, children's soccer leagues, clubs, and civic groups). The advance of healthcare organizations can best be described as rapid and increasingly diverse and complex. Thus, students who intend to become healthcare managers will benefit by studying organization theory, behavior, and development. Understanding healthcare organizations will invariably improve their performance as leaders in their future careers.

■ STUDYING ORGANIZATIONS

Studying organization theory and learning about organization dynamics can be exciting, interesting, revealing, and rewarding. However, it may involve a different kind of learning than some students are used to. This book has many theories, principles, concepts, and abstract ideas—that is the nature of the material. Compared to some subjects and courses, the content is less exact and objective and has fewer absolutes. For example, answers to questions may be "contingent" on context or situations—just like what we experience with organizations in the real world. Students who come from "hard science" backgrounds or clinical professions might have to adjust to become comfortable with ambiguity and the "it all depends" concept. Students can learn about organizations and "bring to life" the conceptual content of this chapter by using methods presented in the rest of this chapter. By using these active learning methods and working with the content of this book, the students will increase understanding of organization theory, behavior, and development. These methods are interactive and may overlap.

Higher-Level Thinking

Bloom's taxonomy of educational objectives identifies six cognitive domains or levels of learning.[2] These are

1. Knowledge (e.g., identify, define, list, describe)
2. Comprehension (e.g., rewrite, explain, predict, summarize)
3. Application (e.g., compute, modify, prepare, use)
4. Analysis (e.g., simplify, outline, examine, diagram)
5. Synthesis (e.g., combine, categorize, develop, plan)
6. Evaluation (e.g., compare, contrast, justify, assess)

Undergraduate education is likely to emphasize lower levels of learning, whereas graduate education should move toward higher levels of learning. Students can develop understanding of organizations by using all of these domains of thinking, especially the higher ones. That will help later in careers, because managing healthcare organizations requires much analysis, synthesis, and evaluation.

Faculty instructors will likely create assignments and class activities that require higher-level thinking. Students will benefit from these and should work hard in completing them. For example, faculty instructors may require students to analyze a local healthcare organization by applying concepts (e.g., mission, goals, structure, and culture) from this book. Students might ask to compare and contrast a primary care medical group with a safety net primary care clinic. These types of learning activities can be done alone or in small groups. The more a student does these assignments and discusses them with others, the more the student will develop the ability to think about organizations (healthcare organizations, in particular).

Besides fulfilling assignments and activities that come from courses and faculty, students may develop their own exercises. Students should get in the habit of examining, analyzing, and evaluating organizations. By doing so, they will begin to develop a mental framework with which they can examine and understand organizations during their careers. Physicians develop a mental framework with which they examine and understand patients. Managers need to develop a mental framework with which they can examine and understand organizations. Students are also urged to reflect on what they learn and then try to link it to their own personal experiences. Students can reflect on organizations they have worked in or interacted with by using theory, principles, and concepts presented in this book: Which of these have they observed in organizations? Which approaches to organization seem most common? Which of these would students prefer in a work situation?

Experiential Learning

Students can strengthen their learning of this book's theories, principles, concepts, terms, and methods by using experiential learning. Didactic classroom learning is important, but it is not sufficient to only learn about organization. Faculty can provide experiential learning opportunities and students should enthusiastically pursue these to more fully learn what is offered in this book. This includes:

1. Problem solving
2. Case studies
3. Organizational analysis
4. Small group discussions (practicing organization behavior)
5. Debate
6. Interviewing healthcare executives

John Dewey reported almost a century ago that an effective way to learn is through solving meaningful problems.[3] Students, with guidance from faculty and others, should engage themselves in solving problems of organizational theory, behavior, and development in healthcare organizations. For example, students can suggest how to apply the concepts and principles in this book to the urgent problem of medical errors and to "cross the quality chasm" in healthcare. Case studies also provide realistic problems for which students can try ideas and discuss them with others to consider various possible solutions. Finally, students might conduct an organizational analysis, in which they analyze a healthcare organization from an organization theory perspective.[4] Students would select a healthcare organization and then use concepts from this book to examine the organization's mission, goals, structure, culture, groups, teams, coordination, learning, and so forth.

Students can develop their understanding through discussion in small groups (in which students may feel more comfortable) and then in the class as a whole. In their discussions, students can practice group skills, reflect on their group's behavior and interaction, and experience organizational behavior principles in their small groups. Students may also debate current issues related to topics in this book: Should healthcare organizations change radically or incrementally? Should organizations empower employees more? After the debate, students can reflect on the process and dynamics of the group activity.

Students can also learn about and study organizations by interacting with managers and clinicians working in healthcare settings. Students tour organizations and then ask healthcare executives specific questions based on chapters and theories in this book. Perhaps, students will also want to "shadow" a manager and observe the organizational behavior first hand. A more substantial approach to applied learning is fieldwork, such as an administrative internship or residency, typically done after coursework is completed.

Competency Development

Health administration education at the graduate level is becoming more competency-based, similar to graduate education in other professional fields. Healthcare organizations' stakeholders expect healthcare managers to demonstrate competencies.[5-7] Employers, professional associations (e.g., Association of University Programs in Health Administration and American College of Healthcare Executives), and accreditors (e.g., Commission on Accreditation of Healthcare Management Education) expect health administration students (especially at the graduate level) to become competent in organization theory, behavior, learning, administration, and management.

Determine students' competencies by multiple factors—including the students themselves. The old saying "you can lead a horse to water but you can't make it drink" applies here. Students themselves must want—and take responsibility—to learn and become competent. Faculty can lead students to the skills, knowledge, and abilities presented in this book. Then students must invest the time, energy, and effort needed to learn, study, practice, think, and eventually develop competencies in organizational theory, behavior, and development. While achievement of competencies will vary based on each student's prior education, experiences, stage-of-career, and other factors, students should approach this book and its academic course with the goal of developing their competencies. This will serve all very well throughout their professional careers.

Integrative Learning

As can be seen in the Table of Contents, organization theory, behavior, and development includes many topics and subtopics. Thus, students are urged to try to integrate these while reading the book and studying organizations. Think about how organization structure is related to the mission, and how those are related to the external environment. Think about how group behavior is affected by organizational culture. Discuss relationships and interactions among the theories, concepts, principles, and ideas in this book. And of course, the topics in this book are only some of what must be learned in a health administration curriculum and its many courses. Students may strengthen their understanding of this book's content by mentally integrating it with the content of other books and courses: How is organizational mission related to financial management? How does human resources management affect organizational development? How does strategic planning influence organizational outcomes? Are there reciprocal relationships? By thinking about these questions and discussing them with others, students can learn about healthcare organizations in ways that are theoretically solid and practically useful.

■ BEYOND THE CLASSROOM

Many often claim that there is nothing more useful than a good theory. Healthcare organizations and their leaders have at their core theories of action that guide them and shape them as they change and develop. The successful manager is a leader who fully understands organization theory, who is a keen observer of organization behavior, and who facilitates change in ways that foster organization development. Each student who reads this book has the opportunity to take a significant step in becoming just such a leader. In fact some of the readers may go on to develop their own theories that can be tested out in the world of practice. This is indeed one way a profession grows and how individuals come to be integral in that growth. Hopefully, the study of organizations will be an empowering experience and a fun endeavor.

References

1. Johnson JA, Breckon DJ. *Managing Health Education and Promotion Programs: Leadership Skills for the 21st Century.* Boston: Jones and Bartlett; 2007.
2. Bloom BS, (ed.). *Taxonomy of Educational Objectives, Handbook I: Cognitive Domains.* New York: Longmans, Green; 1956.
3. Dewey J. *Democracy and Education.* New York: Macmillan; 1916.
4. Olden PC. Teaching organization theory for health care management: Three applied learning methods. *J Health Adm Educ.* 2006; 23:39–52.
5. Bradley E. Use of evidence in implementing competency-based healthcare management teaching. *J Health Adm Educ.* 2003; 20:287–304.
6. Griffith JR. The impact of evidence on teaching health care management. *J Health Adm Educ.* 2003; 20:224–234.
7. Campbell CR, Lomperis AMT, Gillespie KN, Arrington B. Competency-based health care management education. *J Health Adm Educ.* 2006; 23:135–168.

2

Anatomy and Physiology of Theory

M. Nicholas Coppola

Learning Objectives

- Describe the anatomy and physiology of theory.
  - What are the elements and how do they relate?

- Explain the utility of theory in the study of organization behavior.

- Describe a conceptual model.
  - How do conceptual models relate to theory?

- Describe the importance of theory in relation to other chapters in this book.

■ INTRODUCTION

The word theory comes from the Greek word *theorein,* which means "to look at" or, "to contemplate the divine." This chapter discusses the anatomy and physiology of theory while providing important tools and skills that will enable the reader to not only understand, model, and describe complex theories, but also have the ability to deconstruct theory into individual components. This is a very important skill for understanding many of the important concepts in the rest of this textbook. Failing to understand theory and theoretical elements will make it very difficult to understand the meaning of other important concepts presented in this book.

Why Study Theory in Organization Behavior?

Understanding the theoretical properties of complex issues is important to burgeoning executives. This is due to the dynamics of the fast-paced world we live in today. Executives are continually placed in positions where it is necessary to have a greater understanding of complex models that relate to organizational life cycles, bureaucracy, institutional dynamics, employee satisfaction, economic demands, and organizational efficiency, effectiveness, and value—to name only a few leader priorities that theory can help forecast and explain. As a result, understanding the value of theory is significant to the survival of any organization. Furthermore, understanding the complex parts and relationships within theory assists executives in framing problems, developing alternatives, and researching solutions. Without an understanding of theory and the roots therein, researchers, executives, and leaders are forced to make decisions based on opinions and individual heuristics rather than science and literature. Individuals who fail to understand the complexities of theory and how to adequately describe, model, and interpret theoretical models to their advantage will have a distinct disadvantage in the modern workforce. Lastly, an understanding of theory is a necessary precursor to building conceptual models in industry. Model building is a necessary precursor to performance-based management development, system examination, policy formulation, and conducting quantitative analysis. However, understanding the process of building empirically measurable models may be one of the more underrepresented aspects in industry today.

This chapter describes what a theory "is," what the individual parts of theory are (anatomy), and how these elements interrelate within a theoretical model (physiology). This chapter also describes how theories can be used to generate hypothesis, appropriate management research questions, and metrics for benchmarking, and process improvement initiatives. Finally, understanding how theories help in the development of conceptual models, assists in developing organization vision, mission, goal, and benchmarking objectives.

■ WHAT IS THEORY?

Theory is the primordial soup from which research questions, problem statements, and variables of interest are derived. Students should avoid "inventing" their own theory for solving management research. Numerous theories are available in the literature that will help young executives investigate issues relating to organizations, teams, and individuals. This book discusses and describes many such theories.

It is important to know that there is no one accepted definition of theory within the organization behavior literature. In layman's terms, a theory is an advanced form of an idea or an opinion that has some base in the empirical world. A leading theoretical scholar, Samuel Bacharach, has suggested (sic) "that a theory is a statement of relations among concepts within a set of boundary assumptions and constraints." Bacharach also suggests a theory is a coherent narrative composed of assumptions, abstract reasoning, and speculation, which describes and explains observed or experienced phenomenon's constructs, their interrelationships, and their boundaries. Bacharach goes on to suggest that a theory should answer the question of how, when and why, and that a theory should be logically consistent, able to be tested, and subject to disconfirmation (or falsification).[1]

Other authors have suggested that a theory must explain why variables and constructs come about and why they connect, while others suggest that the purpose of theory is to challenge and extend existing knowledge, within the limits of the critical bounding assumptions, through concise organization and clear communication of an idea. Additional authors challenge that the purpose of theory is to bring the components of complex phenomenon together in one understandable whole. Finally, one author has suggested that the purpose of theory is to extend existing knowledge, within the limits of the critical bounding assumptions, through concise organization and clear communication of an idea.[2–4]

Regardless of definition, a theory must be capable of support by qualitative measures or quantitative data. If a theory is incapable of initial development based on qualitative or quantitative properties, the burgeoning theory may not have evolved past the opinion or idea phase and may not be valuable to the profession or the advancement of knowledge.

As the science of organizational behavior has advanced over the last century, scholars have begun to have similar convergent thoughts in reference to theoretical elements and concepts. It is now possible to conceptually represent theory by suggesting biological metaphors. In this regard, elements of theory can be regarded as a biological unit where there is both anatomy and physiology.

Anatomy and Physiology of Theory

The anatomy of theory can be broken down into specific units of analysis. These units include the theory itself, followed by subordinate constructs, variables, and operationalized measures. An environment of discussion surrounds these elements. This enclosure is called bounded rationality. When discussing theoretical constructs, variables, and measures, it is first necessary to frame these elements within a plausible discussion group. By framing constructs, variables, and measures in a bounded rationality, an "out-of-bounds" area is presented that helps researchers stay within certain parameters of discussion.

Contained within this bounded rationality is the physiology of theory. The physiology of theory describes the interaction among constructs, variables, and measures, as well as other elements. In this regard, the interaction of constructs within theory is helpful for developing propositional statements. This is important in the early stages of qualifying theoretical relationships before quantitative data is available for testing or disconfirmation. Forming a more concrete and testable relationship within theory are the relationships between variables known as hypotheses. Propositional and hypothetical relationships are discussed in detail later in the chapter.

Also, contained within the bounded rationality of theory are contextual factors and confounders. Contextual factors are generally known elements that exist in the same environment as constructs, variables, and measures. The interaction of contextual factors on certain constructs and variables may be known in advance and can be controlled for through awareness and intervention. Confounders are properties in the environment that are generally not known in advance and may have interactive effects with theory that are not forecasted—or are difficult to predict.

Figure 2-1 depicts theory as a conceptual model for visual representation and understanding. A conceptual model is a "conceptual description" of the key elements of a study. The conceptual model should be parsimonious (simple) and offer graphic representations of theoretical elements that help outsiders understand the issue(s) being investigated at a glance. A conceptual model may include the actual theory, as well as constructs,

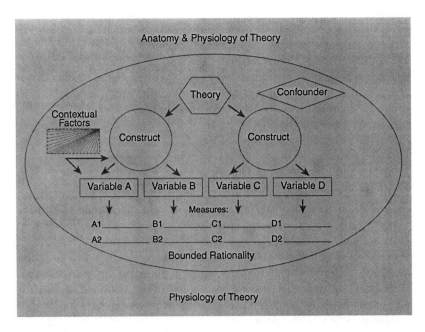

Figure 2-1 Conceptual Model of Theory.

variables, measures, confounders, and contextual factors; however, some conceptual models may only consider specific constructs as well as certain elements specific to the unit of analysis under study. Many of the models presented in this text will include a discussion of the actual theory itself, while other models may only present constructs for discussion.

The modeling of theory in Figure 2-1 is based on the early work on model building suggested by Bacharach, empirical measurement techniques in healthcare suggested by Wan, as well as other authors who have suggested that theoretical models should be simple, elegant, and consistent. This pictorial description and the relationship between theoretical parts will become clearer as the chapter progresses. [5–7]

■ ANATOMY OF THEORY

Constructs

The building blocks of theory are constructs. Throughout this text, students will encounter dozen of constructs. As a result, it is critical to the study of organization behavior to have a clear understanding of what a construct is. Failing to have a clear understanding of constructs will result in an inability to understand many of the concepts in subsequent chapters of this book.

Before defining a construct, it is first necessary to establish a *rule* for how constructs relate to theory. One constraint is that a valid theory must be capable of identification through at least two constructs. Failing to identify a theory by at least two constructs (similar to Figure 2-1), results in what scholars call tautology. Tautology implies a never-ending redundant cycle. The classic tautological statement is, "The sky is blue because it reflects the ocean, while the ocean is blue because it reflects the sky." This statement fails to clarify where the *blue* came from—the sky or the ocean. As a result, we are left in a revolving argument with no resolution. Accordingly, in order to adequately discuss theoretical properties, it is necessary to have two or more constructs in order to properly frame theoretical concepts and issues.

By definition, a construct is a latent variable that lacks empiricism (taste, touch, sight, smell, sound). Elements that are empirical have tangible, physical properties. For example, an apple possesses empiricism insofar that it can be tasted, touched, seen, and smelled. It does not matter that the apple does not make *noise*. Because an apple possesses four of the five empirical senses, we can say that an apple is not a construct because it can be rationalized through empirical properties. Any physical element or property that can be described through at least one of the five senses does not qualify as a construct.

A classic example of a construct is quality. Quality is a construct that cannot be discussed without identifying it through other measurable properties or variables. The classic statement "quality is in the eye of the beholder" generalizes the difficult problem we have describing quality. The discussions of other latent variables (such as efficiency, effectiveness, performance, satisfaction, organizational survival, leadership, success, and motivation) are all examples of constructs. This book discusses many of these constructs that cannot be universally discussed without first assigning empirical properties to them. The empirical property used to describe constructs is variables.

Variables

Flowing from constructs are variables. Variables are empirical units that are capable of identification through one of the five senses. Accordingly, a variable is an element that has precise meaning in the physical world. Generally, variables are universally understood and easily described. *Weight* is a good example of a variable. When discussing the concept of weight with peers or colleagues, universally understood concepts of pounds, ounces, or tons are immediately recognized as valid descriptors of weight. If a variable is incapable of a generalized descriptor, it may cause problems in describing theory. However, if the builder of the theoretical concept makes a careful argument for the use of certain variables—and defines them appropriately—the variable may have utility in helping frame the model. Similar to the tautological rule discussed previously, each construct within a theoretical model must be described using two or more variables.

Measures

Operationalized measures derive from variables. Measures are operationalized descriptions of variables that must be capable of numerical identification. Operationalizing is the process of quantifying a variable using appropriate, numerical-descriptive terms. Additionally, measures must be universally understood and are classically categorized as continuous (1 to n with n equal to infinity), dichotomous or binary (yes or no, on or off, etc.), or finally, categorical (such as Caucasian, African American, Latino, etc.). If measures are incapable of being operationalized through continuous, dichotomous, or categorical identification, the measure may not have enough precise significance to be valid in describing or testing the theoretical model under study.

Variables should be capable of several different methods of operationalization. For example, the variable *age* can be operationalized as a continuous, categorical, or a binary variable depending on how the researcher chooses to define and measure the age variable. The following section discusses this process.

Operationalizing Measures

In order to operationalize the variable age, we first must associate the variable with a specific unit of analysis (such as an organization, team, or individual). Next, we create a brief definition of the variable age that supports the unit of analysis under study. For example, we may say that age is defined as the number of years associated with a human individual's life. This statement includes two important features. One, it qualifies age in terms of years. Secondly, it provides a reference group for age where a potential range for a life span is universally understood. Given this information, it is possible to operationalize age in several different ways: One, as a continuous variable; two, as a binary variable; and three, as a categorical variable, Table 2-1.

In Table 2-1, we arbitrarily establish cutoff points for categorical and dichotomous variables that help support the issue under study. The categorical description of age could have also been classified using quarter century marks or separated by five-year increments. The selection of a category is up to the executive analyzing the data. Finally, if the executive is interested in partitioning Medicare recipients from non-Medicare recipients, the age break at 65 provides opportunity to analyze the two different groups.

Not all variables lend themselves to operationalized measures through all three metrics. For example, the variable *racial category* does not lend itself to a continuous measure. The most appropriate nomenclature for race is a category where the researcher selects racial categories of interest in the study for analysis.

The process of operationalizing measures is critically important in the business world. A requirement to gather, manage, and measure outcomes from data is a continuous process. However, before collecting and analyzing data, operationalize it in a consistent and logical manner. The Balanced Score Card developed by Kaplan and Norton is an example of a quality tool that requires executives to not only select and define constructs of interest to measure, but also, valid and reliable variables capable of identification through operationalized measures that provide meaningful data for trend analysis.

Similar to variables and constructs, at least two operationalized measures should be considered for each variable in order to avoid tautological issues. While oftentimes it may only be necessary to operationalize a variable one way and achieve finality in the measurement

Table 2-1 Operationalized Age Variable
Define age as the number of years associated with a human individual's life.
Continuous: 1 to n.
Categorical: 0–10, 11–20, 21–30, 31–40, 41–50, 51–60, 61–70, 71–80, 81–90, 91–100, $n > 101$.
Binary: Medicare eligible? Yes or No (with Medicare eligibility being 65 years of age or older).

process, it is always a good idea to strategize alternative methods of measurement for each operationalized measure.

Code Sheets

The last step in operationalizing variables is the construction of a code sheet. Whenever testing variables in a hypothetical relationship, it is not the variables being tested but rather the operationalized units of the variables. This is a necessary precursor to loading data into statistical software like SPSS, SAS, Mimi-tab, or Excel. When we operationalize data for statistical software manipulation, we create code sheets.

A code sheet is a very simple explanation of how operationalized units of a variable will be used in the study. The researcher must keep in mind the assumptions of the test when building a code sheet. For example, parametric and nonparametric tests require different assumptions and these should be considered in the code sheet. While there are numerous examples for building a code sheet to demonstrate how data is operationalized in a study, the below table provides one proven example of success. The following code sheet is created for the variable "education" (Table 2-2).

In this code sheet of a single variable, each column contains very specific and mutually exclusive information about the variable that assists in measuring the theory under study.

1. Label: The actual name of the variable used.
2. Description: Define the variable here.
3. Operationalization: How is it coded?

Contextual Factors

Contextual factors are either variables or constructs that exist in the bounded rationality of the theory under study. Contextual factors generally have a known impact on the suggested relationships within the theoretical model. For example, in the proposed example of a conceptual model of nervousness in Figure 2-2, we can suggest that variables of

Table 2-2 Code Sheet Example for Variable Education		
Label	**Description**	**Operationalized**
Education	Highest education degree obtained by member	*Categorical*
		1 = HS
		2 = Community College
		3 = 4 yr College
		4 = Grad School
		5 = PhD
		6 = JD
		7 = MD

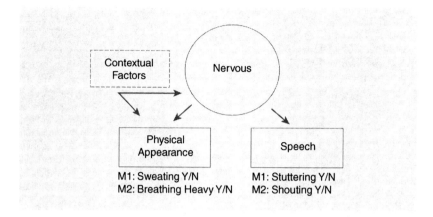

Figure 2-2 Conceptual Model of Nervousness.

physical appearance and an individual's speech pattern may be good indicators of an individual's level of nervousness. We might also suggest that the variables of physical appearance can be operationalized through measures of sweating (individual is or is not) and breathing heavy—a yes or no binary measure as well.

We may continue to suggest that speech is a good indicator of nervousness. If an individual is stuttering (yes or no), and if the individual is shouting (yes or no), the individual may be nervous. It may certainly be reasonable to suggest that if an individual is sweating, breathing heavy, shouting, and stuttering, the person may be nervous.

However, if we fail to take into account contextual factors, such as heat (perhaps it is a 100-degree day), the individual's physical condition (perhaps they are overweight and just walked up several flights of stairs), and the individual's medical condition (perhaps they are hard of hearing and on medication that impairs speech), it is possible to come to a completely incorrect assessment based on physical characteristics. In essence, contextual factors are elements in the environment that affect the outcomes of the constructs or measures we are trying to study. Contextual factors are difficult to identify in advance, but necessary to consider when building conceptual models of phenomenon.

Confounders

Similar to contextual factors, confounders are variables that exist in the bounded rationality of the environment that the researcher is unaware of in advance and cannot control for until after they are identified through alternate means. Confounders are spoilers or wild card factors that are usually identified after a conceptual model is built and testing begins. After confounders are identified through experimental testing or other means, they can be classified as contextual factors and controlled.

The infamous *Butterfly Ballot,* designed in Palm Beach County Florida and used during the 2000 presidential elections, is an excellent example of a confounder when studying voting theory. Local, state, and federal election officials were completely unaware that the unique design of the Butterfly Ballot would result in voter confusion, national controversy, and Supreme Court litigation before it was designed. The fact that it did, classifies the Butterfly Ballot as a confounding variable in the study of voting theory.

The *San Francisco Chronicle* suggested after the 2000 Presidential election that twelve percent of Florida Democrats (over 200,000 individuals) voted for Republican George Bush due to the poorly designed Butterfly Ballot. According to the official 2001 Statistics of the Presidential and Congressional Election of November 7, 2000, George W. Bush beat Al Gore in Florida by 543 votes. Had they discovered this confounding factor and "controlled" for it in advance, the 2000 presidential election would have resulted in a different outcome.

From this example, it is evident that confounding variables can have a significant effect on theoretical and conceptual models. Unfortunately, it is impossible to forecast the grave nature of the effect until after the confounder presents itself. However, once a confounder is identified, it can be recategorized as a contextual factor and controlled for by various means. In the case of the infamous Butterfly Ballot, entire districts in various states moved to completely eliminate paper-voting systems replacing these anachronistic tools with modern electronic voting machines. By doing this, election officials "controlled" for the possibility that voters would punch the wrong hole in a paper record by eliminating the paper record altogether.

The concept of controlling for confounders is a difficult subject and better addressed in a course on experimental design or quantitative analysis. However, an understanding of the likelihood that confounders are present in the environment and can affect assumptive outcomes of models is a necessary tenet of model building.

■ PHYSIOLOGY OF THEORY

Propositions

The physiology of theory can be described in terms of the relationships within the theatrical model. Two of these relationships are expressed in terms of hypotheses and propositions. A proposition is a statement of opinion, based on some degree of preliminary study or heuristics that is offered as a true or valid statement. While the statement may not always be true or valid, it is offered as such until evidence of disconfirmation is provided. The apomorphism that "Time is Endless" is an example of a propositional statement between constructs, (see Figure 2-3). In this example, Time is one construct and is related to a second construct of

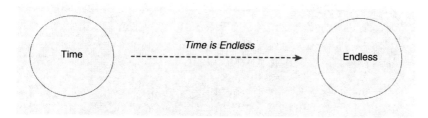

Figure 2-3 Propositional Statement.

Endless in order to form a propositional statement. The propositional statement can be helpful in the development of new opportunities for research and the formulation of new knowledge. The statement also assists in answering questions about the relationships between constructs.

Another classic example of a propositional statement combining constructs is "the right to bear arms." This propositional statement is offered as a statement of fact as is if it was true; however, the interpretive nature of this proposition continues to be readdressed in America every year.

It is no small wonder why the brightest legal minds in our country have debated on the meaning of this propositional statement for over 200 years. This propositional statement has also been interpreted differently by nearly every state in the union. Additionally, there continues to be new interpretive legislation regarding the propositional statement "the right to bear arms" every year (see Figure 2-4).

The difficulty with interpreting this propositional statement is the complex nature surrounding three culturally partisan latent variables of "rights," "bear," and "arms." As an exercise, students are encouraged to try to come up with two variables for each construct in the propositional statement, define each variable with two operationalized measures, and discuss contextual factors and confounders. Students are also encouraged to draw a conceptual model of this propositional statement using the modeling techniques discussed earlier. After this exercise, students will be able to understand the complex nature and difficulty in not only drawing conceptual models, but also operationalizing and defining them.

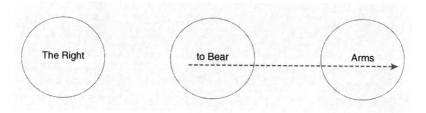

Figure 2-4 Propositional Statement of the Right to Bear Arms.

Although difficult to model and often resulting in different interpretive outcomes, several research articles reviewing healthcare delivery and leadership have utilized the proposition methodology to investigate construct relationships over the years.[8] Recent studies in manager competencies, critical thinking, and quality outcome assessment have also successfully used the proposition methodology to review phenomenon. Although sometimes referred to as concept mapping within the literature, the techniques, and methodologies are similar.[9] Regardless of name, the strength of utilizing the propositional technique is that it assists in generating propositional statements that can be used to guide the development of new variables to help define complex issues.[10]

Hypothesis

A hypothesis is a testable relationship between two variables. Furthermore, the purpose of hypothesis testing is to discover causal relationships between variables. Hypothesis statements are the foundation for all organizational research and form the basis for the advancement of knowledge. When writing a hypothesis, the researcher needs to follow very strict rules of design. From a reductionist point of view, in comparing two variables in a hypothetical relationship, there are generally five common methodologies for analysis.

1. One assumption is that there is no difference between variable 1 and variable 2 (null hypothesis).
2. The second assumption is that as one variable increases the other remains the same (positive relationship).
3. The third assumption is that as one variable decreases the other remains the same (negative relationship),
4. The fourth and fifth assumptions suggest that both variables will increase or both variables will decrease.

There may be some exceptions to these guidelines based on experimental design; however, these five hypothetical relationships form the basis for all hypothesis testing.

As an example, a classic hypothetical relationship may seek to discover the relationship between weight and blood pressure. One potential testable hypothesis may suggest that as weight increases, blood pressure increases. In this instance, weight may be classified as a continuous operationalized measure in pounds (1 to n), while blood pressure may be similarly classified as a continuous measure of systolic and diastolic indicators (again 1 to n). The same relationship can be tested with dichotomous units, a simple yes or no for weight increase, and a similar yes or no for outcome of blood pressure (see Figure 2-5).

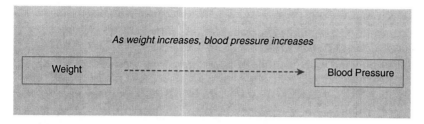

Figure 2-5 Hypothesis example.

In this example, it is first necessary to have a baseline for comparison and capture initial measures for both weight and blood pressure.

Baseline measures: Weight 185 pounds and blood pressure of 120/65 Measure after 6 months: Weight 205 pounds and blood pressure of 135/80

A simple visual inspection supports our initial hypothesis statement. If weight increased, but blood pressure remained the same, or decreased, we would fail to support our hypothesis.

It is incorrect to suggest that the hypothetical relationship is "proved" due to the fact that all hypothetical relationships are supported or not supported. It is incorrect parlance to suggest that a hypothesis is proved.

Hypothesis testing is often the way that the overall theory is falsified. Falsification is achieved through empirical testing of the various operationalized measures in theory. As a result, if a theory is not testable, the theory is not falsifiable in principle, and from an empirical viewpoint, is worthless to the field under study. For this reason, the falsifiability of theory is a necessary property of science. For a more detailed overview of designing and testing hypothetical relationships, encourage students to refer to their course text in research methods or quantitative analysis.

Research Questions

Building conceptual models supports the initial development of research questions. It is never a good idea to use opinions for guiding research questions; rather sound research questions should flow elegantly and easily from a given conceptual model. Similar to theory itself, positing research questions requires the understanding of certain rules and constraints in advance. For example, a research question supporting a conceptual model may include one or more of the following elements:

1. It must include the primary unit of analysis in the statement (i.e., organization, team, or individual).
2. It may include a reference to the environment, a construct, variable, or a contextual factor within the bounded rationality.

3. It may include the methodological tools used for measurement.
4. It must be a simple expression of one statement.

The following is an example of a good research question:

> *How do we measure the efficiency of hospitals*
> *with regression analysis?*

Note this research question has a unit of analysis (hospital), a primary construct (efficiency), and the tool to measure efficiency (regression analysis). Other details reference the research question can be addressed in other parts of the study.

Theoretical Application

Throughout this book, students will have the opportunity to learn about many different theories. Although not all the theories presented in this book lend themselves to easy conceptual modeling through the techniques discussed earlier in the chapter—all are capable of theoretical and conceptual modeling if careful study and analysis of the theory is performed. As a demonstration of the theoretical modeling principles, conceptually model Alderfer's theory of motivation.

In this instance, define motivation as the goal-directed behavior of individuals working in an organization. Alderfer's theory of motivation suggests that if an employer wants to motivate his or her employees that there are three distinct methodologies for doing this. Alderfer suggests that an employer should consider placing emphasis on three things: constructs of affiliation, power, or achievement. For the purpose of this conceptual model, we will only use the constructs of affiliation and achievement to demonstrate the utility of building the model. Remember that conceptual model building is as much an art as a science, so it is not always necessary to model all the parts of the theory.

The first step in the process is to completely define all the parts we are measuring and studying. Since we have already identified the theory, the second step is to identify our constructs. In our model (see Figure 2-6), we define affiliation as the types of opportunities employees have within the organization to join or participate in groups. In our suggested model, we define one group specifically as professional organizations. A professional organization may be something like the American Medical Association (AMA), American College of Healthcare Executives (ACHE), a professional honor society, or some other professional organization. We operationalize professional organizations through two measures of joining (operationalized as a dichotomous variable of yes or no), and advancing in that organization—perhaps to the standing of Fellow (yes or no).

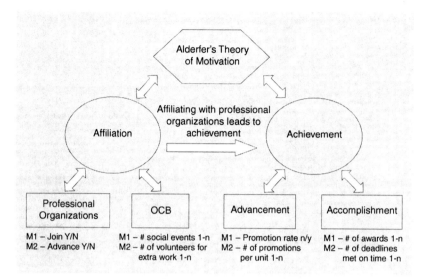

Figure 2-6 Alderfer's application of a conceptual model.

We may also suggest that the affiliation construct can be measured through the number of organization citizenship behaviors (OCB) within the organization. This might be measured by the number of social activities per month the employees in the organization engage in (measured by a continuous variable of 1 to *n*). We can also measure this construct by collecting data on how many people volunteer for extra work within the organization.

Apply the same methodology to the construct of achievement where this construct is measured by two variables of advancement and accomplishment. Define advancement as the promotion rate within the organization and the number of opportunities for advancement. Operationalize accomplishment by the number of awards an individual received and the total number of successful projects met on time.

A suggested propositional statement might be that affiliating with professional organizations leads to achievement. At face value, this propositional statement makes sense because it may be assumed that joining or advancing in a professional organization might make the employee more knowledgeable of job skills and, therefore, more likely to be promoted or become more efficient in his or her job. This may also be called face or construct validity.

As a test of one potential hypothesis, we could suggest the following:

Hypothesis 1: Individuals who join professional organizations have higher promotion rates than individuals who do not join professional organizations.

Once data is collected on each measure, and outcomes are known, this hypothesis can be tested. In this way, the theory can be supported or unsupported by hypothesis testing.

Not represented in this conceptual model are our bounded rationality, possible confounders, and contextual factors. These elements are important to consider when building theoretical or conceptual models, although it is not always necessary to include all parts of the anatomy and physiology of theory in each model. Only the parts necessary to convey the intent of the model are required.

As a teaching tip, students should notice in the aforementioned model that "advancement" is used as a measure of the professional organization variable and as the variable itself for the achievement construct. Similarly, "accomplishment" is used as a variable in this model; however, in a different model accomplishment may be used as a construct. If a construct is defined based on empirical properties, then it can be used as a variable—and sometimes as a measure. It is always incumbent on the builder of the theory to remember that there is both an art and science to model building. The science captures the anatomy and physiology of theory and the rules and constraints therein. However, it is incumbent on the builder to recognize the opportunities and possibilities in applying those elements. As long as elements are carefully defined, and sound research methodologies are used based on literature, the building of conceptual models becomes easy with practice.

■ CHAPTER SUMMARY

This chapter discussed what a theory is, the anatomy and physiology of theory, and provided a short application of model building technique as it applies to Alderfer's theory of motivation. The anatomy of theory includes constructs, variables, measures, confounders, and contextual factors within a bounded rationality. The physiology of theory includes the relationships between constructs called propositions, and the relationships between variables called hypotheses. When properly modeled and operationalized, an aptly built model of theory is essential in falsifying, supporting, and testing the theory.

Review/Discussion Questions

1. How can conceptual model building be used to explain the difficulty in understanding propositional phrases like *the right to bear arms.*?
2. Why is the understanding of confounders necessary in the development of conceptual models?
3. What is the difference between theory and a conceptual model?

4. What are the key differences between the anatomy of theory and the physiology of theory?
5. Why is it possible for a term to be used as a construct, variable, or measure? What must the builder consider before using the selected term?

Learning Activities

Exercise 1

1. Using the theoretical and conceptual modeling techniques you have learned, develop two variables and two measures for the latent variables. See Figure 2-7.

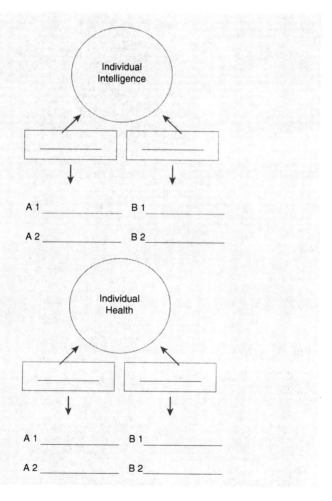

Figure 2-7 Chapter Exercise 1.

Exercise 2

1. Model the theory of motivation using two constructs, four variables, and eight measures. See Figure 2-8.
2. Use your measures to write two hypotheses relating to your theory.
3. Posit a proposition between your two constructs.

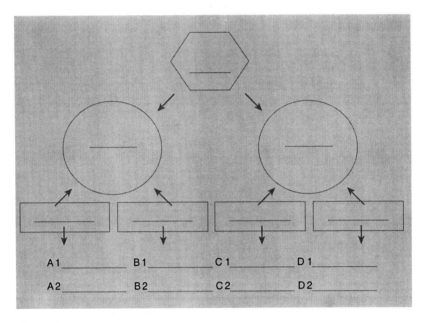

Figure 2-8 Chapter Exercise 2.

    A. Hypothesis 1
    B. Hypothesis 2
    C. Proposition
    D. Question: Where might you get data for these hypotheses?

References

1. Bacharach SB. Organizational theories: Some criteria for evaluation. *Acad Manage Rev.* 1989;14:490–495.
2. Whetten DA. What constitutes a theoretical contribution? *Acad Manage J.* 1989;14:490–495.
3. DiMaggio PJ. Comments on "What Theory Is Not." *Adm Sci Q.* 1995; 40:391–397.
4. Weick KE. What theory is not, theorizing is. *Adm Sci Q,* 1995; 40:385–390
5. Bacharach SB. Organizational theories: Some criteria for evaluation. *Acad Manage Rev.* 1989;14:490–495.

6. Wan TTH. *Evidence-Based Health Care Management—Multivariate Modeling Approaches.* Kluwer Publishers. Netherlands, 2002.

7. Donabedian A. Evaluating the quality of medical care. *Milbank Mem Fund Q.* 1966;44:166–206.

8. Coppola MN. A propositional perspective of leadership: Is the wrong head on the model? *Journal of International Research in Business Disciplines, Business Research Yearbook, International Academy of Business Disciplines.* 2004;11:620–625.

9. Edmondson KM, Smith DF. Concept mapping to facilitate veterinary students' understanding of fluid and electrolyte disorders. *Teach Learn Med.* 1998;10:21–33.

10. Simpson E, Courtney M. Critical thinking in nursing education: Literature review. *Int J Nurs Pract.*, 2002;8:89–98.

CHAPTER

3

Classical Theories of Organization

Peter C. Olden and Mark L. Diana

Learning Objectives

- Trace the evolution of early major theories of organization.
- Understand and explain contributions of scientific management.
- Understand and explain contributions of administrative theory.
- Understand and explain contributions of bureaucratic principles.
- Understand and explain contributions of human relations.
- Understand and explain contributions of administrative behavior.

■ INTRODUCTION

Organizing workers to achieve goals is perhaps as old as the human species, but the development of organization theory is much newer. Classical views of management began in the late 19th and early 20th centuries with the Industrial Revolution. Factories grouped together hundreds and thousands of workers into a much bigger scale of operations than before. Along with larger factories, there came larger universities, government agencies, hospitals, and other businesses and enterprises. This led to new problems of organizing and managing workers for maximum attainment of goals such as efficiency and productivity.

Theories of organization then evolved from different perspectives and schools of thought, and Perrow later grouped them into two broad categories: the mechanical school and the human relations school.[1] The mechanical approach to organizations viewed organizations as machines and emphasized, for example, centralized authority, division of labor, and rules. The human relations approach viewed organizations as groups of people, and emphasized, for example, trust in employees, interpersonal dynamics, and delegated authority. Alternatively, March and Simon divided classical organization theory into two contents—that which focused on physical production (e.g., Taylor's time and motion studies) and that which focused on larger problems of grouping workers and coordinating their work (e.g., Weber's writings on bureaucracy).[2]

The purpose of this chapter is to briefly explain the main contributions of five important approaches to organization theory: scientific management, administrative theory, bureaucratic principles, human relations, and administrative behavior. This is important for understanding the origin and intent of many management practices still in use today, either in part or in whole. The chapter next explains each of these five perspectives and then finishes with a summary, review questions, learning activities, and references.

■ SCIENTIFIC MANAGEMENT

Frederick W. Taylor, in his classic writings on management, stated "in the past the man has been first; in the future the system must be first" to help the worker achieve maximum productivity and efficiency and then be properly rewarded.[3] He believed that better management could help both the employer and the employee achieve greater prosperity while reducing what he perceived to be enormous waste, loss, and inefficiency throughout industries and the United States in general. Taylor argued that rather than management just searching for "better workers," it should apply systematic scientific management. Taylor (1895, 1903, 1911) had come to believe that management was a true science based on defined laws, principles, methods, and techniques, and that this science could be applied to all kinds of activities for big increases in productivity and efficiency. Based on that approach, he led the development of scientific management in the late 1800s and early 1900s.[3-5] His work was extended by Frank and Lillian Gilbreth[6] and Henry Gantt.[7,8]

Taylor argued and demonstrated that individual worker's tasks could be scientifically analyzed to determine how to achieve increased output with decreased energy and resource utilization. He conducted extensive studies of workers manufacturing steel that considered, for example, the design of a tool, availability of a tool for a worker, how a tool was held, how a tool was moved, and so forth. Taylor demonstrated his methods and proved their results, so others came to see his ideas were not unproven theory but instead were proven to work. An early study and experiments at the Bethlehem Steel Plant with pig iron workers became legendary.[3]

In the early 20th century, when Taylor developed his ideas, managers and workers were generally antagonistic toward each other. However, Taylor believed that both groups shared common interests and that each could not succeed without the other. Further, he believed both groups—not just the workers—were responsible for solving productivity and efficiency problems. Thus, he argued that management should assume more responsibility for results than it had previously.

One way Taylor believed that managers could help workers was to help them work in "the one best way." Too often, workers were left to figure out for themselves how to get their work done. Often, the same task might be done in dozens of ways—with some ways more efficient than others. Taylor believed there was "one best way" and one best tool or implement to perform a task, and he applied scientific methods to find it. The "one best method and best implement can only be discovered or developed through a scientific study and analysis of all of the methods and implements in use, together with accurate, minute, motion and time study . . . and the gradual substitution of science for rule of thumb."[3] This approach to management (sometimes called "Taylorism" or the Taylor System) required more planning and designing of work, and then training of workers to perform work in "the one best way."

Although Taylor's ideas began by focusing on individual workers, they expanded to management and led to new management processes and methods. Taylor expected managers each day to plan and write out in detailed instructions the next day's work tasks, methods, tools, time allowances, and so forth to enable workers to be more productive with less effort and waste. Further, the managers were to establish methods, rules, standards, actions, physical motions, tools, techniques, and systems—"the best way"—and then help workers understand all of this. In this way, managers and workers would be cooperative partners in achieving improved results. Managers were expected to pay higher wages to the laborers, so that everyone would gain from the higher productivity and output. Rue and Byers noted that piecework schemes (that pay workers based on the number of items produced regardless of the time taken to produce them) had been tried in production previously.[9] Those payment plans were mostly unsuccessful, because rates were based on weak standards and tradition. Taylor based rates on scientific empirical analysis and measurement that workers felt were fair, and Taylor expected this approach to be embraced by workers and managers alike.[3]

Taylor identified several main principles of scientific management:

1. Managers develop a science to determine the best way to perform each element of work.
2. Managers scientifically select the best worker for each job.

3. Managers scientifically educate, train, and develop the worker for the job.
4. Managers cooperate with workers and assure work follows scientific methods.
5. Managers share almost equally with workers the responsibility for work results.[3]

Taylor's work became known as scientific management, which was very different for managers and workers, and it led to better understanding and cooperation between both groups, because they used empirical measurement, the scientific method, experimentation, and research management to maximize output and minimize effort. This approach was applied to work conditions, equipment, procedures, and employee selection. It led to more worker specialization, which created the need for coordination, departmentalization, and other administrative principles discussed later. It also led to management control, because once work standards were set and agreed upon, managers could measure actual work achieved by an employee and compare it to standards. In this way, Taylor's focus on the specifics of the one best way to work also led to numerous changes in management and structure within the organization.[3]

Scientific management studied repetitive, simple, physical tasks in factory production or clerical work that could be clearly broken down and identified, and which had few mental or cognitive elements. The Gilbreths sought to further deconstruct work into basic activities—grasp, reach, turn, etc.—and established time standards.[6] However, this was confounded by the realization that the time to perform such actions depended on many other factors. They also analyzed muscle fatigue, speed, effort, skill, and other factors of human performance. Later disciples of Taylor (e.g., Henry Gantt and Carl Barth) expanded scientific management and applied it to other businesses and types of organizations, including those in municipal government and education.

The scientific management approach became widespread early in the 20th century, replacing traditional methods and "rule of thumb" standards. Many managers accepted it. However, some did not accept it because they felt it interfered with or reduced managers' role, judgment, and ability. As Scott points out, these studies and changes led to higher-level studies and changes in how work was organized, how tasks were sequenced and assigned, who was selected to perform particular tasks, and how production could be maximized.[10] To do this, managers had to look at not only individual tasks and workers, but also at how those tasks and workers were connected to others, which meant rationalizing, coordinating, and sequencing communication, processes, and many aspects of production. The work of laborers was changed and so too was the work of managers. Managers' decisions no longer were personal or arbitrary;

they were based on scientific analysis and experiments that led to more output and productivity.

Along with some managers, some workers resented this new approach because it standardized and proscribed much of their daily work. March and Simon stated that it studied men as accessories to machines for routine productive tasks and tried to prescribe their work to increase production. This approach sought to improve productivity of an inefficient organism (person) by carefully prescribing precise steps and methods of work. This converted a "general-purpose mechanism, such as a person, into a more efficient special-purpose mechanism,"[2] and thus was a form of mechanization and automation. March and Simon believed that part of scientific management was concerned with utilization of human beings in organizations. They referred to scientific management as "physiological organization theory" because it included analysis of employees' physiological constraints of production.[2] Morgan argued that the scientific approach to management mechanized people and de-humanized the workplace.[11] Further, it separated the "hand" of workers from the "brain" of managers. However, others (e.g., Rue and Byars) believed Taylor was concerned about helping both managers and employees improve production while improving work conditions and pay for employees.[9] Indeed, Taylor advocated higher rates of pay for workers who increased production.

Perrow identified several problems of the scientific management school. First, labor and labor unions gained power, which led management to cooperate and share more with employees and move away from rigid views of people as machines. Second, changing markets required businesses to adapt and change to meet new customer preferences. Frequent and sometimes rapid change did not work well with rigid scientific management. Third, social ideas and political viewpoints emerged that did not support the harsh authoritarian management that existed in some businesses imbued with scientific management. Finally, the search for leaders of large growing organizations increased the realization that people, leaders, and organizations were not machines but social systems involving human relationships.[1]

■ ADMINISTRATIVE PRINCIPLES

While the scientific management approach advanced the performance of individual tasks in an organization, not much theory had yet been developed for organizing different tasks into jobs, jobs into work units, and work units into departments. Minimizing the cost of production would require an organization to consider relationships, coordination, and possible synergies among tasks, jobs, work units, and departments. Further, it would depend on the volume of work and whether there was enough need for a particular task to make it a full-time job or combine it with other tasks to make a full-time job. Principles for developing these kinds of structures emerged in the work of Fayol and Gulick and Urwick among others.

Based on his experience in management, Henri Fayol developed a more complete theory of administration and is often considered the first writer to do so.[12] Unlike Taylor, who examined work from the level of the individual employee, Fayol examined organizational management from the perspective and role of top managers. Thus, his work is more about managing an organization than just managing a worker. His classic book *General and Industrial Management* published in 1916, and a revised translation of it by Gray, explains Fayol's fourteen management principles that are considered universally applicable to managing organizations. Drawing from Fayol, Gray, and Rue and Byars, these principles are summarized below:[9,13,14]

1. Division and specialization of work
2. Authority, based on the formal position rather than the person
3. Discipline, based on obedience and respect
4. Unity of command, so an employee takes orders from only one boss
5. Unity of direction, coming from one boss and plan for activities that have the same objective
6. Placing group interests above individual interests
7. Pay, based on factors that are fair, uniform, and understood
8. Centralization, based on the situation, authority, and communication channels
9. Line of authority or scalar chain, to show formal communication channels
10. Order, with a place for everything and everyone
11. Equity, based on kindness and justice
12. Stability of personnel and personnel planning
13. Individual initiative, to plan and then help implement the plan
14. Esprit de corps, harmony, unity in the organization

Fayol believed management was a process based on these principles and that these principles are applicable to all types of organizations. Thus, his ideas form a general theory of administration that sought to form broad principles of administration to guide the management of organizations. These were "top down" rather than the "bottom-up" approaches of Taylor. Two important concepts—specialization and coordination—were emphasized. As can be seen, these principles helped form organizational design based on hierarchical levels and chain of command for control, with workers having a single boss, jobs being specialized by tasks and activities, and then jobs being grouped into departments. Line and staff work was distinguished from each other, in which line work contributed directly to achieving organizational goals, while staff work supported the line work. These principles were to be flexible; Fayol expected managers to adapt them to particular situations.[13]

Gulick and Urwick (1937, p. 22) also developed administrative principles by describing administrative concepts including division of work, coordination of work, span of control, unity of command (one boss), top-down and bottom-up approaches to designing organizations, and executive functions. In doing so, they helped build on—and corrected problems of—Taylor's work. For example, their unity of command principle was developed because multiple bosses caused inefficiency and conflict. They claimed that even "Taylor fell into this error in setting up separate foremen to deal with machinery, with materials, with speed, etc., each with the power of giving orders directly to the individual workman."[14]

They did much work to develop departmentalization and grouping of work units both vertically and horizontally, realizing that both should be considered. Departmentalization of work units could be based on *purpose* and *process*, and the work itself could be grouped based on purpose, process, clients, or location. When grouping work by purpose—group all tasks, jobs, resources, etc. needed to completely accomplish a certain purpose—then the work is self-contained within a single department. Self-containment means everything (labor, resources, etc.) needed by a work unit to accomplish its work (purpose) is contained within that work unit, so it can achieve its purpose independently of what happens elsewhere in the organization. This approach has advantages. It helps assure completion of a particular purpose or project by putting it completely under the control of a single person (department director) who has control over all necessary staff, experts, services, and workers needed to accomplish the entire project and purpose. The department does not have to depend or wait for others outside of the department director's control. It does not have to deal with inter-departmental conflicts, which might have to be resolved by a higher-level manager, and in any event would cause delays and interference. It minimizes coordination time, cost, and energy. More self-containment means less coordination with other work units in the organization. However, there is less specialization, which increases costs, as discussed next.

Grouping work based on process is basing work on skills and the types of work performed. When grouping all secretarial work in one department, economies are achieved by having a highly specialized focused department. However, when grouping work based on specialized processes, increased coordination is required with other work units that need the specialized work to complete their purpose. These potential economies are lost when work of various skills are grouped together based on purpose (rather than process). So, an organization must decide how much to group work based on process (specialized jobs) versus purpose (self-containment). More self-containment means less coordination cost—but also less economy of specialization.

Gulick and Urwick also helped form the executive function by identifying and describing the work of the chief executive. They asked what work does a chief executive perform? They then answered "POSDCORB". That was their acronym for planning, organizing, staffing, directing, coordinating, reporting, and budgeting. These seven functions may be subdivided so that the work is organized and performed by more than one person if necessary. When an organization is large, these functions should be divided among subparts of the organization.[14]

This approach continued to evolve with contributions from other writers. For example, Mooney further developed principles including coordination, scalar (hierarchical) levels of authority and responsibility, delegation, staff work, and function (duties).[15]

While these principles helped formulate a theory of management and organization, some of them were criticized as being too simplistic, contradictory, and based on dubious assumptions.[16,17] At this point in the development of organization theory, "there is a tendency to view the employee as an inert instrument" without consideration of individual behavior, motivation, and variability."[2] Despite these shortcomings, these administrative principles helped develop organization theory, structure, and design. The criticisms led to the realization that broad principles may not apply to every situation or organization—there are limits to the applicability of principles—they are contingent on factors.

■ BUREAUCRATIC PRINCIPLES

Concurrent with development of scientific management and administrative principles was the work of Max Weber in developing bureaucracy theory. Weber was a sociologist, economist, and political scientist who studied civilization and society. He wrote in the early 20th century in German; his work was translated by Gerth and Mills (1946) and Henderson and Parsons (1947) and brought to the United States. Weber strongly believed in the bureaucratic form of organization that included hierarchical structure, promotion based on merit rather than personal relationships, impersonal rules, and other principles of organization. He believed this was superior to prior forms of organization such as feudalism or patrimony.[18,19]

Weber began by identifying three types of legitimate authority based on three different views of what was legitimate:[19]

1. Rational (legal authority)—based on the "legality" of normative rules and on the right of those in authority under those rules to give commands.
2. Traditional (traditional authority)—based on the sanctity of long-standing traditions and the legitimate status of those who use authority under those traditions.
3. Charismatic (charismatic authority)—based on devotion to exceptional heroism, sanctity, or character of a person and the normative patterns of that person.

Weber thought the traditional and rational-legal forms were the most stable for administrative structures because charismatic leaders eventually lose influence or pass away. The rational grounds for authority rest "on a belief in the 'legality' of patterns of normative rules and the right of those elevated to authority under such rules to issue commands (legal authority)."[12]

"In the case of legal authority, obedience is owed to the legally established impersonal order. It extends to the persons exercising the authority of office under it only by virtue of the formal legality of their commands and only within the scope of authority of their office."[12] This contrasted to authority based on feudalism's tradition, religion's charisma, or heredity's charisma. "Bureaucratic administration means fundamentally the exercise of control on the basis of knowledge. This is the feature of it, which makes it specifically rational."[12] This knowledge includes, of course, the technical knowledge that is the basis for selection into an office. But, there is also knowledge from knowing the history and experience in an organization and having access to knowledge in office files.

The purest form of exercised legal authority is found in a bureaucratic administrative staff. It is an ideal form, with these principles:[19]

1. Staff are free personally and subject to the organization's authority only for their impersonal official work.
2. Staff are organized in a clear hierarchy of offices (bureaus) with a higher level one controlling those beneath it (rather than control based on personal loyalty of people).
3. Each office has clearly defined division of labor and duties and competencies, and it is managed based on written documents in files.
4. An office is filled by open free selection and appointment rather than election.
5. Staff are selected and appointed based on technical qualifications and ability, rather than personal loyalty and relationships.

6. Staff are paid by fixed salaries based largely on rank in the hierarchy and responsibility.

7. An office is the sole or main occupation of a person in that office.

8. An office is part of a career in which someone can be promoted up the hierarchy based on achievement and/or seniority.

9. Staff employment in an office is separate from ownership of rights, property, equipment, and other means of work production in that office; the office (not the hired worker) owns the means of production and rights of an office.

10. Staff are subject to strict systematic rules, norms, discipline, and control of their work, decisions, actions, and performance in that office and must obey impersonal orders given by officials in their official positions; these systematic rules were known and fairly stable (rather than vague and subject to arbitrary change).

These principles were interrelated so that they combined to form a system of administration. Weber believed, once a bureaucracy was established, it would likely remain permanent since it would be difficult to destroy such an organization. Bureaucratic principles comprised a tool for leaders to have their legitimacy supported by rules and law. Bureaucracy had rules, procedures, and preset routines in a defined administrative system. This approach was both rational and legal and carried the force of rational thought and the laws.

While Weber considered this the ideal organization for efficiency, he realized it had shortcomings. The bureaucratic form of organization has precision, unity, continuity, is unambiguous, and is thus technically superior to other organizational forms the way a well-designed machine is technically superior. However, to do this, the bureaucracy must eliminate human emotions such as love and hate from business. Bureaucracies thus become dehumanized. Rules are valued and followed closely to the point of minimizing creativity, individuality, and initiative. In this way, Weber himself realized the human aspects of work were reduced as administrative work became mechanized the way machines mechanized production. "The individual bureaucrat cannot squirm out of the apparatus in which he is harnessed. . . . He is only a single cog in an ever-moving mechanism, which prescribes to him an essentially fixed route of march" in an impersonal methodically integrated organization of official functions.[18] Also, like previous writers and theories, Weber and his work were criticized later for having too many unproven propositions that were taken for granted rather than being tested.[20,21] His work was further criticized for not distinguishing between two sources of authority—line authority based on position and staff authority based on special expertise.[22,23] Nonetheless, he contributed much to the development of organization theory.

■ HUMAN RELATIONS

A catalyst for the human relations movement was the Hawthorne Studies, which began in 1924 and studied how physical working conditions affected worker productivity. Investigators conducted experiments by adjusting lighting, rest periods, and other factors at the Western Electric Hawthorne Plant near Chicago. As Western Electric executive C. G. Stoll stated in the classic book on the Hawthorne Studies, the "work described in this volume grew out of our experience in other investigations, which revealed a considerable deficiency in our knowledge of the intangible factors in the work situation that affect the morale and productive efficiency of shop workers. . . .[24] The human reactions, of people engaged in productive work, have a much more important effect on their morale and efficiency than had previously been realized."[25]

Like in scientific management, the unit of analysis for the human relations approach was often the individual worker, though work groups and cliques were later studied. During more than 10 years of study, the research used observations, experiments, and interviews. No clear relationship was found between working conditions and worker productivity. In some cases productivity improved even when work conditions worsened (e.g., less lighting), and sometimes productivity improved for both the test group and the control group. Psychologists, who then joined the study, concluded that other factors beyond the physical working conditions—such as peer norms, recognition, teamwork, participation, and cooperation—affected workers and their productivity. Behavioral and social sciences offered insights and theories to better understand workers and organizations, and management of them. Organizations now had further reason to think workers were not just economically motivated—they were also socially and psychologically motivated. Workers were more complex than previously realized and were not always "rational." Thus, the Hawthorne Studies helped launch the human relations approach to management, although their methods and conclusions were later questioned by some.

Trained in listening, interviewing, and helping others express themselves, Hawthorne researchers, over a period of years, interviewed thousands of workers who spoke confidentially and eagerly. It was realized that workers as individuals want to confidentially express their thoughts and feelings about things in their lives—personal and work-related—to someone (in this case, researchers) who would listen with care and interest.[26] Human relations theory thus evolved to include the idea that managers should pay attention to workers' complaints and warnings that workers are upset about something, though not necessarily what it is they are upset about.

In these studies, groups and their informal social control of work and work behavior were found to be important for both the internal workings of the group and how the group externally interacted with other parts of the organization. The industrial organization was a social organization. Work cliques, through their norms, roles, and memberships, affected workers' attitudes and productivity. Commenting on studies of wiremen at the Hawthorne plant, "their behavior at work could not be understood without considering the informal organization of the group and the relation of this informal organization to the total social organization of the company.[25] Further, "the behavior of no one person in an industrial organization . . . can be regarded as motivated strictly by economic or logical considerations. . . . Non-economic motives, interests, and processes, as well as economic, are fundamental to behavior in business, from the board of directors to the very last man in the organization."[25] Elton Mayo interpreted the results of the Hawthorne studies and generally concluded that in the work setting of the Industrial Revolution, workers lost a feeling of security, camaraderie, informal membership, and group belonging.[10] When mechanical processes, new technology, and engineered job design were implemented, workers' social relationships at work changed and became unstable and insecure.

Barnard helped advance human relations by writing about his experiences as president of the NJ Bell Telephone Company. He viewed the entire organization and believed in hierarchy, authority, and clear formal communication. His views and theory emphasized the cooperative social relations among human beings in an organization, and he conceptualized organizations as systems that integrate the cooperative purposeful efforts of its individual workers. Barnard articulated the need for individuals to cooperate with others in order to accomplish things they could not do alone. Creating cooperative relationships formed a system of parts (people) that, to survive, had to meet the purposes of the cooperative and of the individuals in the cooperative. Barnard believed this required that people accept the cooperative purpose, be willing to cooperate, and communicate effectively with other parts (people) in the cooperative unit. Those three conditions were the necessary and sufficient conditions to have an organization, and they become the basis of Barnard's theory of formal organization.[27]

Barnard had been a student at Harvard and afterwards maintained his relationship with the Harvard faculty conducting the Hawthorne experiments. They all came to see that man was not just an economic man— there were also social, psychological, and behavioral dimensions of the worker. The necessary cooperation had to be developed and fostered by organizational leaders using social, behavioral, and moral motivators and rewards (not just material rewards). Barnard's theory of administration also placed importance on the informal organization and extensive communication throughout the organization. He wrote in detail about conditions necessary for effective communication with authority and leadership. Together, these approaches created interpersonal relations, cohesion, and motivation for workers to stay and work toward the organization's overarching purpose. Humane leadership and fair treatment of employees was another aspect of Barnard's work.[27]

Flowing from all this came organizational research investigating culture, behavior, groups, leadership, workers' personality traits, supervision, worker satisfaction, job design, and participation in decision making.[25,28–31] Research found that some elements of the mechanistic approach—specialization, routinization, and centralization—negatively affected employee morale and loyalty. Employee autonomy, creativity, and freedom gained credence.

■ ADMINISTRATIVE BEHAVIOR

Herbert Simon was skeptical of earlier work by Fayol and Taylor, criticizing some of the writing as based on faulty, limited assumptions. He also disliked commonly used administrative principles that to him were mere proverbs with terms (e.g., "purpose" and "centralization") that lacked rigorous definition and conceptual meaning.[2,17] Consequently, they were not universally applicable. After dissecting four administrative principles and showing how they contradict themselves in some situations, Simon concluded "none of the four survived in very good shape, for in each case there was found, instead of a univocal principle, a set of two or more mutually incompatible principles apparently equally applicable to the administrative situation."[17]

Unlike Taylor, who considered "economic man" as fully informed and able to calculatedly make the best economic decision for his own self-interests, March and Simon assumed that man was limited in his ability to identify and evaluate alternatives and thus would settle for an acceptable choice solution rather than a best solution or decision.[2] They theorized administrative behavior by the "administrative man" rather than economic behavior by the "economic man." Earlier work (e.g., by Taylor) assumed that when facing a situation that required a decision, managers were rational people who could conceive of the possible alternatives, identify the consequences of each alternative, calculate the utility of alternative choices, and then choose an optimal decision. March and Simon thought otherwise. They believed man had limited ability to obtain all necessary information, identify all appropriate alternatives, objectively determine consequences, and rationally evaluate choices. Human beings instead had "bounded rationality" because they were only capable of mentally processing a limited amount of information. Further, available information, perceived alternatives, and anticipated consequences were partly determined by the social and organizational environment, which therefore should be included in a theory of managerial decision making. Managers—and people in general—usually select a satisfactory alternative rather than going through the much more difficult process of searching for and determining an optimal (best choice) decision.

Another contribution of March and Simon was their distinction between routine and non-routine problem solving.[2] When problems arise that have been repeatedly encountered before, the person or organization will quickly form a problem definition, possible responses, and a process for selecting a response. Organizations may form written policies and procedures for how to handle routine situations and problems in order to simplify and expedite how they are handled. These routine problems are handled easily with established processes, checklists, forms, procedures, and so forth. However, when a new or uncommon problem arises, the person or organization must develop a problem definition, search for alternatives, gather information for a decision, and form a decision-making process. All of that requires time, resources, and other costs, so the organization must also decide how much time, effort, and resources to expend to make a decision. This often leads to satisficing— accepting the first satisfactory solution that can be found rather than continue to spend resources searching for and evaluating other choices.

A second aspect of this was Simon's theory of hierarchical goals in which one level's means were a lower level's ends. The work performed at the lowest level of the organization was just a means to accomplish the end purpose of the second-most lowest level, whose work was just a means by which to achieve the end purpose of the next higher level of the organization. These hierarchical means-ends relationships among organizational levels guided the decisions made by each worker, work unit, department, division, etc., so that decisions made at one level (e.g., a worker or department) would help achieve the end purpose of the next higher level. In this way, each worker and work unit sufficiently focused toward the end purpose of the organization. These approaches to decision making were necessary because of people's bounded rationality or limited cognitive ability.[2] This view reflected that organizational life had too many alternatives that required too much information to fully process if a person were to consider all possible alternatives for a decision. Thus, organizations set rules, premises, and boundaries in which decisions must be made. Like the nested means-ends sequences, they helped to rationalize decision making in organizations and integrate the many decisions that are made each day throughout an organization.

"Administrative theory is peculiarly the theory of intended and bounded rationality—of the behavior of human beings who satisfice because they have not the wits to maximize."[17] A person's rationality is limited by a triangle of three factors: mental habits, abilities, skill, and speed; values and motives; and knowledge of the immediate problem and of how to make a decision. These factors will vary for a person over time and in different situations. Thus, all of these factors must be included in administrative theory for decision making.

■ CHAPTER SUMMARY

Theories of organization began to develop in response to the large businesses and factories of the Industrial Revolution. Taylor's scientific management applied scientific methods, analysis, and measurement to work in order to improve productivity and efficiency. Additionally, scientific management expected managers to plan and organize tasks more efficiently so that individual workers could perform their work more efficiently. Fayol's administrative principles created a theory of administration for grouping tasks into jobs, jobs into work units, and work units into departments; his approach emphasized specialization and coordination. Gulick and Urwick extended administrative theory by developing departmentalization based on purpose, process, clients, time, and location. Weber created bureaucratic principles based on rational legal authority of a position (office), which made organizations impersonal. These principles formed a stable system of organizational administration based on hierarchy, division of labor, systematic rules, impersonal orders, and files (records) for each office.

The human relations movement (of the Hawthorne Studies and later Barnard) recognized that workers were human beings with feelings, personal needs, and variable performance that was influenced by psychosocial factors in the work setting. Simon's administrative behavior theory of decision making assumed that managers had limited cognitive ability to evaluate alternatives, thus they would "satisfice" (accept the first satisfactory solution available).

Taylor, Simon, and the human relations school focused largely on the individual worker, whereas Fayol and Weber addressed the organization. Focus on the individual assumed that improving the ability of the individual to work would lead to increases in performance and productivity. Similarly, an organizational focus assumed that the proper structure would improve performance and productivity. Scientific management, administrative principles, bureaucratic principles, and administrative behavior assumed organizations could be made rational by applying (impersonal) structures, hierarchies, goals, principles, plans, positions, legal-rational authority, rules, and controls. The human relations approach, while focused on the individual, was also concerned with other (not necessarily rational) aspects of an individual's participation in organizational life. This included study of such things as leadership, job redefinition, participatory decision making, motivation, and morale.

Review/Discussion Questions

1. How are scientific management, administrative theory, bureaucratic principles, and human relations similar? How are they different?
2. Which principles and theories in this chapter assume "the economic man?" What other assumptions of human behavior influenced early organization management theory?
3. How did criticisms of some classical management theories lead to new theories?
4. Which principles of classical management theory are still used today?

Learning Activities

1. Reflect on the word "bureaucracy." Which images come to mind? How similar are those to what Weber originally envisioned?
2. Arrange to tour a local health organization and interview one of its senior managers. Try to learn which principles of classic organization theory are used in this healthcare organization.

References

1. Perrow C. The short and glorious history of organization theory. *Organization Dynamics*. 1973;2:3–15.
2. March JG, Simon HA. *Organizations*. New York: John Wiley & Sons, Inc.; 1958.
3. Taylor FW. *The Principles of Scientific Management*. New York: Harper & Brothers Publishers; 1911.
4. Taylor FW. *A Piece Rate System*. NY: McGraw Hill; 1895.
5. Taylor FW. *Shop Management*. New York: Harper and Row; 1903.
6. Gilbreth FB, Gilbreth L. *Applied Motion Study*. New York: Sturgis & Walton Company; 1917.
7. Gantt H. *Organizing for Work*. New York: Harcourt, Brace and Howe; 1919.
8. Gantt H. *Industrial Leadership*. New York: Association Press; 1921.
9. Rue LW, Byars LL. *Management Theory and Application*. 4th ed. Homewood, IL: Richard D. Irwin, Inc.; 1986.
10. Scott WR. *Organizations, Rational, Natural, and Open Systems*. 5th ed. Upper Saddle River, NJ: Prentice Hall; 2003.
11. Morgan G. *Creative Organization Theory*. Newbury Park, CA: Sage Publications, Inc.; 1989.
12. Boone LE, Bowen DD. *The Great Writings in Management and Organization Behavior*. New York: Random House; 1987.
13. Fayol H. *General and Industrial Management*. London: Pittman; 1916.
14. Gulick L, Urwick L. *Papers on the Science of Administration*. New York: Institute of Public Administration, Columbia University; 1937.
15. Mooney JD. *The Principles of Organization*. New York: Harper & Brothers Publishers; 1947.
16. Massie JL. Management theory. In: JG March, ed. *Handbook of Organizations*. Chicago: Rand McNally; 1965.

17. Simon HA. *Administrative behavior*. 2nd ed. New York: Macmillan; 1957.
18. Weber M. *Essays in Sociology*, translated and edited by H Gerth, CW Mills. New York: Oxford University Press; 1946.
19. Weber M. *The Theory of Social and Economic Organization*, translated by AM Henderson, T Parsons, T Parsons, eds. New York: Oxford University Press; 1947.
20. Blau PM, Scott WR. *Formal Organizations*. San Francisco: Chandler; 1962.
21. Udy SH. "Bureaucracy" and "rationality" in Weber's organization theory. *Am Sociol Rev.* 1959;24:791–795.
22. Dalton M. Conflicts between staff and line managerial officers. *Am Sociol Rev.* 1950;15 (June):342–351.
23. Thompson VA. *Modern Organization*. New York: Knopf; 1961.
24. Carey A. The Hawthorne studies: A radical criticism. *Am Sociol Rev.* 1967;32 (June):403–416.
25. Roethlisberger FG, Dickson WJ. *Management and the Worker*. Cambridge, MA: Harvard University Press; 1939.
26. Mayo E. *The Social Problems of an Industrial Civilization*. Boston: Graduate School of Business Administration, Harvard University; 1945.
27. Barnard CI. *The Functions of the Executive*. Cambridge, MA: Harvard University Press, 1938.
28. Homans GC. *The Human Group*. Harcourt, Brace. New York; 1950.
29. Katz D, Kahn R. Some Recent Findings in Human Relations. In: E Swanson, T Newcomb, E Hartley, eds. *Readings in Social Psychology*. New York: Holt, Reinhart, and Winston; 1952.
30. Lewin K. *Resolving Social Conflicts*. New York: Harper & Brothers; 1948.
31. Stogdill RM, Coons AE. *Leader Behavior: Its Description and Measurement*. Columbus, OH: Columbus Bureau of Business Research, Ohio State University; 1957.

CHAPTER

4

Modern Theories of Organization

Mark L. Diana and Peter C. Olden

Learning Objectives

- Distinguish between open and closed systems and between rational and natural systems.
- Understand and explain contributions of general systems theory.
- Understand and explain contributions of contingency theory.
- Understand and explain contributions of transaction cost economics.
- Understand and explain contributions of resource dependence theory.
- Understand and explain contributions of institutional theory.
- Understand and explain contributions of population ecology.

■ INTRODUCTION

Most of the organization theorists discussed in Chapter 3 examined and thought about organizations as entities closed off from their environments. Suchman phrased it this way: "Resources materialized at factory gates, production technologies 'revealed' themselves to engineers, and products evaporated off loading docks. . . ."[1] These early theorists generally viewed organizations as rational entities seeking improved efficiency and performance, which resulted in classifying their theories as rational systems models. There were two important exceptions to this pattern. The human relations school viewed organizations as organic entities concerned with workers' needs and wants more than with efficiency and performance; thus, it is classified as a natural system model. Administrative behavior, which introduced the concept of bounded rationality, was the first theoretical framework to suggest that organizations might be influenced by events outside of their boundaries.

Beginning in the 1960s and continuing to the present, organizational scientists began to develop models that explicitly incorporated the environment. Scott and others have classified these theories as open systems models.[2,3] Scott's classification scheme follows the development of organizational theories through two phases that each have two sub-phases. The two phases are the closed-systems model and later the open-systems models. The two sub-phases took place twice—once during the closed-model phase and then again during the open-model phase. These sub-phases were the transition from rational models to natural models. Thus, there were closed-rational systems models followed by closed-natural systems models. Then, after acknowledging the environment, there were the open-rational systems models followed by the open-natural systems models. This chapter next explains the theories that fall under these last two categories, specifically the general systems theory, contingency theory, transaction cost economics, resource dependence theory, institutional theory, and population ecology.

■ GENERAL SYSTEMS THEORY

General systems theory was founded in the late 1950s by Ludwig von Bertalanffy to develop an approach to systems that crossed disciplinary boundaries.[4] Bertalanffy believed that the various scientific disciplines, in developing their own theoretical frameworks, became isolated from each other with communication between them increasingly difficult. Further, he believed there were common elements in many of these frameworks that crossed the boundaries between biology, physics, psychology, sociology, and so on. The common element these scientists studied was systems.

A system can be defined as a set of interdependent parts.[5] Boulding developed a systems typology with nine levels of increasing complexity.[6] In general terms, the simpler or less complex a system is, the more tightly connected the component parts are and the more specific and constrained their behavior is. Alternatively, the more complex the system, the looser the connections between parts, which lends more flexibility to the system. In addition, the types of flows between the system's parts, and between the system and its environment, change as the complexity of the system changes. In general, system-flows move from materials and energy in less complex systems to information in more complex systems. Systems that are more complex are also capable of renewal, self-maintenance, growth, and change.

One more important concept that is a part of Boulding's typology is that systems are hierarchical. That is, as systems become more complex, they incorporate the characteristics of the less complex systems below them in the typology. The following is a summary of Boulding's typology:

1. Frameworks—the structural components of systems; the "geography and anatomy of the universe—the patterns of electrons around a nucleus, the pattern of atoms in a molecular formula" all the way up to "the mapping of the earth, the solar system, the astronomical universe."[6, p. 202]

2. Clockworks—simple dynamic systems that function like a clock, such as the motion of the planets and moons in the solar system.

3. Thermostat or cybernetic systems that maintain an equilibrium, but the equilibrium point can be changed within the limits of the system.

4. Open systems—self-maintaining structures that utilize a throughput of resources from their environment. "This is where life begins to differentiate itself from not-life . . . the existence of even the simplest living organism is inconceivable without ingestion, excretion and metabolic exchange."[6, p. 203]

5. Genetic-societal (plants)—systems that have developed a division of labor with differentiated and mutually dependent parts, and that have separated their appearance (phenotype) from their genetic makeup (genotype); also called blueprint growth systems, as they reproduce using preprogrammed instructions (through seeds or eggs) rather than duplication.

6. Animal—have highly specialized information processing capabilities (eyes, ears, etc.) and a highly developed nervous system that organizes the information into an image or knowledge structure of the environment as a whole.

7. Human—possess self-consciousness; ". . . he not only knows but knows that he knows,"[6, p. 204] and characterized by the capacity for speech.

8. Social—"The unit of such systems is not perhaps the person—the individual human as such—but the 'role'—that part of the person which is concerned with the organization or situation in question, and it is tempting to define social organizations, or almost any social system, as a set of roles tied together with channels of communication."[6, p. 205] The person can also affect the role, so this level ". . . is human life and society in all its complexity and richness."[6, p. 205]

9. Transcendental—". . . the ultimates and absolutes and the inescapable unknowables, and they also exhibit systematic structure and relationship."[6, p. 205]

Boulding thought most social science research focused on level two of his typology, with some work at level three, although the subject matter involved level eight. Because of the hierarchical nature of systems, however, studying a system at a lower level is still useful to understanding the system. For example, many managerial control systems within organizations function as cybernetic systems. In addition, highly complex systems can be broken down into component sub-systems to make the complexity more manageable.

General systems theory helped to propel organization theory into the open systems era, where the environment plays a prominent role. Katz and Kahn were instrumental in bringing general systems theory approaches to organization theory by including it in the first edition of their textbook written in 1966.[2,7]

■ CONTINGENCY THEORY

Lawrence and Lorsch coined the term contingency theory in 1967, although the prior work of Burns and Stalker and Woodward helped to lay the foundation.[8-10] Subsequent work by Galbraith and Donaldson expanded the framework.[11-13] The underlying theme of contingency theory is that there is no one best way to organize but instead features of the environment within which an organization exists determine the structure that will enable it to perform best. In other words, the best structure for an organization is contingent on aspects of its environment. These aspects are called contingencies, or contingency variables, and include, for example, size, technology, geography, and uncertainty. Aspects of the organizational structure that are contingent upon these environmental characteristics include the degree of formalization, differentiation, decentralization, and integration.

Lawrence and Lorsch proposed that the whole organization did not necessarily face the same contingencies, but instead various sub-units within the organization faced differing environments and contingencies.[8] Thus, structural features should also differ. The greater the variation of environments faced by individual sub-units within the organization, the greater the need for differentiation, and so the greater subsequent demand on coordination and control. Lawrence and Lorsch therefore saw contingency theory operating at both the sub-unit level and the organization level.

Galbraith focused more on the demand for information processing within the organization as the complexity and uncertainty of the environment increased.[11,12] The more complex and uncertain the environment, the greater the demand on the organization for effective information processing that would lead to better decisions and increased performance. Structural features of the organization—including formalization, hierarchy, and decentralization—would need to be designed to maximize information processing.

Donaldson developed a variation of contingency theory that proposed an adaptive response of the organization to its structural fit with its environment.[13] In this model, an initial state of fit exists between the organization and its environment. When a contingency variable changes, misfit occurs between the organization and its environment and the organization then adapts its structure to improve fit with the environment. Donaldson labeled this model the structural adaptation to regain fit (SARFIT) model.

The notion that there is no one best way to organize contrasts with ideas of early theorists, some of whom searched for that one best way. Though compelling, contingency theory is not without its problems. Chief among criticisms of contingency theory are: (1) a focus on the reaction of the organization to its environment with a seeming lack of acknowledgment that the organization can alter its environment; (2) a proliferation of contingency variables, many of which are not well defined; (3) a poor definition of the concept of fit; and (4) a poor definition of what constitutes improved organizational performance.[14]

■ TRANSACTION COST ECONOMICS

Transaction cost economics (TCE) was first proposed by Coase and then developed more fully by Williamson.[15–19] Transaction cost economics, as its name implies, has its origins in economics rather than sociology, and it focuses on individual transactions or exchanges of goods or services between buyer and seller. An organization has three choices when it comes to obtaining a good or service: purchase it on the market, produce it internally, or some combination of the two, such as a joint venture. Managers must decide which of these approaches to use, but because of *bounded rationality* (the concept developed by March and Simon), there are conditions under which managers cannot account for all possibilities.[20] Williamson argues that the costs of transactions are useful in helping managers make this decision.

Transaction costs arise from the need to monitor the other party in the transaction. This need to monitor stems from both bounded rationality and *opportunism*. This latter concept is the possibility that the other party may behave opportunistically, a behavior Williamson characterizes as "self-interest seeking with guile." The potential for opportunistic behavior depends on the nature of the transaction. In situations where the exchanged good or service is generic in nature and there are many sources of the good or service, there is little potential for such behavior, and the parties to the exchange do not need to know anything about each other's needs. In such cases, the transaction costs are low and the good or service can be purchased in the market with little concern for monitoring. If, on the other hand, the good or service is highly specific to the buyer's needs, there are likely to be fewer sources, and the buyer becomes susceptible to opportunistic behavior and higher transaction costs. In such cases, Williamson argues that the organization can reduce its susceptibility to opportunism and enforce monitoring of the transaction more economically by internalizing the exchange, or producing the good or service itself rather than purchasing it outside. Thus, an organization adds structures that define its boundaries in response to the need to reduce transaction costs, which helps to explain why vertical integration takes place. Williamson calls this internalization *hierarchy*.

Transaction costs were difficult to measure, so Williamson added factors to the threat of opportunism that indicate the transaction cost: the type of transaction and the degree of uncertainty. Determine the type of transaction by its *asset specificity* and *frequency*. Asset specificity refers to the degree of substitutability of the transaction, or how easily it can meet the needs of different organizations. The more specific the asset, the higher the transaction cost. Frequency simply refers to the number of times a transaction takes place. The more frequent the transaction, the higher the cost. Uncertainty increases the cost of transactions because it worsens the effect of bounded rationality. Williamson developed a framework that incorporates these elements that can be used to predict under what conditions organizations will conduct transactions externally and when they will internalize transactions. When asset specificity is low, always leave transactions to the market, regardless of the amount of uncertainty or other characteristics of the transaction. When all asset specificity, uncertainty, and frequency are high, do transactions internally. Intermediate levels of these variables can lead to forms of organization other than markets or hierarchies, such as joint ventures.

Transaction cost economics does not directly address issues of organization structure and performance. Williamson's argument is that the need to reduce transaction costs explains why not all transactions take place in the market, and thus gives rise to hierarchies or organizational structures that allow for monitoring and control of these transactions. Therefore, organizations arise from a rational approach to economizing on transactions, rather than through a conscious management decision to organize in a certain fashion. Further, Williamson argues that reducing transaction costs results in a more efficient organization that can be more successful than otherwise.

There are many criticisms of TCE, perhaps most notably those of Perrow and those of Ghoshal and Moran.[21,22] Perrow's critique consists of two main points. First, he argues that all of the factors that contribute to increased transaction costs in the market—opportunism, uncertainty, bounded rationality, and so on—also exist within the firm. In fact, Perrow points out that Williamson acknowledges this explicitly in *Markets and*

Hierarchies.[16] However, once acknowledged, Williamson does not return to this problem, and essentially leaves the matter of the ability of an organization to reduce internal transaction costs as a given, primarily through fiat. Second, Perrow argues that the motivation for vertical integration is market power and dominance, not efficiency gains through reduced transaction costs.

Ghoshal and Moran's critique focuses on the concept of opportunism.[22] They argue that Williamson's formulation of opportunism does not adequately address its components, specifically the differences between the tendency to behave opportunistically and opportunistic behavior itself. Further, they argue that the ability of organizations to control opportunistic behavior through fiat and other types of rational controls may actually lead to increased levels of opportunistic behavior within the organization. The result is a self-fulfilling prophecy and an endless feedback loop between the level of opportunistic behavior and the controls instituted to prevent it. Ghoshal and Moran argue that this situation could well result in sapping the competitive ability of the organization.

More recently, Slater and Spencer have criticized TCE on the basis of the apparent contradiction between the notion of bounded rationality on the one hand, and the elaborate system for efficiently organizing transactions on the other.[23] How is it that managers, so constrained by bounded rationality, cannot determine all of the potential pitfalls of conducting transactions but are able to analyze the characteristics of those transactions and determine the most efficient governance structure for organizing those transactions? Despite these criticisms, there is much empirical research to support transaction cost economics, particularly in the case of the relationship between asset specificity and vertical integration.[24]

■ RESOURCE DEPENDENCE THEORY

Pfeffer and Salancik developed the resource dependence theory primarily in their 1978 book *The External Control of Organizations: A Resource Dependence Perspective.*[25] The book's title makes it clear that Pfeffer and Salancik viewed the external environment as capable of exerting control over the organization. This external control is exercised through the organization's need for resources that are controlled by external entities. All organizations require resources to function, because they are open systems, and no organization can internally provide all its needed resources. This need to acquire resources from external entities makes the organization dependent on those outside entities. The degree of dependency varies with both the importance of the resource to the organization and the scarcity of the resource (how many suppliers there are).

Resource dependence theory offers a framework for understanding and predicting the actions of organizations to environmental pressures.

More specifically, resource dependence theory suggests that organizations will take actions to secure the resources needed to function and survive. Resource dependence theory views organizations as existing in open systems within which they must contend with other organizations and entities for needed resources. Thus, control of the organization shifts from within the organization to outside the organization reducing organizational control to the extent that other entities control access to the needed resources.

Resource dependence predicts that organizations will consciously scan the environment and adopt strategic responses to better manage acquisition of resources. Usually the goal is to improve the performance of the organization, either as outcomes, products, or some form of change. The focus of the theory is on resources and the organization's behavior in its attempts to acquire those resources. A fundamental proposition of the theory is that an organization cannot supply all of the resources needed for its survival and so must enter into relationships with entities in its environment to obtain those resources. Pfeffer and Salancik term this interdependence.

The theory predicts organizational behavior by analyzing the degree of control the organization has over resources held by other entities, the degree of need for those resources, and the degree of access to alternatives. When needed resources are scarce or not under the control of the organization, the organization must act upon the environment to secure the resources or it will cease to exist. Another way to view this is that external entities will be able to exert control over the organization under these conditions:

1. The resource is critical to the operation of the organization.
2. The external entity controls the resource and there are few or no alternative sources for the resource.
3. The organization does not control resources critical to the functioning of the external entity.
4. The outputs of the organization are visible enough for the external entity to be able to judge compliance with its demands.
5. Satisfaction of the demands of the external entity does not face legal restrictions and does not conflict with satisfaction from other components of the environment with which the organization is interdependent.
6. The organization does not control the formulation of the external entity's demands.
7. The organization is capable of meeting the demands.

These conditions clearly demonstrate Pfeffer and Salancik's view of organizations as interdependent.

Therefore, this dependence on the environment gives power and influence over the organization to those external entities possessing control over needed resources. The degree of control relates to the degree to which the external entities are able to control the resources needed by the organization, along with the other conditions listed above. Conceivably this control could reach the level of direct administrative control, where the external entity makes managerial decisions for the organization. The result is that organizations will develop strategies that minimize dependence on others or increase dependence of others on them. To be effective, organizations must satisfy the demands of those in its environment from which it requires support, in the form of needed resources.

There are two primary methods that organizations will use to manage resource dependency. They can stockpile resource inventories and thereby reduce dependence on external entities, although this does not alter the underlying insecurity. Or, they may seek to establish some type of inter-organizational relationship to increase resource stability and predictability. To ultimately obtain resources needed for continued survival, resource dependence theory then predicts that organizations will undertake a variety of inter-organizational relationships to gain some control over their environment. These relationships can take the form of joint ventures, associations, diversification, vertical integration, mergers, and co-optation of those that control needed resources. This view of organizational action in response to the environment requires that managers be proactive in scanning the environment to detect resource risks and opportunities, and that they take actions to reduce resource uncertainty and dependence.

■ INSTITUTIONAL THEORY

Institutional theory developed out of the work of Meyer and Rowan, Meyer and Scott, and DiMaggio and Powell, and it attempts to explain organizational behavior from a cognitive and cultural viewpoint.[26-28] This is in sharp contrast to contingency theory and resource dependence theory, both of which take a strategic view of organizational behavior. All three theories are open-systems theories and as such, they acknowledge the role and influence of the environment on organizational behavior. They also allow for adaptive responses to the environment by the organization. Contingency and resource dependence theories are rational systems models, however, which pre-suppose the organization's responses to the environment are based on objective environmental scanning and rational responses chosen to improve efficiency. In contrast, institutional theory is skeptical of this rational model, and proposes instead that organizational responses are often based on factors that have little or no relationship to organizational efficiency.

The concept of an institution is central to institutional theory. The word institution has several meanings. Institutional theory refers to the meaning of something that is well established or has been established for a long time and in place for many years. This leads to institutionalism, which generally can be defined as support for institutions, or belief in the merits of established customs and systems. Scott and Meyer developed the following definition of institutions: "Institutions are symbolic and behavioral systems containing representational, constitutive, and normative rules together with regulatory mechanisms that define a common meaning system and give rise to distinctive actors and action routines."[29, p. 68] Scott gives a similar definition: "Institutions consist of cognitive, normative, and regulative structures and activities that provide stability and meaning to social behavior. Institutions are transported by various carriers—cultures, structures, and routines—and they operate at multiple levels of jurisdiction."[30, p. 34]

These regulative, normative, and cognitive elements are central to both of these definitions. Scott refers to these as the Three Pillars of Institutions. The regulative pillar refers to how institutions constrain and regulate behavior. Regulation is coercive through the application of rules, laws, and sanctions. An organization that does not abide by these regulatory constraints will have its legitimacy challenged through legal sanction. The normative pillar refers to ". . . normative rules that place prescriptive, evaluative, and obligatory dimensions on social life."[30, p. 37] Normative pressures are applied through social obligation, or the belief by the organization that it will be viewed as acting inappropriately if it does not comply with these norms, and thus it will not be considered legitimate. The cognitive pillar refers to the ". . . rules that constitute the nature of reality and the frames through which meaning is made."[30, p. 40] This refers to the idea that organizations should look and behave like other similar types of organizations.

Scott nicely synthesizes these concepts, and this synthesis makes evident the power of institutions in shaping organizational behavior in a variety of ways. Institutions give rise to a rationalized image of the legitimate structure and appearance of organizations in the same field. An organizational field is defined as ". . . those organizations that, in the aggregate, constitute a recognized area of institutional life: key suppliers, resource and product consumers, regulatory agencies and other organizations that produce similar services or products."[31] These rationalized images are referred to as *rationalized myths* because they focus on external legitimacy rather than internal efficiency. In fact, adherence to these myths may adversely affect technical efficiency. However, the institutional forces are so powerful that failure by the organization to adhere to the image of a legitimate organization may threaten its access to needed resources and support, both internal and external, and threaten its very survival. If organizations act in generally unacceptable ways, as defined by the institutions in the environment that the organization is subject to, their resources and support may be threatened or withdrawn. Because highly institutionalized organizations may have significant conflict between the need for both external legitimacy and technical efficiency, organizations will attempt to decouple elements of their production structure from their legitimizing activities. This decoupling serves to insulate the technical core of the organization from the activities of the organization focused on gaining external legitimacy. The result is there may be a difference between what an organization does and what it portrays itself as doing.

Institutional pressures cause organizations in the same field to become similar over time in a phenomenon called isomorphism. DiMaggio and Powell cite this homogeneity in organizational forms and practices as one of the driving forces behind the development of institutional theory.[31] They argue that in the early stages of the life cycle of an organizational field, there may be a considerable diversity of form and approach, but that as a field becomes well established, homogeneity develops. This inexorable move toward isomorphism is driven by three mechanisms discussed below: coercive forces, mimetic pressures, and normative pressures.

First, coercive isomorphism is the result of formal and informal pressures exerted by other organizations. These organizations may be governmental and regulatory agencies that make and enforce laws and rules the organization must comply with or face some sort of penalty. Coercive forces may also arise from higher levels of the organization, as in the case of standardized policies and procedures enforced by the parent organization of a multi-level system. Second, mimetic isomorphism occurs when organizations model themselves on other organizations that externally are favorably viewed. This behavior is a response to uncertainty. When uncertainty is high, organizations will mimic the structures and behaviors of other organizations that appear successful, assuming these other organizations face the same type of uncertainty. Mimetic behavior can also be an effort to gain legitimacy. Third, normative isomorphism arises primarily from professionalization in two ways. Formal education instills a common cognitive reference that becomes viewed as legitimate, and, therefore, other approaches are to be considered illegitimate. And, the extensive professional network that develops with these professions serves to disseminate normative rules across the profession.

■ POPULATION ECOLOGY

Population ecology has been developed through the work of Hannan and Freeman and Aldrich.[32–36] Based on natural biological selection theories and the work of Charles Darwin, population ecology assumes that organizations have life cycles including birth, growth, maturation, decay, death, and distinction. This theory holds that some processes of change in organizational populations parallel processes of change in biologic populations. It focuses on the issue of organizational survival rather than efficiency and argues that organizations are powerless to control their destiny because the environment selects out organizations best suited to survive. A striking difference between this and other organization theories is that population ecology focuses on populations of organizations rather than single organizations or people inside organizations.

There are four key assumptions to this theory. First, it assumes that the environment differentially selects organizations for survival based on "fit" between organizational forms and environmental characteristics. Second, new organizations are always appearing, which leads to continuous changes within organizational populations. Third, organizations are subject to inertial pressures, meaning it is difficult for organizations to change. Finally, it assumes that organizations must struggle to remain competitive in the marketplace and survive.

Population ecology argues that populations of organizations evolve through four different life stages. First, a large number of variations (analogous to mutations in biology) appear in a population of organizations. These variations add to the scope and complexity of organizational forms in the environment. Next, selection occurs in which some organizations find niches and survive while others do not and die. Market forces, competition, and/or internal structural characteristics determine whether specific organizations find niches. When insufficient demand for a firm's product exists in the market, and when insufficient resources are available, the environment selects organizations out of the population that die. Third, retention occurs and a few organizations grow large and become institutionalized in the environment. That is, those that "fit" with the current environment survive, reproduce, and transmit their values. Certain technologies, products, and services become highly valued by the environment and others do not. The environment is always changing and if the dominant organizational forms fail to adapt to external changes, other organizations gradually replace them. Finally, adaptation occurs. Organizations are subject to inertia according to this framework; that is, those that do not "fit" with the environment grow old, lose energy, and often cannot adapt quickly enough to survive.

Hannan and Freeman propose that organizations operate under internal or external constraints that impede their adaptation to a changing environment.[32,33] These constraints result in structural inertia, a central concept in population ecology. Structural inertia occurs because organizations must produce services and products reliably and account rationally for their decisions and actions. These pressures result in highly standardized routines that inhibit organizational change.

Population ecology also assumes that environmental resources are structured niches, whose existence and characteristics organizations cannot affect. Each population of organizations must find a niche sufficient to support it, or else it will decline and eventually fail or give way to new organizational forms. Population ecologists maintain there are definite limits to the degree to which autonomous strategic choices are available for organizations. They view organizations as severely limited in their ability to adapt to different niches. As a result, organizations are at the mercy of their environments, since they either "fit" into a niche and survive, or are "selected out" and fail. This clearly relegates the managerial role to that of an observer on the sidelines at the mercy of the environment, unable to do anything much to enhance the organization's chances of survival.

Population ecologists also propose that newer organizations will fail more frequently than older ones. This liability of newness results from the costs of learning new roles and tasks, capital constraints on new roles, a lack of information about normal procedures, and unstable links to clients, supporters, and customers. Further, the growth of organizational populations follows a distinct pattern that depends on population density. Early in the development of a population, new organizations are created slowly and fail at high rates. As the number of organizations in the population increases, competition eventually causes consolidation and higher failure rates, slowing the growth and leading eventually to a gradual decline in the population. This density dependence results in a curvilinear growth curve for new organizations.

■ CHAPTER SUMMARY

Modern theories of organization are open-systems theories that made the same transition from rational models to natural models as the earlier closed-system theories made. General systems theory is a meta-theory that attempts to apply general characteristics of systems to theories in a wide variety of disciplines, including management. Contingency theory is a rational model that maintains there is no one best way to organize, but that the best structure for an organization depends on its fit with its environment. Transaction cost economics is also a rational model that focuses on transactions between buyers and sellers. According to this approach, the nature of the transaction determines whether it is best for the organization to conduct the transaction in the marketplace, internally, or some combination such a joint venture.

Resource dependence theory is a rational model that focuses on the resources an organization needs, and which entities control those resources. The more control external entities have over important resources, the more control they have over the organization. The organization responds to external control by trying to reduce its dependence on the resource, or by gaining control over the resource itself.

Institutional theory is a natural model that focuses on the impact of institutionalization on the way organizations structure themselves and behave. The institutional pressures come from normative, cognitive, and coercive sources, and these pressures tend to make organizations in the same organizational field resemble each other over time.

Population ecology is a natural model that examines populations of organizations, rather than individual organizations. Population ecology is modeled after biological theories, and it argues that organizations are subject to similar forces of adaptation, selection, and retention as are living organisms. Population ecologists argue that organizations are difficult to change, and that the environment is beyond the control of managers to understand, so managers have little effective ability to determine the survival of entire populations of organizations.

Review/Discussion Questions

1. How are general systems theory, contingency theory, transaction cost economics, resource dependence theory, institutional theory, and population ecology similar? How are they different?
2. Which theories in this chapter assume a "rational model," and which assume a "natural model?"
3. Which modern organizational theories assume managers can strategically direct their organizations, and which assume managers essentially cannot?
4. Which principles of modern management theory do you see in use today?

Learning Activities

1. Think about the relationship between management, the environment, and the different theories discussed in this chapter. Which theories assume the greatest ability of managers to act strategically to affect the organization, and which assume the least? Which theories assume the ability of the organization to affect the environment and which do not?
2. Arrange to tour a local health organization and interview one of its senior managers. Try to learn which principles of modern organization theory are used in this healthcare organization.

References

1. Suchman MC. Managing legitimacy: Strategic and institutional approaches. *Acad Manage Rev.* 1995;20:571–610.
2. Scott WR. *Organizations: Rational, Natural, and Open Systems.* 5th ed. Upper Saddle River, NJ: Prentice Hall; 2003.
3. Thompson JD. *Organizations in Action: Social Science Bases of Administrative Theory.* New York: McGraw Hill; 1967:192.

4. Bertalanffy LV, Rapoport A, eds. *General Systems Theory*. General Systems: Yearbook of the Society for the Advancement of General Systems Theory. Vol. 1. Ann Arbor, MI: The Society; 1956.

5. Nicholson N, Schuler RS, Van de Ven AH, eds. The Blackwell Encyclopedic Dictionary of Organizational Behavior. In: CL Cooper, C Argyris, eds. *The Blackwell Encyclopedia of Management*. Oxford: Blackwell Publishers; 1998.

6. Boulding K. (1956). General Systems Theory: The Skeleton of Science. *Manage Sci*. 1956;2:197–208.

7. Katz DN, Kahn RL. *The Social Psychology of Organizations*. 2nd ed. New York: John Wiley; 1978.

8. Lawrence PR, Lorsch JW. *Organization and Environment: Managing Differentiation and Integration*. Boston: Graduate School of Business Administration, Harvard University; 1967.

9. Burns T, Stalker GM. *The Management of Innovation*. London: Tavistock; 1961.

10. Woodward J. *Industrial Organization: Theory and Practice*. London: Oxford University Press; 1965.

11. Galbraith J. *Designing Complex Organizations*. Reading, MA: Addison-Wesley; 1973.

12. Galbraith J. *Organization Design*. Reading, MA: Addison-Wesley; 1977.

13. Donaldson L. *American Anti-Management Theories of Organization: A Critique of Paradigm Proliferation*. Cambridge, New York: Cambridge University Press; 1995:263.

14. Hrebiniak LG. The organization and environment research program: Overview and critique. In: AH Van de Ven, WF Joyce, eds. *Perspectives on Organization Design and Behavior*. New York: John Wiley & Sons; 1981.

15. Coase RH. The nature of the firm. *Economica*. 1937;4:386–405.

16. Williamson OE. *Markets and Hierarchies: Analysis and Antitrust Implications*. New York: The Free Press; 1975.

17. Williamson OE. Transaction cost economics: The governance of contractual relations. *J Law Econ*. 1979;22:233–261.

18. Williamson OE. The economics of organization: The transaction cost approach. *AJS*. 1981;87:548–577.

19. Williamson OE. *The Economic Institutions of Capitalism*. New York: Free Press; 1985.

20. March JG, Simon HA. *Organizations*. New York: John Wiley; 1958.

21. Perrow C. Markets, hierarchies, and hegemony. In: AH Van de Ven, W Joyce, eds. *Perspectives on Organization Design and Behavior*. New York: Wiley; 1981:371–386.

22. Ghoshal S, Moran P. Bad for practice: A critique of the transaction cost theory. *Acad Manage Rev*. 1996;21:13–47.

23. Slater G, Spencer DA. The uncertain foundations of transaction cost economics. *J Econ Issues*. 2000;34:61–87.

24. David RJ, Han S-K. A systematic assessment of the empirical support for transaction cost economics. *Strategic Management Journal*. 2004;25:39–58.

25. Pfeffer J, Salancik G. *The External Control of Organizations: A Resource Dependence Perspective*. New York: Harper & Row; 1978:300.

26. Meyer JW, Rowan B. Institutionalized organizations: Formal structure as myth and ceremony. *AJS*. 1977;83:340–363.

27. Meyer JW, Scott WR. *Organizational Environments: Ritual and Rationality*. Beverly Hills, CA: Sage; 1983.
28. DiMaggio PJ, Powell WW. The iron cage revisited: Institutional isomorphism and collective rationality in organizational fields. *Am Sociol Rev.* 1983;48:147–160.
29. Scott WR, Meyer JW. *Institutional Environments and Organizations: Structural Complexity and Individualism*. 1st ed. Thousand Oaks: Sage Publications; 1994:328.
30. Scott WR. *Institutions and Organizations*. 1st ed. Thousand Oaks: Sage Publications, Inc.; 1995:178.
31. DiMaggio PJ, Powell WW. The iron cage revisited: Institutional isomorphism and collective rationality in organizational fields. In: WW Powell, PJ DiMaggio, eds. *The New Institutionalism in Organizational Analysis*. Chicago: The University of Chicago Press; 1991:63–82.
32. Hannan MT, Freeman J. The population ecology of organizations. *AJS.* 1977;82: 929–964.
33. Hannan MT, Freeman J. Structural inertia and organizational change. *Am Sociol Rev.* 1984;49:149–164.
34. Hannan MT, Freeman J. *Organizational Ecology*. Cambridge: Harvard University Press; 1989.
35. Aldrich H. *Organizations Evolving*. Thousand Oaks, CA: Sage; 1999.
36. Aldrich HE. *Organizations and Environments*. Upper Saddle River, NJ: Prentice Hall; 1979.

5

Complexity and Postmodern Theory

Reuben R. McDaniel, Jr. and Michele E. Jordan

Learning Objectives

- Understand assumptions and ideas about healthcare organizations shared by complexity science and postmodernism, and compare those assumptions with modernist and Newtonian models of healthcare systems.
- Describe key characteristics of complex adaptive systems and develop a mental model of healthcare organizations as complex adaptive systems.
- Develop implications of complexity science and postmodernism for those who manage health care organizations,
- Identify major changes a traditional manager or leader might have to make if they wished to adopt a postmodernist and complexity science view of healthcare organizations.

■ INTRODUCTION

Typically, people viewed healthcare organizations through the lenses of modernist philosophy and Newtonian (classical) science, which has led to understandings of these organizations as machines that should be well run, well oiled, and well managed. There has been a focus on information gathering, correct decision making, and "doing the right thing." Healthcare researchers and healthcare managers have often adopted a reductionist approach to understanding organizations, analyzing pieces and fitting them together, predicting future outcomes of managerial behavior, and controlling the behavior of workers. Under these two traditional paradigms, organizational problems are dealt with by finding the "weak link" in the chain, and fixing the part of the system that "broke." These theoretical perspectives have also driven the clinical side of healthcare as physicians train to provide the proper diagnosis and proper treatment, and nurses train to help patients in a prescribed manner.

Previous chapters in this book have done an excellent job of articulating the modernist and classical science views of organizations. We plan to present an alternative view; one that we think is particularly useful in today's highly volatile and ambiguous healthcare environment. The past few decades have seen medicine and healthcare management influenced by the rise of new philosophical and scientific paradigms, most notably complexity science and postmodernism.[1,2] These new theoretical lenses offer insights that enable innovative approaches to managing healthcare organizations.

"Complexity science is the study of complex systems and the phenomena of complexity and emergence to which they give rise."[3, p. 166] Complexity science is an observational-based science that emerged in the early 1900s. It has proven itself useful in fields as disparate as physics, biology, cosmology, psychology, sociology, and anthropology for understanding a multitude of phenomenon from immune systems and spread of diseases to ecosystems and social economic systems. It was probably in the late 1980s that complexity science was brought to the attention of the general public and researchers in domains outside of the physical and biological sciences when books such as Gleik's *Chaos* and Waldrop's *Complexity* became available to the general public.[4,5]

It was at this time that organizational theorists began using concepts from complexity science in their attempts to understand organizational design, the evolution of organizations, and the dynamics and structure of specific types of organizations such as high reliability organizations. At the present time there is considerable work in healthcare using complexity science as a grounding theory. This work has been used to help us understand hospitals, nursing homes, clinical specialty systems, and family healthcare practices. Complexity science has brought to the forefront of organization science a better understanding of the uncertain nature of reality and the implications of that uncertainty for managerial action. It also led us to understand that the nature of relationships was critical, and that by focusing on those relationships, new alternatives for management made themselves apparent. These organizational insights arrived on the scene just as crises in healthcare organization management became apparent. The healthcare community was ready for some new ways of thinking about the issues they faced, and James Begun was one of the first organizational scholars to indicate our need to attend to these new sciences in our thinking about these issues.[6,7]

Postmodernism is an umbrella term for a group of philosophical ideas that challenged the assumptions of modernism and the resultant social and historical viewpoints. Postmodernism avoids definitions that claim to be the final word on issues and generalizations that claim to be all encompassing, and it denies the existence of universal truths or absolutes.[8] For the postmodernist, all models are only partial descriptions of reality, and scientific models are shaped not only by traditional scientific processes, but also by political, social, and personal interest.[9] Postmodernists focus on the role of social construction in understanding reality and emphasize the central place that language, discourse, and culture have in the knowledge and meaning construction process. This causes them to attend to the subjective and interpretive nature of knowledge. Philosophers such as Derrida, Foucault, Baudrillard, and Deleuze, and sociologists such as Latour, Laclau, and Mouffe are often associated with postmodernism.[10,11] Although some very extreme views of postmodernism have been used in organizational analysis, in this chapter we use moderate postmodernist views to help us understand healthcare organization.[12]

Though some people see complexity science as a model-centered science with close ties to modernism, the ontology and epistemologies of complexity science are more often compared with and linked to postmodernism, particularly to "affirmative postmodernism."[13,14] It is at the points where postmodernism and complexity science dovetail that we will spend our time. Our purpose is not to compare and contrast complexity science with postmodernism, nor is it to provide a primer of postmodernism or complexity science. Rather our purpose is to highlight some major ideas from these two frameworks and show how they inform organizational theory. By the end of the chapter, we hope you will find theories of postmodernism and theories of complexity science useful in understanding healthcare organizations and in developing strategies and tactics for improving them.

In the remainder of this chapter, we first explore the intersections of postmodernism and complexity science, applying their assumptions to healthcare organizations and explicating ways in which these two theories help us understand healthcare organizations differently than either modernism or classical science. We follow that with a more detailed description of one branch of complexity science, complex adaptive systems theory, which has provided unique insights for organizational theory and organizational management. We describe key characteristics of complex adaptive systems and examine how each characteristic is exemplified in healthcare organizations. We outline managerial implications suggested by these understandings and focus on those things a healthcare manager might do to help his or her organization provide services, achieve goals, and contribute to its community.

■ SHARED NOTIONS AND COMMON FOCUS

Though complexity science and postmodernism were founded in different domains and followed different evolutionary paths, they both address problems grounded in the disparity between what people observe and the way they think things should be. They share certain views of reality, and how one comes to know reality. *Both complexity science and postmodernism focus attention on similar aspects of the world, and therefore, viewing healthcare organizations through this joint lens can illuminate critical issues.* In the following section, we discuss six insights/aspects of organizations that complexity science and postmodernism perspectives might call to the attention of healthcare managers.

Limits of Knowability

Postmodernism and complexity science share the notion that at least some segments of the world are unknowable. Postmodernism addresses the limitations of our ability to understand the world through its belief that all knowledge is necessarily subjective and a reduction of reality.[15] Though some worldviews tend to dominate in specific cultural settings, this domination is not due to any inherent and essential truth of that worldview. Complexity science addresses the unintended consequences, unpredictable outcomes, and emergent properties that can result from nonlinearity and multiplication of effects even in fully deterministic systems.

Both theoretical frameworks conclude that no one is smart enough to figure out exactly where the healthcare system is going at any level. Both address the question, "What can we know if part of the world is unknowable?" There are limits to what people can know in healthcare organizations, and these limits cannot always be overcome by getting more information or waiting longer. For example, estimating nurse availability is often impossible, as is determining the impact of a new heart hospital on a family practice. Likewise, changes in reimbursement strategies will often affect the administrative processes in unexpected ways.

The Importance of Relationships

Both postmodernism and complexity science adopt principles consistent with the essentially interconnected nature of the world. Postmodernists stress the primacy of the social in the ability of the individual to acquire identity and make meaning of experience. As an example, postmodernists often cite the effect of the Information Age on people's fundamental understanding of the world (exchange models of communications to dispersed and emergent communications). Complexity science focuses on the importance of connections and interdependencies for creating emergent order in networked systems.

The quality of relationships within a healthcare organization may be more important than the quality of the people, because healthcare organizations are essentially relational in their structures, processes, and functions.[16] It is not simply the sum of the individual behaviors and actions within healthcare organizations that give them their identity, but the connections between them that are critical. For example, the interaction of value systems within a hospital influences the adoption of EMRs.[17] Trust is an essential ingredient in the use of telemedicine.[18] Conceptions of healthcare organizations as collections of parts has led to silos of expertise, compartments, and departments, and may lead to things such as the scheduling of nurses in ways that may break up well-functioning teams. Conceptualizing of healthcare organizations as *collectives* rather than collections causes us to focus on such things as the interdependencies among all of the clinical areas and the way in which culture sets bounds on behavior.

History Dependence

Postmodernism and complexity science both lead us to a deeper understanding of how history constrains and enables possible futures. For postmodernists, perceptions and experiences are always situation dependent; the present influence of powerful *discourses* historically derives rather than originates from any innate natural order. Complexity science stresses how the state of a system at a given time is a nonlinear function of the state of the system at some previous time. Another way to put this is that the possible futures of a system are path dependent and irreversible.[15]

For healthcare organizations, choices made in the present are going to influence what the organization can do and what it can become in the future. You cannot get every place from where you are. The difficulty that many hospitals have experienced in opening nursing homes is a manifestation of path dependence; the cultures of hospitals and nursing homes are so incongruent that although it appears that the same operational abilities are required, it turns out that this is not true. Furthermore, predicting the importance of any one decision may be very difficult, as something may appear to be unimportant and turn out to be very important. For example, the casual assignment of diagnostic codes can run a hospital into bankruptcy.

Structure as Dynamic

Postmodernism and complexity science both recognize that structure is an ongoing, generative process rather than a stable entity. Postmodernism accepts that even personal identity is a fluid, unstable quantity that is always in flux due to changing social and cultural influences. Complexity science sees structure as emerging from decentralized, bottom-up processes of adaptation, learning, and evolution.[3] Structure is not a priority or externally given, but arises in systems in which some degrees of freedom are constrained within boundaries. These boundaries connect the system with its environment and are themselves emergent structures. Hierarchical structures are also necessary in order to generate order in a system and are too often transformed.

People in healthcare organizations organize themselves in an ongoing basis. This may seem very disruptive to the manager of a healthcare system and to patients, families, and workers. It is, however, an inevitable reflection of the nature of these organizations. Created explanations of structure organize our actions. Often the outcomes of these actions, such as quality of care in hospitals, and even the ability of surgical teams to incorporate new methods, are the result of dynamic characteristics of structure.[19,20]

The Inevitability of Change

Both postmodernism and complexity science see change as the inevitable product of their dismissal of the notion of equilibrium. Both postmodernists and complexity scientists believe that the search for equilibrium, a balance, a stable state, is futile. Postmodernism arrives at this conclusion through its focus on the interdependencies of past and present perspectives. The fragmented perspectives that one has do not come together in any unified and coherent manner. Complexity science says that because systems are open to exchanges with the environment, they continuously adjust to moment-by-moment perturbations and other inputs from within the system and from without.

Both theoretical frameworks recognize that the definition of organizational success is an emerging property of any healthcare system.[21] Healthcare systems are continuously looking for higher peaks on a fitness landscape in response to continuously evolving environments. The roles people play in healthcare organizations continuously change, so when you think of an organization as a set of roles, that is correct, but who plays them and what those roles are is continuously subject to change. Efforts to contain or constrain system evolution might waste a lot of energy. Because we tend to see what we expect to see, we may also fail to see a lot of the change and this failure limits our ability to respond flexibly. As the healthcare system has gotten more resource poor, managers have been able to shape more of the basic care delivery functions.

Issues of Power

Power differentials and power exploitation are big ideas in postmodernism. Postmodernism points to the propensity for power bases generated by information asymmetries to increasingly monopolize and exploit the environment. Bases of power do not necessarily thrive because of the inherently elite characteristics they possess, rather they often exist because they overpower all else.[10] The complexity science position is that power is created from one's location in the chain of information exchanges and from the capacity to provide unique information or points of view.[22]

Traditional healthcare systems locate power within the legitimacy of the roles people play, and power is often granted through externalities and rules of conduct. But, because healthcare organizations are such information-dependent systems, then the significant information asymmetry in healthcare organizations between care clinicians, patients, and managers greatly shapes relationships. In most healthcare settings, the information power of the physician is symbolized by the white coat culture. The implementation of electronic medical records is reorganizing information asymmetries and thereby calling into question the monopolistic power of the white coat.

Both postmodernism and complexity science are at the same time more optimistic and more pessimistic than either modernism or classical science. Neither accepts the world as it is; rather, both believe in the transformative power of events and ideas, "opening the space for" possible futures, because neither accepts the world as it is, as some sort of inevitable thing.

■ CHARACTERISTICS OF COMPLEX ADAPTIVE SYSTEMS

This chapter focuses on a single branch of complexity science, complex adaptive systems (CAS) theory, first, for the sake of simplicity, and second, because it best describes healthcare organizations. When we view healthcare organizations as CAS, new organizational characteristics come to the forefront. This approach to describing the characteristics of CAS draws on several sources of understanding including: Waldrop, 1992; Capra, 1996; Cilliers, 1998; Leventhal and Warglien, 1999; Chu, Strand, and Fjelland, 2003; Beinhocker, 2006; Marguire, McKelvey, Mirebeau, and Oztas, 2006; McDaniel and Driebe, 2001; and McDaniel and Driebe, 2005.

Agents

CAS makes up of a large number of diverse agents that are information processors. There must be adequate diversity within the group of agents to enable the group to develop new solutions to problems and to make decisions in unique circumstances. In CAS, agents have the capacity to exchange information among themselves and with their environment and to adjust their own behavior as a function of the information they process. In a healthcare organization, all the players count; not only does each person contribute their talents, but they must also help others contribute. The management of such a diverse and changing cast of agents is one of the more difficult tasks in healthcare management.

Interconnections

The essence of a CAS is captured in the nonlinear relationships among agents. Inputs are not proportional to outputs; small changes can lead to big effects and big changes can lead to small effects. The way in which clinicians interact with each other, coupled with the way they interact with non-clinicians, is often a key determinant of a healthcare organization's ability to succeed. Everyone is busy and everyone has his or her job to do. But, CAS theory teaches us that the successful healthcare manager pays more attention to the relationship system than to the individual agents.

Self-Organization

CAS theory teaches us that order in a system may well be a result of the properties of the system itself, rather than some intentionality on the part of some external controller. Rather than hierarchical control, CAS are characterized by "decentralized, bottom-up process of co-design."[3, p. 166] New structures and new forms of behavior spontaneously emerge as agents self-organize themselves into relatively stable patterns of relationships. No matter how hard a nursing home manager tries to control certified nursing attendants, the attendants will organize themselves to do their job in the way that they see fit. Efforts to help them see the job better and to develop better skills at organizational analysis are likely to pay higher dividends than efforts to get them to toe-the-line.

Emergence

The behavior of a CAS cannot be obtained by summing the behaviors of the constituent parts, but emerge as the result of the pattern of connections among diverse agents. Emergence is a source of novelty and surprise in CAS. When we treat safety and clinical success as emergent properties of the system, then we are more likely to be able to learn from the past behaviors of the system and develop alternative strategies for achieving our goals.[20]

Co-Evolution

CAS does not simply change; it changes the world around them. CAS and its environments co-evolve such that each fundamentally influences the development of the other. The organizations act and others react, often in unexpected and unpredictable ways. When a healthcare organization even begins to investigate the purchase of some new information technology, the potential ramifications will almost immediately come to the fore in the decision-making process. And when a big payer decides that you should be paid by a system using diagnostic related groups (DRGS), then you will figure out a way to code the illness of your clients in a way that is profitable to you.

CAS theory tells us that successful understanding of healthcare organizations and the development of successful management strategies will involve the study of patterns and relationships rather than objects and substance, because it is the quality of the relationships among agents and between agents and their environment that most affect the quality of the system. CAS theory also tells us that successful management strategies will involve the study of wholes instead of parts because the effect of nonlinear interactions at all levels of the system mean that the whole is greater than the sum of the parts. Lastly, CAS theory tells us that an astute manager will recognize that the trajectory of a healthcare organization is unpredictable because CAS is a non-equilibrium-seeking system that continuously evolves. The goal is not to always be able to anticipate the future, but to always be organized in such a way as to respond appropriately to the future as it unfolds.

■ MANAGING HEALTHCARE ORGANIZATIONS AS POSTMODERNIST COMPLEX ADAPTIVE SYSTEMS

If we accept the assertions of postmodernism and complexity science that the world is essentially unknowable in many of its aspects and fundamentally relational in its nature, then we are standing at the precipice of several prescriptions for managing healthcare systems. In the following section, we address eight sets of things that managers should focus on as leaders in complex postmodernist organizations.

Uncertainty Reduction and Uncertainty Absorption

Modern healthcare systems have focused on uncertainty reduction as a strategy for better management. Uncertainty reduction involves collecting information to understand clearly the risk that is involved in any situation. This helps us to understand, for example, the present push for EMR adoption. Newer management perspectives would suggest that the successful manager will also concentrate on uncertainty absorption; developing a posture and organizational structure that allows confident action even when risk might be poorly understood.[23] Healthcare managers in the modern context must think about how they can organize their systems to be more able to operate effectively in the presence of uncertainty. Time and opportunity must be provided for reflection and careful consideration of alternatives. Trust will become a key component, as members of the team understand that nobody "knows" what to do, but as a team, they can discover an effective course of action. It is clearly important that today's manager and his or her management team have a deep knowledge of computerized information systems and how to effectively use these new forms of communication. It is even more important that the effective manager look at things from a variety of positions, paying careful attention to tacit knowledge and being confident but not overconfident. Pay attention to both uncertainty reduction and uncertainty absorption. The adoption of new clinical technologies often leads to uncertainty about roles and responsibilities. To write flawless job descriptions, we can never know enough about new technology or about all of the circumstances that surround its use. But, we can provide an environment of psychological safety that will help workers develop an attitude toward innovation that enables them to act with a presumption of personal and professional confidence.[24]

■ DECISION MAKING AND SENSEMAKING

Healthcare managers are traditionally taught to make good decisions, by which is often meant collecting information required to identify relevant choices and to make the "correct" choice among them. It is almost as though the question before the manager is clear to all observers and the task is simply developing a strategy for choosing. Postmodernism and complexity science alert us to the fact that situations are never clear and that the world may well not make sense when initially confronted. This means that sensemaking must take a prominent position in organizational action. A primary role of the manager is to help people make sense of the world as it unfolds.[25,26] Managers must be willing and able to share much more information about situations than they have traditionally shared. They must also be prepared to invite people with very different perspectives of the world to look at any specific situation because diversity improves sensemaking. For example, both doctors and nurses need to be involved in the adoption of new surgery technologies.[20] Good healthcare managers dedicate adequate time to those conversations that lead to good sensemaking. Postmodernists often stress narrative, fiction, and rhetoric as avenues for making meaning of the world, along with dialogue, discourse, and just plain talk. Because sensemaking is a social act, such interaction helps people make better sense and improves their ability to take action.[27]

While decision making has a ring of finality and closure, sensemaking is an ongoing process and therefore more closely matches the dynamic world posited by postmodernism and complexity science. While decision making implies the ability to predict how decisions will be implemented and the affects of implementing those decisions, sensemaking recognizes that one continually makes sense in order to act in the face of uncertainty: People make sense, take action based on the sense they made, observe as the world unfolds, and make further sense. It is not a question of either decision making or sensemaking. Rather, managers can improve their decision making by recognizing the need to improve the sensemaking capacity of their organizations.

Problem Solving and Dilemma Resolving

Managers have traditionally been taught to be good problem solvers: find out what is wrong and fix it.[28] Complexity science and postmodernism suggest that managers are faced with dilemmas much more often than they are faced with problems. A dilemma is a set of circumstances in the world that has no correct answer, but is rather a circumstance where differing points of view and issues of concern come to the table together. Healthcare managers can reduce their tendency to ask, "What is the right thing to do?" and increase their tendency to ask, "What is the thing to do that will enable us to learn and to enhance our potential for goal achievement?" Complexity science and postmodernism support that we stop asking, "Is it this or that?" and rather start asking, "How do we achieve this *and* that?".[29] In many ways, the development of the role of hospitalists and nurse practitioners were resolutions of dilemmas through the creation of new ways of viewing the world.

Knowing and Learning

Whereas healthcare managers are often taught to think of learning as something we do in order to know; from the perspective of postmodernism and complexity science, knowing and learning switch places: Knowing is something we do in order to learn. Because the future is uncertain, knowing based on prior experience must be "held loosely." We learn, not so that we will "know," but so that we can act more effectively in situations we have not seen before. Not only can healthcare managers learn to learn themselves, but they can also increase their skills at helping others learn to learn. There is a tendency to treat workers as if they do not learn. Once they have been taught their jobs and socialized into the dominant culture, it is assumed that that is the end of their learning. But, we know that people get wiser as they have more experience on the job and that they develop their own insights into the nature and meaning of their work. Managers must develop strategies for taking advantage of this ongoing learning and for shaping that ongoing learning in order to avoid pitfalls and missed learning. The most important learning may not be learning for preparation for action, but learning while action is going on. As noted by Stacey, "The most important learning we do flows from the trial-and-error action we take in real time and especially from the way we reflect on these actions as we take them."[30, p. 17] This suggests that healthcare managers and healthcare workers need to attend to multiple interpretations of unfolding events and pay careful attention to various ways that others might perceive the world.

Planning and Improvisation

Postmodernism and complexity science make it clear that management and operational strategies that depend on forecasting are likely to be futile.

Traditional healthcare theories have highlighted planning as a managerial strategy for preparing for the future. However, planning focuses on the capacity to forecast with confidence. Because the future is still unfolding and is unknowable, this tool is of limited utility for deciding on action alternatives, particularly at the strategic level.[31] While healthcare managers can and should capitalize on the potential of planning as a strategy for legitimizing the organization in the eyes of stakeholders, they will find it much less useful as a strategy for figuring out what to do next. When you do not know what you are going to get, you need to be prepared to use what comes.[32] Managing in the face of the unexpected requires skills at improvisation; the ability to make it up as you go and to respond with flexibility and creativity to chance happenings within a loose structure. Effective managers become bricoleurs, people who are able to use whatever tools are at hand, pay attention to small wins,[33] and learn from small failures[34] in order to accomplish the goals of the organization. They must treat mistakes as platforms for future action and ideas instead of as things to be fixed. Rather than seeking to eliminate uncertainty, managers must be willing to embrace its transformational possibilities.[35] Healthcare managers who wish to capitalize on improvisation must create a culture that fosters willingness to experiment; a culture in which people are encouraged to play around with ideas, bounce ideas off others, and imagine scenarios of possible futures. Improvisation is often considered an act engaged in individually and is not recognized as a group activity. But people in healthcare organizations improvise collectively, and thus they must gain skills in continuously negotiating and assessing as they spontaneously make decisions and take action. Learning to respect that improvisation is enhanced by diversity; it is not unification of perspectives that is sought in group improvisation, but an *integration of multiple perspectives*.[9]

We used to think that what was needed to deal with the uncertainties of the healthcare environment was a well-shaped script. Postmodernism and complexity science tell us that what is needed is the ability to use a script as a springboard for creating new potential in real time. The culture of healthcare organizations tends to be such that the typical responses to an unforeseeable future is to "do what you need to do in order to do what others expect you to do." Too many healthcare organizations are managed by great planners. This has led to a situation in which many great plans gather dust because the situations they were created for either never happened or changed too quickly to allow implementation of the plan. Improvisation, on the other hand, allows an organization to constantly negotiate and assess, to learn while in the middle of action, and to change a plan into an enabling structural tool.

Controlling (Steering) and Observing (Awareness and Reflection)

Having an organization that runs like clockwork is sometimes seen as the ideal endpoint of management; the objective of managing is to be in control and know what is going on. To do this, managers depend on strategies such as privileging policies to maintain physician quality, regulating and monitoring professional development hours, and gathering information about unit performance. Postmodernism and CAS theory recognize that what is in short supply is not information, but attention.[28] Rather than watching as a strategy for gaining and keeping control, managers should observe in order to learn what is happening in real time, reflect on that, and develop shared strategies for enhancing performance. Often healthcare organizations are managed in ways that hinder the ability of the people in them to observe and pay attention. For example, the high level of specialization in healthcare settings as well as the tremendous time pressures often limits workers' ability to observe the world as it unfolds. Managing in order to control the system may lead one to paying attention to the wrong things. For example, often we set up control systems and end up watching the control system instead of the system.[36] Awareness and reflection enable managers to deal more effectively with the turbulent healthcare environment while attempting to steer a healthcare organization often leads to disaster.

Exercising Power and Providing Leadership

There are many factors in the healthcare environment that cause patients and providers to seek the seat of power in the healthcare encounter. People are often faced with critically important circumstances where they feel "out of control." While recognizing the psychological need for the safety vested in the powerful other, modern science suggests that this safety is illusive and in the final analysis provides less psychological comfort than expected. Trying to determine how to provide leadership instead of exercise power in these circumstances is difficult. There are many ways to think about this, but one is to think about leadership as the legitimization of doubt.[37] Another is to think about leadership as an emerging property arising from the interactions in the system.[38]

Traditionally, managers in healthcare organizations have been imbued with legitimate power based on their position. But, access to mass media and information technologies have undermined traditional power bases of expertise, creating a situation in which power and leadership are both distributed in a decentralized system. Rather than relying solely on their ability to exercise power, healthcare managers need to pay attention to the ways that traditional bases of power interrelate with each other and with those with less power. For example, the traditional dual hierarchy that separated power and authority between clinicians and non-clinicians in a healthcare setting is breaking down. It sometimes seems as though a treatment for a diagnosis is as much a function of what the insurance company will pay for, as it is what the patient needs.

While authority based on legitimate power and reward power is important and meaningful, accomplishment of goals beyond the mundane requires leadership that extends beyond the correct, responsible, moral exercise of power. Leadership skill involves the ability to help people be reflective about the situations in which they find themselves and their organization.[16] Good leaders in healthcare organizations recognize that reflection requires time; therefore, they provide workers with adequate time to reflect, show them how to reflect, and make it a requirement that they do so. Successful leaders of healthcare organizations help people ask questions, because they recognize that part of being able to figure out an answer is being able to ask the right questions. Good leaders help everyone bring their unique perspectives to the table, recognizing that power can emerge from the interaction of multiple worldviews.

Achieving the Expected and Creating and Releasing Potential

Classical views of the world led to the assumption that the "correct performance" was the best performance that could be expected. The paradigms that we have explicated here acknowledge that the best that can be expected is, in fact, an unknown. While given our present understanding of a system, we may believe we can estimate what that system will achieve in some given timeframe, we are always being surprised as rehab workers become the center of a patient's clinical improvement, kitchen staff attract a team of workers committed to organizational success, or physicians develop insights across specialties that lead to new clinical processes. In other words, we're always being surprised by the unanticipated competencies of our organizations.[39]

Healthcare managers often find themselves in a trap of trying to accomplish is expected of them. They concentrate attention on keeping accreditation and meeting other standards and legal mandates and raising their average standing in comparison to similar organizations on issues, such as average expenditures for dietary services, infant mortality rates, and unnecessary readmissions. In an uncertain and changing world, the ability to respond creatively to unexpected events may be a very important skill, being curious combines with being critical as a managerial response to unanticipated events. Create an environment where the unexpected is not shunned, but is welcomed, where people feel free to discuss both the positive and negative outcomes of unintended events, and where the sharing of ideas is seen as a way to leverage new things in unexpected ways and to create new fabric. But, creating and responding to the unexpected may require that managers learn a different set of reactions than just following rules, procedures, and instructions and doing what is expected of them. Complexity science and postmodernism concentrate on "transforming the space of the possible."

Rather than asking people in their organizations, "Did you do this?" managers should ask instead, "What did you do?" When people walk into the healthcare setting, we often assume that they leave their intelligence behind. We act as if people in authority must make all decisions, and then complain because patients "don't take responsibility for their own health." New approaches may be required such as the approach exhibited by a clinic that does not weigh women because weight is such a sensitive issue for them. If you consider different questions than the ones given, expected, or assumed, you are likely to open up the organization to new ways of envisioning the past, present, and future.

■ WHAT DOES THIS ALL MEAN?

Relating, connecting, reflecting, and creating are the ongoing actions that successful managers keep at the forefront of their thoughts. The eight tensions described previously bring us back to new managerial postures. These postures are not things a thoughtful healthcare manager does, but rather things a thoughtful healthcare manager *is doing*. While unfolding and developing these postures, one will find that they have an emerging and receding horizon; deeper engagement with them will always reveal more intricacies and complexities.

Because our models are incomplete we should indulge in "creative actions" in order to find out more about what might happen and in this way increase our possible choices of action and improve the scope of our models."[15] In order to be a successful healthcare manager, you have to face up to the fact that being good at your job involves creativity, not just knowing what to do. Imagining the future: "Creatively should not (only) be understood in terms of flights of fancy or wild (postmodern) abandon, but also in terms of a careful and responsible development of the imagination. Imagining the future will involve risk, but the nature of this risk will be a function of the quality of our imagination. It is important that we start imagining better futures and for that we need better imaginations."[12,10] Good management is about getting good people to do great things. Most management is about getting great people to do mediocre things.[40] This is not accomplished by motivating workers to work harder, but by giving them better tools that help them make sense of the world, think about learning and reflecting, and be creative.

The posture a manager must take might look something like that of a top-notch jazz group. Wynton Marsalis said in an interview with David Frost, "The thing about Jazz is that it requires that . . . you have empathetic listening. You're endowed with the power to create what you want to play and you have to monitor yourself and play something that will fit with the group. And also you're not in control of what is going on; the whole group is in control of it. And you're constantly trying to negotiate and assess."[41]

■ CHAPTER SUMMARY

Complexity science (CS) and postmodernism (PM) have brought to the forefront of healthcare management a better understanding of the uncertain nature of reality and the implications of that uncertainty for managerial action. These approaches have led us to understand that the nature of relationships is critical, and that by focusing on those relationships new alternatives for management make themselves apparent. CS and PM focus attention on similar aspects of the world and therefore, viewing healthcare organizations through this joint lens can illuminate critical issues such as the history dependence, dynamic structures, inevitability of change, and issues of power. Also CAS theory calls our attention to the diversity of agents in the system and their capacity to learn, as well as the importance of the nonlinear interdependencies between these agents. Nonlinear interdependencies generate self-organization, emergence, and co-evolution leading to unpredictable future states and, at the same time, order and structure; thereby suggesting that managers focus on emergent patterns rather than focus on stable states.

Managing healthcare organizations as postmodernist complex adaptive systems requires attention to eight pairs of leadership actions:

1. Uncertainty reduction and uncertainty absorption
2. Decision making and sensemaking
3. Problem solving and dilemma resolving
4. Knowing and learning
5. Planning and improvisation
6. Controlling and observing
7. Exercising power and providing leadership
8. Creating the expected and creating and releasing potential

Managing healthcare organizations requires enabling creative action, helping good people do great things, and assuming a posture of continuous negotiation.

Review/Discussion Questions

1. What are some assumptions about the nature of the world that complexity science and postmodernism share? What are the implications of these assumptions for understanding the nature of healthcare organizations?

2. On what characteristics of their organizations does this chapter suggest that healthcare managers focus their attention?

3. What managerial actions are suggested by complexity science and postmodernism that are different from those suggested by traditional management approaches?

4. Describe the posture that healthcare managers should take toward their organizations.

5. What are the most critical elements of a healthcare system from the standpoint of complexity science and postmodernism?

6. What are some of the differences between modernist healthcare models and models derived from postmodernist and complexity thinking?

7. What are some implications of complexity science and postmodernism for those who manage healthcare organizations?

8. What explanations would complexity science give for a lack of effectiveness of planning and control methods for managing healthcare organizations?

9. What are some key attributes of leadership when one recognizes that healthcare organizations are complex postmodernist systems?

10. Why do you think someone, trained as an excellent problem solver, might run into difficulties when attempting to manage a complex adaptive system?

11. What is the value of diversity in an organization's workforce from the standpoint of complexity science and postmodernism?

12. If a manager attempted to adopt a postmodernist/complexity science stance, what conflicts might he/she anticipate with traditional clinicians?

13. What are major changes a traditional manager might have to make if he/she adopted key views from postmodernism and complexity science?

Learning Activities

Exercise 1: Surprises from Complex Adaptive Systems

Because of the nature of CAS, they are always presenting managers with surprises. Definitions of surprise range from "an attack made without warning" to "a taking unawares." When we are surprised, we are struck with wonder or amazement, or are impressed forcibly through unexpectedness or unusualness. "Unexpectedness, rather than novelty, unfamiliarity, or uncertainty, elicits surprise."

Below is a list of specific surprises that have been identified in organizational settings. Each represents a situation that any manager in a healthcare organization might face. While these may seem clear when stated and may seem like "common sense" at the time the research was done, these findings were contrary to conventional wisdom and often viewed as radical. Think about what we know from this chapter that might help us understand these surprises. Though modernism and classical science might consider these surprises as problems to avoid or solve, we are asking you to look at them from the standpoint of postmodernism and CAS theory. Based on the material presented in this chapter, develop management strategies and tactics suggested by the surprises presented.

1. Participation of clinicians in hospital strategic decision making is more helpful in terms of bottom line performance than the participation of middle managers.[42]
2. Organizations engaged in effective, fast decision making use just as much information as slow decision makers but information of a different kind.[43]
3. Safety on aircraft carriers is a function of the development of shared understanding of situations rather than simply a function of the development of well-articulated procedures.[44]
4. Homes that want to improve quality care can use Registered Nurse participation in strategic and tactical decision making to make performance improvements without significantly increasing costs.[45]

Exercise 2: Error Avoidance in CAS

One advantage of the joint postmodern/complexity lens is that managers might avoid some errors that would otherwise be pitfalls. Some of these are identified in the following list. From the perspectives outlined in this chapter, why are these errors? How might the ideas presented in this chapter help you avoid these errors?

- Failing to account for employees' ability to learn safe machine operation methods by experimenting on their own with ways to speed up production and thereby reduce the effort they are required to use.
- Putting all employees through the same orientation program regardless of differences in cultural interpretations of organizational hierarchies and thereby missing the potential for conflict among employees and between employees and management caused by different expectations of roles.
- Disciplining one employee, expecting a modest change in that employee's behavior but getting a massive union response.
- Changing a work process without considering the role of communities of practice on work performance.
- Assuming that employees will not reallocate work assignments based on their perception of the best arrangement even after receiving work allocation assignments from management.
- Ignoring the speed with which the informal organization can transmit messages and, therefore, failing to manage rumors in a productive manner.

- Failing to treat the organization's dominant logic as an emergent property of the system and, instead, treating it as something that can be imposed on the system.
- Looking for one bad apple in a group as a strategy for improving work quality, when the quality of output may be an emergent property of the group.
- Conducting careful market analysis to determine whether to release a new product but ignoring the fact that the release of the new product may change the market in such a way as to make the market analysis incorrect.
- Offering a premium to internal workers for extra production without expecting the change in reward structure to affect relationships with suppliers

Exercise 3: A Case in Point

It would be instructive to consider a specific case in point. Readers should be able to use material from this chapter to understand what went on in the case and how the organization might learn from the events of the case. Readers should also be able to identify possible actions that might be taken now to manage future situations of this type.

The fall 2002 issue of *Frontiers* (a well-known healthcare journal) was devoted to a discussion of "When Disaster Strikes: Healthcare's Response." One of the lead articles in that discussion was by David J. Campbell, FACHE, "9/11: A Healthcare Provider's Response" (pp. 3–13). This case outlines the response of Saint Vincent Catholic Medical Centers' (SVCMC) eight hospitals to the attack on the World Trade Center. St. Vincent's Manhattan was the nearest level 1 trauma center to the disaster and, as such, was centrally involved in the immediate aftermath of the bombings.

St. Vincent's had a diverse set of agents that interacted to respond to various events. The team of clinicians, called upon to speak to the press, represented a wide variety of specialties, and was able to create a comprehensive and trusting relationship with the media (p. 11). Volunteers flooded the hospital to offer their services (p. 4). The situation demanded not only acute care physicians, but also behavioral specialists to deal with the multiple effects of the tragedy (p. 5).

The role of the family center shifted from a source of information to providing counseling to families and friends of victims (p. 5). The behavioral staff found itself serving not only the direct victims of the tragedy but hospital employees as well (p. 5). People from a wide variety of hospital sections organized to meet the emerging communication needs on a 24-hour-a-day basis (p. 11). Systems properties emerged as the overwhelming need of people for information and relief from horrors that had been witnessed became a priority (p. 5). SVCMC's computers emerged as the consistent communication link when telephone service was disrupted (p. 4). The city provided water to compensate for broken water mains (p. 4) and the New School University provided space to relieve an impossibly crowded family center (p. 5).

The first "lesson learned" reported in the article had to do with the need for regional planning for a regional response to disasters, and the critical need to have appropriate liaison strategies developed before they are needed (p. 6). The Greater New York Hospital Association is in the process of developing a comprehensive emergency contact directory so that organizations can be of assistance to each other (p. 8). SVCMC has built on "its history of community outreach, its preexisting relationships, and the skills, ability, and dedication of its staff to address [the issues of behavioral trauma]" (p. 10). Respectful interaction, mindfulness, and collective mind can be clearly seen in SVCMC's response to the psychological needs of those directly affected by the tragedy (p. 5). They can also be seen in the response to the need to provide accurate and timely information to the media (p. 11). Surprises occurred—some positive such as the influx of volunteers and donations that flooded the system (p. 4), and others more problematic, such as the torrent of families and friends searching for loved ones that threatened to overwhelm the hospital (p. 5) and they had to be managed.

References

1. West BJ. Where medicine went wrong: Rediscovering the path to complexity. *Studies of Nonlinear Phenomena in Life Science*. Vol. 11. Hackensack, NJ: World Scientific Publishing Co.; 2006.
2. Zimmerman B, Lindberg C, Plsek P. *Edgeware: Insights from Complexity Science for Health Care Leaders*. Irving, TX: VHA Inc.; 1998.
3. Maguire S, McKelvey B, Mirabeau L, Oztas N. Complexity science and organization studies. In: Clegg SR, Hardy C, Lawrence TB, Nord WR, eds. *The Sage Handbook of Organization Studies*. 2nd ed. London: Sage Publications; 2006:166.
4. Gleick J. *Chaos: Making a New Science*. New York, NY: Penguin Books; 1987.
5. Waldrop MM. *Complexity: The Emerging Science at the Edge of Order and Chaos*. New York, NY: Touchstone by Simon & Schuster; 1992.
6. Plsek P. Redesigning health care with insights from the science of complex adaptive systems. *Crossing the Quality Chasm: A New Health System for the 21st Century*. Vol Appendix B. Washington DC: National Academy Press; 2001:322–335.
7. Begun JW. Managing with professionals in a changing health care environment. *Med Care Rev*. 1985;42:3–10.
8. Fleener MJ, Merritt ML. Paradigms Lost? *Nonlinear Dynamics Psychol Life Sci*. 2007;11:11–18.

9. Giere RN. *Science without Laws*. Chicago, IL: University of Chicago Press; 1999.

10. Alvesson M, Deetz SA. Critical theory and postmodernism approaches to organizational studies. In: Clegg SR, Hardy C, Lawrence TB, Nord WR, eds. *The Sage Handbook of Organization Studies*. 2nd ed. London: Sage Publications; 2006:255–283.

11. Bereiter C. Implications of postmodernism for science, or, science as progressive discourse. *Educational Psychologist*. 1994;29(1):3–12.

12. Cilliers P. Complexity, deconstruction and relativism. *Theory, Culture & Society*. 2005;22(5):255–267.

13. Morcol G. What is complexity science: Postmodernist or postpositivist? *Emergence*. 2001;3(1):104–119.

14. Cilliers P. *Complexity and Postmodernism: Understanding Complex Systems*. New York, NY: Routledge; 1998.

15. Allen PM, Varga L. Complexity: The co-evolution of epistemology, axiology and ontology. *Nonlinear Dynamics Psychol Life Sci*. January 2007;11(1):19–50.

16. Stroebel CK, McDaniel RR, Crabtree BF, Miller WL, Nutting PA, Stange KC. How complexity science can inform a reflective process for improvement in primary care practices. *Jt Comm J Qual Patient Saf*. August 2005;31(8):438–446.

17. Seligman LS. *Perceived Value Impact as an Antecedent of Perceived Usefulness, Perceived Ease of Use, and Attitude: A Perspective on the Influence of Values on Technology Acceptance*. Ann Arbor, MI, The University of Texas at Austin; 2001.

18. Paul DL, McDaniel RR, Jr. A field study of the effect of interpersonal trust on virtual collaborative relationship performance. *MIS Quarterly*. June 2004;28(2):183–227.

19. Weick KE, Sutcliffe KM. Hospitals as cultures of entrapment: A re-analysis of the Bristol Royal Infirmary. *Calif Manage Rev*. 2003;45(2):73–84.

20. Edmondson AC, Bohmer RM, Pisano GP. Disrupted routines: Team learning and new technology implementation in hospitals. *Adm Sci Q*. 2001;46(4):685–716.

21. Cilliers P. Boundaries, hierarchies and networks in complex systems. *International Journal of Innovation Management*. 2001;5(2):135–147.

22. Capra F. *The Web of Life*. New York: Anchor Books Doubleday; 1996.

23. Boisot M, Child J. Organizations as adaptive systems in complex environments: The case of China. *Organization Science*. May/Jun 1999;10(3):237–252.

24. Edmondson AC. Learning from mistakes is easier said than done: Group and organizational influences on the detection and correction of human error. *J Appl Behav Sci*. March 1996;32(1):5–28.

25. Weick KE. The collapse of sense making in organizations: The Mann Gulch disaster. *Adm Sci Q*. 1993;38(4):628–652.

26. Weick KE. *Sense-Making in Organizations*. Vol 3. Thousand Oaks, CA: Sage Publications; 1995.

27. March JG, Sproull LS, Tasmuz M. Learning from samples of one or fewer. *Organization Science*. 1991;2(1):58–71.

28. Simon HA. *Information, Technology and Computers in Management. Lecture at the Graduate School of Business*. The University of Texas at Austin; 1991.

29. Kelso JAS, Engstrøm DA. *The Complementary Nature*. Cambridge, MA: The MIT Press; 2006.

30. Stacey RD. The science of complexity: An alternative perspective for strategic change processes. *Strategic Management Journal.* 1995;16(6):477–495.
31. Crossan MM, Sorrenti M. Making sense of improvisation. *Advances in Strategic Management.* 1997;14:155–180.
32. Erickson F. *Talk and Social Theory.* Oxford: Polity Press; 2004.
33. Weick KE. Small wins: Redifining the scale of social problems. *Am Psychol.* 1984;39(1):40–49.
34. Sitkin SB. Learning through failure: The strategy of small losses. *Research in Organizational Behavior.* 1992;14:231–266.
35. Merry U. *Coping with Uncertainty: Insights from the New Sciences of Chaos, Self Organization, and Complexity.* Westport: Praeger; 1995.
36. Weick KE. Cosmos vs. chaos: Sense and nonsense in electronic contexts. *Organ Dyn.* 1985;14(2):51–64.
37. Weick KE. Leadership as the legitimation of doubt. In: Bennis W, Spreitzer GM, Cummings TG, eds. *The Future of Leadership.* San Francisco, CA: Jossey-Bass; 2001:91–102.
38. Goldstein JA, Hazy JK. Editorial introduction to the Special Issue: From Complexity to Leadership and Back to Complexity. *Emergence: Complexity and Organization.* 2006;8(4):v–vii.
39. McDaniel RR, Jr., Jordan ME, Fleeman B. Surprise, surprise, surprise! A complexity science view of the unexpected. *Health Care Manage Rev.* 2003;28(3):266–278.
40. Pfeffer J, Sutton RI. *Hard Facts, Dangerous Half-Truths, and Total Nonsense.* Boston, MA: Harvard Business School Press; 2006.
41. Marsalis W. Talking with David Frost: Wynton Marsalis. PBS VIDEO, 1997.
42. Ashmos DP, Huonker JW, McDaniel RR, Jr. Participation as a complicating mechanism: The effect of clinical professional and middle manager participation on hospital performance. *Health Care Manage Rev.* May 1998;23(4):7–20.
43. Eisenhardt KM. Speed and strategic choice: How managers accelerate decision making. *Calif Manage Rev.* 1990;2:39–54.
44. Weick KE, Roberts KH. Collective mind in organizations: Heedful interrelating on flight decks. *Adm Sci Q.* 1993;38(3):357–381.
45. Anderson R, McDaniel RR, Jr. RN participation in organizational decision making and improvements in resident outcomes. *Health Care Manage Rev.* 1999;24(1):7–16.

Organization Behavior and Dynamics

"It is the theory that decides what is to be observed."

Albert Einstein

6

Individual Behavior and Motivation

Mary S. O'Shaughnessey

Learning Objectives

- To become familiar with theories of motivation.
- To identify different types of motivation.
- To understand the effects of motivation on behavior.

■ INTRODUCTION

Individual behavior and motivation has been and continues to be a conundrum for most people. We wonder why did that person do what he/she did? Why does that student study 4 hours a day and another student never take home a book? Why does that team always seem to win while others always seem to lose? Some individuals dedicate their lives to a profession or a sport, while others have the talent or intelligence but do not spend the time or energy to develop the skills necessary to succeed. What is the difference between these individuals? The key to understanding the reasons for the different behaviors is motivation. Motivation is important to everyone involved in leading others and encouraging them to act. This chapter will explore some of the theories of motivation and the behaviors that result from the different types of motivation. As you read this chapter, consider the reasons for your behavior and the reasons that you are reading this book.

■ THEORIES OF MOTIVATION

Abraham H. Maslow's Theory

In 1943, A. H. Maslow published the article "A Theory of Human Motivation" in the journal *Psychological Review*.[1] He began with an overview of 13 propositions that he stated must be included in a definition of motivation and followed the overview by presenting his theory, which is composed of a hierarchy of five goals or basic needs. At the bottom of the hierarchy, as seen in Table 6-1, is the lowest level, which addresses physiological needs, such as food, water, and shelter. The second level represents safety needs, which are often fulfilled in a civilized society, but are more evident in war, natural disasters, and other emergencies. The third level represents social needs, which correspond to the human being's need for love and affection. At the fourth level is esteem needs, the desire for respect from others and for independence and freedom. At the top of Table 6-1 is self-actualization, which is the need to be fulfilled or maximizing one's potential and fulfilling one's passion.[2]

If needs at the lowest level are not satisfied, an individual will seek to have them satisfied before any others at the higher levels are satisfied. For example, if a person is hungry, especially if the person is starving, he or she will do almost anything to satisfy the need for food. The other needs will be unimportant. However, if the physiological needs are met, the next level of needs becomes prominent. As the needs at one level are met, the person will be motivated to reach satisfaction at the next higher level until reaching the top. At this level, people will have different types of self-actualization. Some will aspire to be an athlete, a lawyer, or even a teacher. In order for self-actualization to occur, the preceding levels must be satisfied. However, the lower level needs, such as the physiological needs, may take prominence at various times until they are satisfied, at which time the individual will resume activities designed to satisfy needs at a higher level. Maslow determined that the three lower level needs were extrinsic, from outside the individual, while the top two levels were intrinsic, that is within the individual.[1,3]

Table 6-1 Maslow's Hierarchy of Needs

Level Five: Self-Actualization Needs

Level Four: Esteem Needs

Level Three: Social Needs

Level Two: Safety Needs

Level One: Physiological Needs

Behavioral Implications

If a person has physiological needs, the need for food or water becomes paramount. All other needs become unimportant until this need is satisfied. Consider a newborn infant's need for food. If the infant is fed, then he or she sleeps or is calm because those needs have been met. The same outcome occurs when a hungry or starving adult is fed. After that need is fulfilled, the adult's attention moves to higher levels.[4] As each level is met, behavior is directed at the next need or goal. An individual seeking self-actualization might pursue a college degree in order to become a professional, or enroll in a comedy club to become an entertainer, or attend a technical school to learn a skilled trade. Whatever the interest of the individual, the motivation drives the person to follow a path leading to the desired goal or outcome that fulfills that specific need.

Employees in healthcare organizations represent a variety of professionals and staff who are dedicated to providing health services to patients. Their motivation to attain the skills and knowledge necessary to achieve this level of proficiency is evident by their past dedication to academic study and acquisition of specific competencies. Because of the continual improvements in technology and the development of new or enhanced diagnostic tools, healthcare professionals often must learn new skills in order to provide the most up-to-date service. Training and continual education have become part of the healthcare professionals' career. Maintaining a position within a healthcare system requires learning new skills and ensures that the second level of the hierarchy, safety, which refers to job security, becomes satisfied. The camaraderie among employees fulfills the social need for belonging to a group. As employees become more skilled, they also add to the fourth level, self-esteem, because they become more valuable to the organization. Thus, Maslow's theory regarding different levels of motivation may be demonstrated by the behaviors of healthcare providers. When the lower levels are satisfied, healthcare professionals are motivated to provide excellent care through self-actualization.[1,3]

Frederick Herzberg's Theory

In 1959, Frederick Herzberg along with Mausner and Snyderman published *The Motivation of Work*, which classified Maslow's hierarchy into two levels—the three lower levels are known as the hygienes, and the top two levels are the motivators.[5] This theory became known as the Two-Factor Theory. The authors proposed that employees need to be satisfied with the hygiene factors, even if the higher-level factors are in place. If lower-level factors such as pay, incentives, and the work environment are improved, employees will quickly become satisfied. Employees will then want more because the motivating factors are not satisfied. The employer must emphasize intrinsic motivators, such as the need for more challenging work, that offer the opportunity for the employee to achieve a level of competence, which leads to self-actualization. Herzberg's theory postulates that the employee derives satisfaction from the achievement, which is the motivation to do the job well.[3]

According to Herzberg's theory, extrinsic motivation is not as powerful as intrinsic motivation. Many psychologists have tested his assumptions and reported the results of their studies. Muchinsky[6] reported two criticisms of the theory. The first involved the method of data collection, which could have been slanted in favor of the two factors. The second criticism was that other studies have not been able to replicate the results. However, Martin Wolf reported that the motivators or content components were more able to predict job satisfaction than were the hygiene or context components.[7] Wolf also contended that Herzberg was incorrect "equating 'satisfaction' with 'motivation.'"[7]

Behavioral Implications

The Two-Factor Theory implies that utilizing rewards that only meet the hygiene needs will not completely satisfy employees. Researchers have found that both factors are important in meeting the employees' needs and goals. In order to have satisfied employees, organizations must provide the environment that encourages achievement, allows employees to reach self-actualization, and recognizes employees' accomplishments.[3,7] Satisfied employees remain with organizations that provide this level of motivation. In order to have a satisfied and stable workforce, healthcare leaders must strive to provide employees with challenges and opportunities for improvement.

Edward Deci's Theory of Motivation

Edward Deci proposed a theory of self-determination in *The Psychology of Self-Determination* in 1980.[8] The Self-Determination Theory (SDT) espouses that intrinsic motivators "relate to the experience of being competent and self-determining."[9] People are motivated by their past experiences and the outcomes of those experiences. Both intrinsic and extrinsic motivators cause people to behave in different ways. Deci indicated that those who are intrinsically motivated demonstrate improved effectiveness, inventiveness, and accomplishment as compared to those who are extrinsically motivated. The SDT identified different types of motivation, depending on the particular type of motivation that causes a person to act. The different types include cognitive evaluation theory, organismic integration theory, and basic needs theory.

Cognitive Evaluation Theory

Within SDT are elements that address the differences in motivation due to social and environmental influences. The cognitive evaluation theory suggests that forms of communication, such as feedback, increase the individual's level of competence, which also increases that person's motivation for that event. Positive remarks encourage individual motivation in contrast to negative comments that weaken individual motivation. In addition, individuals need to feel that they are in control or caused the action in order to have intrinsic motivation enhanced. Relatedness, or connection with others, such as a mother with her infant, may also be significant in strengthening intrinsic motivation. Of course, these concepts only apply to those that have the interest and the intrinsic motivation to reach a specific goal.[10]

Contrasted to intrinsic motivation is extrinsic motivation, which also is considered in the SDT. An individual's behavior in response to extrinsic motivation depends upon previous experiences. Deci explains extrinsic motivation as an activity that is executed in order to achieve an outcome in contrast to intrinsic, which is performing the activity for the pleasure of doing it. For example, extrinsically motivated employees may do their work because their job requires them to complete assignments in order to earn a salary. Intrinsically motivated employees provide service because they enjoy personal fulfillment in the work. The two groups differ in that the first group is responding to a requirement, whereas the latter group has chosen to perform the activity, which also indicates more autonomy among these employees.

Organismic Integration Theory (OIT)

The OIT provides information about various "forms of extrinsic motivation"[11] along with elements that influence integration and internalization. Figure 6-1 illustrates a continuum that displays various types of motivation from non-self-determined to self-determined. Moving from left to right the continuum illustrates the changes from external regulation to integrated regulation as the motivation becomes less extrinsic and evolves into intrinsic motivation. Extrinsic motivation lies between intrinsic motivation and lack of motivation, or as Deci describes the concept, amotivation. At the far left of the extrinsic motivators are factors regulated by outside forces, such as supervisors, regulatory agencies, governments, etc. In these situations, the motivator is outside the control of the individual. Moving along the continuum to the right is introjected regulation, which

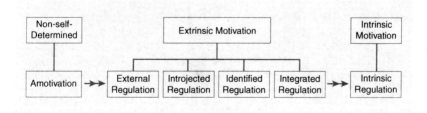

Figure 6-1 Motivation and Regulation Flowchart.

Source: Adapted from "Self-Determination Theory and the Facilitation of Intrinsic Motivation, Social Development, and Well-Being" by Ryan, M.R. and Deci, E.L.

refers to the ability to internalize the activity, but not fully invest in it as an intrinsic motivator. The cause here remains external to the individual, however, the concept is moving toward being internalized. Between introjected and intrinsic motivation is integrated regulation, wherein an individual accepts the regulation and values it as significant. The control has moved to more of an internal regulation. When the regulation becomes intrinsic, individuals discover an increase in autonomy along with personal satisfaction.

Basic Needs Theory

Ryan and Deci report that basic needs include physiological and psychological needs, which are competence, autonomy and relatedness. These needs must be satisfied for an individual to enjoy well-being. Culture plays a role in determining the manner and extent to which an individual's psychological needs are satisfied. However, the processes by which one acquires this satisfaction do appear comparable.

Behavioral Implications

The SDT addresses motivation as a composite of a variety of motivators. Inherent in the Cognitive Evaluation Theory is that individuals, who feel they are competent, must believe that they caused the event or action. By experiencing the combination of competence along with autonomy and possible relatedness, individual's intrinsic motivation will be enhanced. The resulting behavior will be demonstrated by increased performance, persistence, and creativity along with a feeling of comfort and an increased sense of worth.[10] For example, students taught by a very controlled approach do not learn as productively and suffer a decline in initiative when compared to students taught through a less controlled approach. Parents, who exert control over their children, raise offspring who are less intrinsically motivated than parents who support autonomy. Intrinsic motivation that is supported by autonomy results in behaviors that encourage persistence and competence.

The OIT suggests that behavior can be enhanced when extrinsic motivators become more intrinsic. This change is noted in children as they age and assert more control over their behavior. Students, who were more interested in school, enjoyed the experience, and had more coping skills, exhibited introjected regulation. Patients with chronic medical conditions were more compliant with medications when they internalized the regulations and valued the need for adherence to the regimen.[10] Integrating the regulation involves individuals understanding the reasons for the regulation and incorporating it as a part of their own value systems.

The basic needs theory proposes that people have needs for competence, autonomy, and relatedness. If these needs are not met, mental health can suffer and determination and performance can diminish. These needs are psychological, rather than physical, and thus contribute to an individual's performance. If the social environment supports the three needs, intrinsic motivation is maintained or strengthened, extrinsic motivation becomes more intrinsic and life goals are bolstered. Conversely, not fulfilling these needs leads to a reduced level of intrinsic motivation, lack of motivation, and an increase in extrinsic motivation. These changes result in poorer performance and a reduction in wellness.[10]

Steven Reiss's Theory

Dr. Steven Reiss stated that Maslow's theory of motivation does explain much of people's behavior.[12] The desires that Dr. Reiss describes are consistent with the thoughts of William James and William McDonald ". . . that our basic needs are genetically determined."[12] In his text *Who Am I? The 16 Basic Desires That Motivate Our Actions and Define Our Personalities,* Reiss lists the 16 desires, which are in included in Table 6-2.

Although almost everyone can relate to the 16 desires, the intensity is different within each person. This difference is due partially to the genetic diversity among individuals. For example, your mother may exhibit the desire "order," but you do not exhibit that desire. In fact, you may have a very weak desire to maintain a clean room, but your mother may have

Table 6-2 Reiss' 16 Basic Desires That Motivate Our Actions and Define Our Personalities

Basic Desire	Definition	Behavior
Power	Desire to influence others	Leadership, achievement
Independence	Desire for self-reliance	Self-reliance
Curiosity	Desire for knowledge	Truth-seeking, problem solving
Acceptance	Desire for inclusion	Assertive behavior
Order	Desire for organization	Makes many rules, clean, "perfect," compulsive
Saving	Desire to collect things	Collecting, frugality
Honor	Desire to be loyal to one's parents and heritage	Character, morality, principled behavior
Idealism	Desire for social justice	Social causes, fair play
Social Contact	Desire for companionship	Party, join clubs/groups
Family	Desire to raise one's own children	Parent, homemaker
Status	Desire for social standing	Concern with reputation, showing off
Vengeance	Desire to get even	Revenge
Romance	Desire for sex and beauty	Sex, courting
Eating	Desire to consume food	Eating, dining, cooking
Physical Activity	Desire for exercise of muscles	Physical exercise, participatory sports
Tranquility	Desire for emotional calm	Avoid stressful situations

Reiss, S. (2000). *Who Am I?: The 16 Basic Desires That Motivate Our Actions and Define Our Personalities.* New York, NY: Penguin Putnam, Inc.

a strong desire to see it clean. Individuals will also differ in the hierarchy of their desires. One person may consider honor as the most important desire while another person has status at the top of his list. Because people are born with these genetic predispositions, these desires remain fairly constant throughout life.

Behavioral Implications

Power

The desire for power involves mastery and/or competence, motivating people to pursue challenges. Satisfying the need for power often results in people accomplishing a difficult task, such as Lance Armstrong winning seven Tour de France races. Leadership is often a method of satisfying this desire and can result in people who are dominant, overbearing, and manipulative. Usually people with this desire are obstinate and headstrong. The desire for power and the behavior resulting from it is often intermittent, occurring in some situations, such as at work, but not in others, such as at home. If you are determined, strive to be in command and often control others in social situations with peers, you likely have a strong desire for power.

Independence

The desire for independence reflects the need to be free and self-reliant, not depending on others to assist you, especially if you can do or manage the activity yourself. If others help, the independent person may resent the help. Often elderly people who must live in nursing homes detest living there, because they must be dependent on others, proving every day that they are no longer able to care for themselves and be independent. As in the previous example of power, independence does not have to be a total lack of dependence. In some situations, such as in a partnership in a corporation, or in a marriage, people with a strong desire for power will become interdependent to compensate, or balance the freedom they experience elsewhere. People who have a strong desire for independence often refrain from taking advice from others. Some of their happiness results from being secure and self-reliant.

Curiosity

Reiss describes curiosity as ". . . one of the great joys in life" because it reflects the amount of joy that a person receives from the learning process.[12] Curious people want to know the truth, to be able to distinguish it from fiction, and often are dedicated to learning and analyzing the events not only around them but in the world. If an individual displays a strong desire to learn and is curious, searches for answers wherever he/she is, has a passion for scholarship, and uses discretionary time to consider what is true, that person exhibits a strong desire for curiosity.

Acceptance

Acceptance refers to the desire to be included and respected for his/her own unique capabilities and personality. Individuals who lack self-confidence and avoid conflict often have a strong desire to be accepted. Behaviors, such as not speaking in class, withdrawing from activities in which they may be evaluated, and not asking for promotions at work, are suggestive of a strong desire for acceptance. People who demonstrate this desire set goals that are easy to accomplish, do not persist at tasks that are difficult, and are very sensitive to criticism.

Order

People who are highly organized make lists, plan, and clean their surroundings. They dislike clutter because they prefer the stability of an orderly environment. If a person displays a very strong desire for order, they may exhibit an obsessive-compulsive disorder (OCD) which may interfere with the ability to perform daily activities. The famous aviator, Howard Hughes, had OCD and lived the last years of his life in seclusion due partly to this obsession. The desire for order can be expressed through exhibiting excessive organization, exorbitant cleaning, and strict adherence to rules.

Saving

The desire to save is rooted in the animal kingdom and seen in humans as collecting. Animals will hoard food while humans will collect antiques, money, stamps, and a myriad of other items. The amount of money saved depends on your previous experiences and the culture in which you were raised. In a marriage, how money is spent and how much money is spent can precipitate arguments because each person may have different ideas as to the amount to save and the amount to spend. Saving is very important to you if you are a collector, are frugal, and do not spend money easily, even when you have sufficient funds.

Honor

Honor represents the desire to be dutiful to one's heritage, family, and country. The desire for honor in this theory represents loyalty to family and friends and does not extend to loyalty beyond the immediate support structure. A strong desire for honor is seen in people who are categorized as highly principled and very loyal.

Idealism

The next desire, idealism, reflects people who are motivated by social justice and are committed to helping the underserved. Some people have a strong motivation to help others, such as Mother Theresa, while others have little to no motivation, such as those who steal or betray the trust of others. Individuals who display a strong desire for idealism commit themselves to causes that help humanity, often volunteer, and contribute to organizations that provide support to those less fortunate.

Social Contact

Social contact involves spending time with others whom you enjoy and share common interests. Gregarious people enjoy being around others and look for fun. They do not want to be alone very often as contrasted with people who would rather be alone more of the time than socialize. The amount of socializing desired varies with each individual. Isolating oneself can be a sign of mental illness as seen in clinical depression. The desire to be social is strong in people who need to be around others in order to be happy and who are recognized as playful.

Family

The desire for family reflects the need to raise and love your own offspring. Some parents devote their entire lives to their children, working many jobs to provide a better life for them. Other parents do not enjoy raising their children and hire others to fulfill this obligation. If your happiness is dependent on raising your children, and you spend considerably more time with them than other parents do, you have a strong desire for family.

Status

The desire for prestige is manifested in status, seen in people who are impressed with things that the wealthy have, such as large homes and expensive vehicles. They are very conscious and concerned about their reputations and what others think about them. Those with low status are not concerned about what others think about them. In societies such as India, the caste system is built on status and dictates the employment positions people can obtain, the food they can eat, the friends with whom they socialize, and the people they can marry. In the United States, people are very aware of status, which is evident by the titles of their positions within a company, the parking space allotted, and the size of their offices. People who have a strong desire for status often want to buy the very best, try to impress others with things they have purchased and devote much time to joining or maintaining memberships in prominent establishments.

Vengeance

The desire for revenge can cause aggression and competitiveness. People's responses to treatment they perceive are unfair, or delayed, may range from anger to retaliation. A University of Michigan study and studies from Great Britain, Finland, and Sweden reported that aggressive children grew into aggressive adults. People look for revenge in a variety of situations, such as filing a claim against someone in a court of law, or shooting the people that they dislike. The desire for vengeance is strong in people who have difficulty with anger management, are aggressive, are competitive, and spend time and energy pursuing retaliation.

Romance

The strong desire for romance, also categorized as sex and beauty, is influenced by genetics as well as by cultural perceptions of beauty. Romance also involves beauty in the forms of art and music. In order to look attractive, people spend hours and a great amount of money to improve their looks and appeal to others. Consistent with the previous desires is the variability that people experience in their desire for romance. Some people have a strong desire for romance as noted by frequently pursuing it, having sex with multiple partners, and difficulty controlling the desire for sex.

Eating

Eating is a biological need, but has no psychological significance. Eating involves time to shop for food, cook it, and then eat the meal or snack. People who are overweight or obese have difficulty controlling their behavior, because they think about food more often than thin people do, eat faster, and eat larger portions. At the other extreme are people who are anorexic or bulimic and will either starve themselves or rid their bodies of any food that they have eaten before it can be absorbed into the body. Both the extremely overweight and underweight individuals are in perilous health states and often require outside intervention to change their eating habits. People who exhibit a strong desire for eating eat more and diet more than people who are the same age.

Physical Activity

The desire for physical activity ranges from very little, as exemplified by the couch potato, to the professional athlete and the individual who regularly pursues exercise. Athletic ability is different from the desire for physical activity. One only has to go to the local golf club to see that many people enjoy playing golf, but do not play well or to the standards of a professional golfer. These people intrinsically enjoy the game and the physical exercise. Those who have a strong desire for physical activity exercise routinely and consider sports an important facet of their daily lives.

Tranquility

Reiss defines this desire ". . . as the absence of disturbance and turmoil, or the absence of anxiety, stress and fear."[12] Some people, such as relief pitchers, are able to tolerate stress and have a low desire for tranquility. Their confidence in their ability to produce reduces the stress that others try to avoid as evidenced by drinking excessively or taking medication. People's desire for tranquility is determined by their response to anxiety, stress, and pain. If they believe that anxiety and stress are harmful, they have a strong desire for tranquility. Other determinants of a strong desire for tranquility are repeated panic attacks and usually feeling fearful and timid.[12]

■ MOTIVATION IN THE WORK ENVIRONMENT

Supervisors often have the task of motivating their employees to increase production, improve a product or a service, deliver it more efficiently, or work more cooperatively with others. In order to accomplish these tasks, employees must have the required skills and the appropriate work environment as well as the motivation to perform well. Although an employee may be motivated to accomplish these tasks one time, the level of motivation may not be sufficient to improve performance consistently because of changes in the environment or other factors. The behavior is similar to that seen in Maslow's hierarchy of needs, wherein a person may be at the self-actualization level until he becomes hungry. The individual will need to satisfy the lower level need before he can resume activity at the higher level. This section of the chapter will explore motivation and behavior in the work place.

Theories of Motivation at the Workplace

Many psychologists have attempted to describe reasons for the motivators that explain the behaviors seen in the workplace. No one theory has emerged that explains all the factors involved in motivation, however, many theories do address some of the factors that are inherent in motivation. Author Paul Muchinsky describes theories of work motivation in his book *Psychology Applied to Work*. Muchinsky's theories are need, intrinsic motivation, expectancy, goal setting, equity, and reinforcement. The need and intrinsic motivation theories postulate that people have internal motivation that causes individuals to behave in ways that are enjoyable and ones that the people can control. The expectancy and goal-setting theories are based on the premise that people are rational and choose behaviors that will result in the outcomes that are desired. The equity and reinforcement theories assert that external factors are the motivating factors. Equity theory involves motivation caused by perceptions of inequities. Reinforcement theory is predicated on rewarding individuals on a scheduled basis. Therefore, motivation may be intrinsic, that is, inside of us, or a result of our desires or "a result of things that are 'done' to us."[6]

Another theory espoused by K. Sheldon, R. M. Ryan, E. L. Deci, and T. Kasser concerns the differences between extrinsic and intrinsic goals as they relate to well-being. Extrinsic goals are reported to be negatively correlated with well-being because those who focus on fame, wealth, and beauty report more symptoms of mental illness. The research does appear to be evidence that the goals individuals choose can be the underlying foundation that influences their future well-being.[13]

Behavioral Implications

Which theory is the best one to apply to the work environment? Which theory will the employees respond to in the most positive way? The answer is that there is no one theory that will be effective all the time. The need theory indicates that we are different in our motivators and that physiological needs must be satisfied before other needs are addressed. The equity theory recognizes that people are social and that other people influence us in many ways. Expectancy theory describes motivation based on the benefits to be gained by devoting time and energy to a project. If there are no rewards, the individual will lose motivation. Goal setting involves working toward a set goal by establishing specific objectives and working without distractions. Reinforcement theory suggests that motivation is increased when people are rewarded on specific defined performances rather than on time. People who have intrinsic motivation are said to behave in ways that give them feelings of personal control and their ability to perform a task or service.[6]

In response to the question of, "How does a supervisor motivate an employee?" one needs to consider the various theories of motivation and to discuss potential motivators with the employee. Because of the differences in people and in situations, one theory will not be effective all the time and likely not effective with everyone. Consideration must be given to all the theories, and the most appropriate theory applied to the current situation.[6]

Job Satisfaction

In a 2006 report, L. Kimball and C. Nink state that there is an increasing number of dissatisfied employees. The relationship between the employees and their supervisor was found to be a critical factor in the length of time they remained employed with the organization and with their level of productivity. When workers are satisfied, or in this report, "engaged," their productivity and commitment to the organization are increased. One suggestion for managers to improve employees' engagement is to match the job with the strengths of the employee because those employees will demonstrate high performance, are innovative, and endeavor to become highly efficient. Managers who canvassed employees about what they wanted and what was important to them were more effective in improving employees' productivity.[14] By engaging the employees, managers were able to discover the employees' motivations and to respond to those desires.

Further support of this approach in motivating employees was noted in a study by Baard, Deci, and Ryan that showed that intrinsic need satisfaction at work was highly correlated with performance.[15] As noted, the self-determination theory contends that individuals have three psychological needs, which are competence, autonomy, and relatedness. Competence refers to the capability of the individual to achieve the objectives they wanted. Autonomy is related to being the generator of one's behavior, while relatedness addresses forming a relationship with others that demonstrates mutual regard and dependence. After testing for the three needs, the authors investigated the relevance of a self-determination theory in terms of its applicability to workplace motivation. The study supported the theory that satisfaction of an individual's intrinsic needs is reflected in job performance. Managers who support autonomy also influence employees' perceptions of satisfaction.[15]

Job satisfaction was linked to job motivation by Martin Wolf.[7] He reported that context elements, such as job security, technical supervision, and interpersonal relationships with peers are not related to motivation in the workplace because an employee is not able to change or improve them. However, content elements, for example, achievement, recognition, and advancement closely relate to job motivation because an employee can increase the amount of his or her satisfaction by increasing the amount of work done. The strength of the motivation relates to the outcomes that are expected from the increase in work. This concept is also reflected in the expectancy theory as ascribed by Vroom and summarized by Muchinsky.[6]

Measuring Work Preference

The Work Preference Inventory (WPI) as described by Theresa Amabile, Karl Hill, Beth Hennessey, and Elizabeth Tighe in the *Journal of Personality and Social Psychology* was developed to evaluate the differences in adults' perceptions of their intrinsic and extrinsic motivators.[16] The authors wanted to discover whether or not intrinsic motivation and extrinsic motivation are compatible. They described extrinsic motivation as a focus on ". . . money, recognition, competition, and the dictates of other people."[16] In contrast intrinsic motivation involves ". . . challenge, employment, personal enrichment, interest and self-determination."[16] Note that self-determination is the same concept proposed by Edward Deci. The WPI was highly correlated with other questionnaires used previously to measure motivation.

After the WPI was administered to over 1300 undergraduate students and more than 1000 employed adults, results indicated that the WPI does provide information on individuals' motivation. The authors concluded that extrinsic motivation and intrinsic motivation are different procedures. Neither classification appears to affect the other in a negative way. This tool may be appropriate in assigning adults to the proper work sites within the healthcare environment.

■ CHANGES IN MOTIVATION

As stated by many researchers, motivation differs from individual to individual and individuals display varying levels of motivation. Authors Carol Sansone and Dustin B. Thoman suggest that a self-regulation process is helpful in comprehending the differences among people's interest levels as they pursue goals.[17] If a goal is not interesting, a person's motivation to reach the goal must be greater than the interest level itself. People may choose to quit working toward the goal or may choose behaviors that enhance the experience as they work toward accomplishing the goal. Thus, individuals are motivated by the outcomes and the process that occurs in reaching the outcome. Each area of motivation is self-regulated in order for individuals to cope with the daily trials of life. Understanding differences among individuals and the influences that these differences have on behaviors is important to predict future actions.[17]

■ MOTIVATION AND LEARNING

Healthcare organizations often provide opportunities for clinical and administrative staff to learn new methods and acquire new skills. In the fast-changing world of medical care, it is imperative that healthcare employees understand the necessity of continually improving the provision of care and assessing the impact of the improvements. One method is to utilize Maslow's model and follow the path from physiological needs to self-actualization. Wages are considered to be at the lowest level, but if an employee is not satisfied with the pay, focus may be on locating a new job or the inequities in pay. The next highest level concerns safety, which can be satisfied by providing a safe work environment, such as having sharps containers in hospital examination rooms, as well as providing sufficient benefits and training, which increase the employee's skill and value to the organization. The third level is social belongingness, which can be enhanced by presenting training that involves employees from a variety of areas. Self-esteem is strengthened by attending training which in turn may lead to rewards and positive recognition. At the very top of the hierarchy is self-actualization, which is reinforced by the individual striving to acquire new skills and improve confidence.[18]

Employee Involvement in Learning

Creating a successful learning culture requires that employees and management commit to development that encourages and enhances skill development. Hiring employees that have demonstrated prior interest in development is important as is keeping current employees motivated to learn and apply new information. Employees who are motivated to advance in their careers often view learning as a means to acquire skills and knowledge that will lead to additional responsibilities and promotions. They may believe that participating in learning activities will make work more engaging and inspiring, which is consistent with intrinsic motivators being important in encouraging individuals to work toward a goal. The benefit to the organization is that employee retention is greater for those individuals who feel and experience that learning contributes to retention by providing growth opportunities and work that is challenging. In contrast, extrinsic rewards, such as pay, were not nearly as important in retention as were the presence of learning opportunities. Factors that contributed to an employee's development include positive learning experiences in the past, comprehension of the need for learning, confidence in his/her ability to learn, realization of intrinsic benefits from learning, and support by those internally in the work environment and externally to the work environment.[19]

A meta-analysis of the variables that correlate with training revealed that motivation to learn was relevant along with skill development and performance on the job after completing training. Personality variables, job investment, and career planning were also important factors as were individuals' positive attitude toward their own capabilities and intelligence. Positive learning appears dependent on the individual's motivators as well as adequate resources, feedback, and favorable outcomes as a result of applying the newly acquired skills and knowledge.[20]

■ IMPACT OF AGE AND CULTURAL FACTORS ON MOTIVATION AND LEARNING

The large number of baby boomers who are nearing retirement is projected to have an enormous impact on the economic climate of the United States. Many baby boomers indicate that they are not ready to retire to a porch swing, but have the motivation and desire to continue working in some capacity. Employers who want to retain this experienced workforce are faced with challenges in developing older workers' skills. The older employees may not be interested, may not have the motivation to learn new skills, or may face discrimination from younger workers.[19] However, if older workers, those 40 years of age and older, are presented with relevant benefits, their motivation to learn may be enhanced. When a training session was described as work rather than play, older workers achieved the same level of skill as did younger workers.[21]

Culture does influence both intrinsic and extrinsic motivation. For example, Canadian athletes preferred more democratic behavior from coaches and positive feedback whereas Japanese players liked "... more ... control-oriented behavior from coaches."[22] A study by Ivengar and Lepper investigated the concept of choice as a motivating factor for Asian-American and Anglo-American children.[23] The results indicated that Anglo-American children preferred to make their own choices, whereas Asian-American children performed better when the choice was made by respected adults, especially in this study, by a parent. The indication from these studies is that extrinsic motivation, that is behavior driven by outside influences, can be as motivating or more motivating for some cultures than others.

Markus and Kitayama propose that the cultural influences inherent in the people of North America and Western Europe seek independence and prefer to make their own choices.[24] In contrast is the Asian culture in which motivations are based on conforming to social requirements, such as respecting the wishes of one's family to excel in scholastic achievement. This difference is also noted in the workplace. In Western cultures, leadership success is based on relationships among the leader, the followers, and the tasks. In Eastern cultures, leadership success is fostered by the employee's obligation to the leader.

Behavioral Implications

The United States has been referred to as a "melting pot" because people from a variety of cultures have migrated from their countries to live in the United States. One only has to visit a metropolitan airport within a large city to observe the diversity amongst the travelers who are arriving and departing for locations within and outside the United States. The diversity of cultures is important to note because the people who are, and will be, working in healthcare exemplify the various cultures. They bring with them the variety of motivators and behaviors that are inherent in their backgrounds and experiences. Healthcare organizations and administrators must acknowledge these differences, so that they provide environments that allow managers to respect and understand these employees' motivations in order to meet the employees' goals and the goals of the organization.

■ MOTIVATION AND SPORTS

An increasing number of television broadcasts of sporting events are seen throughout the industrialized nations of the world. During the world soccer games in 2006, Italians pulled televisions and chairs into the streets to sit with friends and cheer for the Italian soccer team. Throughout the United States, cable television broadcasts sports events almost continuously. From the time some children are able to understand even the nuances of a game or a sport, they are organized into teams or enrolled in lessons to instruct them on the rules of the sport and the techniques to play at their highest level. Many adults continue to play sports into their 80's and a few into their 90's. A few very talented individuals will eventually become professional athletes. What motivates the children as they grow into adults to become professional athletes? What motivates them to keep playing a sport? Are the motivators intrinsic or extrinsic?

As children acquire more skill, they become more proficient and experience greater enjoyment from the sport. They perceive a feeling of personal achievement and enjoy the physical exercise, the contest, and the team synergy. These intrinsic motivators have been reported to be more effective than external motivators, such as awards.[9] College athletes who receive scholarships view their sport as work as compared to athletes who did not receive scholarships.[25] However, as a child grows into an adult and becomes a professional athlete, the extrinsic rewards, such as fame and wealth, become more influential.[9]

Other factors that influence motivation are whether or not the athlete receives feedback and whether or not there was competition. As expected, positive feedback increased intrinsic motivation while negative feedback had the opposite reaction. Competition was of greater interest to males than females perhaps due to greater ego involvement and evidence of self-worth for males as compared to females.[9]

Behavioral Implications

What does motivating an athlete have in common with motivating health-care employees? The answer is that there are some commonalities that can be applied in both environments. The athlete is motivated by positive feedback, as is the employee. Intrinsic motivation is inherent in both individuals because they desire to fulfill Level Five in Maslow's hierarchy—self-actualization. They are self-determined as displayed by their need for competence, autonomy, and relatedness. Most athletes play on a team, which is similar to the healthcare provider who works with a team of providers to deliver patient care. The athlete enjoys competition and winning while the healthcare employee enjoys curing patients, thus defeating the illness. Thus, the motivators and the resulting behaviors are comparable in both groups.

■ CHAPTER SUMMARY

Maslow's hierarchy described five levels of needs ranging from the basic physiological needs to self-actualization. Maslow's needs were further classified into intrinsic and extrinsic motivators. Herzberg used Maslow's theory of motivation as a foundation for the Two-Factor Theory. Additionally, Deci and Ryan proposed the Self-Determination Theory, which built on the foundation of intrinsic and extrinsic motivators. Intrinsic motivators appear to lead to an increase in competence and self-worth as opposed to extrinsic motivators. Reiss's list of 16 desires that provides a framework to analyze behaviors and define individual motivators underlying these behaviors. It can be said that motivation in the workplace is dependent on the employee's intrinsic and extrinsic needs or goals, as well as his/her age, cultural background, and motivation to learn. Ultimately, the athlete and the healthcare provider are motivated by similar needs and display behaviors that reflect those common factors.

Review/Discussion Questions

1. Describe Maslow's hierarchy. Which need best describes your current motivational stage?
2. Name one of the psychologists other than Maslow and describe the author's theory of motivation.
3. Define intrinsic and extrinsic motivation. What is the major difference between them?
4. Why is culture an important factor in understanding an individual's motivation and behavior?

Learning Activities

1. Using the 16 basic desires that Dr. Reiss has described, rate your desires with the most prominent being first. Explain the reasons for your selection of the first three items.

2. Choose a classmate to be your partner, preferably someone that you know well. Try to predict his/her top three desires as described by Dr. Reiss. Exchange lists with your partner and discuss the choices that you each have made. Support your choices based on the behaviors that you demonstrate.

3. Intrinsic motivators are reported to have more impact on employee retention than extrinsic motivators, such as salary. Would you stay in a position that you did not like because it paid a high salary? State the reasons for your answer.

4. What cultures do you see represented in your workplace, in your community and in your class? What are the differences and the similarities between your culture and one of your classmates or co-workers from another culture or country? How might the differences affect the classroom or work environment?

Case Study

Setting: A large community hospital is located in a low socio-economic neighborhood and provides services to the people living in the surrounding area. The hospital employs 15 respiratory therapists to service the inpatients. At least one therapist has to be available at all times to meet the demand of the patients in the emergency room and those in intensive care.

Problem: One of the therapists is not able to respond to the demands of the position because of difficulty in providing services to patients in a timely manner. Floor nurses and charge nurses complain when this therapist is on the midnight shift because she does not respond quickly, and the lack of a quick response could compromise patient care. The supervisor has talked with the employee about the problem, but there has not been any change in the therapist's behavior. The therapist does not seem motivated to do a good job, in part because she knows that her skills are in demand and she could find another position in another facility. Also, the therapist had a recent divorce and now has custody of her small son. The supervisor wants to retain the therapist and provide the appropriate environment and assistance so that the employee will perform at or above expectations.

Alternatives Considered: The supervisor has consulted with colleagues about the situation and they offered the following suggestions:

- Terminate the employee because she is not capable of meeting the demands of the job.

- Develop an action plan to assist her in better time management.
- Encourage her to see an Employee Assistance Counselor to help with family problems.

Actions Taken: The supervisor did not want to terminate the employee because of her excellent skills and because it is quite difficult to find therapists willing to come to that part of the city. However, the supervisor did develop an action plan with the employee to improve her time management skills. She paired the therapist with a senior therapist who followed her and gave her suggestions on better ways to manage her time and still complete the required documentation. The supervisor arranged for the employee to receive additional training on the hospital computer system, which improved her ability to document the care she provided and see patients more efficiently and expeditiously.

After the supervisor and the therapist discussed the recent change in her family status, the supervisor scheduled the employee to meet with a member of the human resources staff and discuss the Employee Assistance Program (EAP). The supervisor was concerned that the therapist was so focused on the basic needs of her family that she could not concentrate on the patients and her work.

Outcome: After a few days of working with the senior therapist, the employee was able to integrate more efficient techniques into her therapy and respond more quickly to requests from hospital nurses. The therapist began counseling through the EAP, which assisted her in obtaining reputable care for her son when she had to work a late night shift. Within 6 weeks, the therapist's behavior changed and she demonstrated more interest in her position and her patients. Her intrinsic motivation had moved from the lower levels to the higher levels as noted by Maslow. She was now feeling self-actualized because her physiological and safety needs were satisfied.

References

1. Maslow AH. A theory of human motivation. *Psychological Review*. 1943; 50:370–396.
2. Johnson JA, Breckon DJ. *Managing Health Education and Promotion Programs: Leadership Skills for the 21st Century*. Sudbury, MA: Jones and Bartlett; 2007.
3. Dessler G. *Human Resource Management*. Upper Saddle River, NJ: Pearson Education; 2005.
4. Stephens DC (ed.), Maslow AH. *The Maslow Business Reader*. New York: Wiley & Sons, Inc.; 2000.
5. Herzberg F, Mausner B, Snyderman BB. *The Motivation of Work*. New York:Wiley; 1959.
6. Muchinsky PM. *Psychology Applied to Work. An Introduction to Industrial and Organizational Psychology*. Pacific Grove, CA: Brooks/Cole Publishing; 1990.

7. Wolf MG. Need gratification theory: A theoretical reformulation of job satisfaction/dissatisfaction and job motivation. *J Appl Psychol.* 1970;54:87–94.

8. Deci EL. *The Psychology of Self-Determination.* Lexington, MA: Lexington Books, D.C. Heath and Company; 1980.

9. Deci EL, Ryan RM. *Intrinsic Motivation and Self-Determination in Human Behavior.* New York: Plenum Press; 1985.

10. Ryan MR, Deci EL. Self-determination theory and the facilitation of intrinsic motivation, social development and well-being. *Am Psychol.* 2000; 55:68–78.

11. Deci EL, Ryan RM. The "what" and "why" of goal pursuits: Human needs and the self-determination of behavior. *Psychol Inq.* 2000;11:227–268.

12. Reiss S. *Who Am I?: The 16 Basic Desires That Motivate Our Actions and Define Our Personalities.* New York, NY: Penguin Putnam, Inc.; 2000.

13. Sheldon KM, Ryan RM, Deci EL, Kasser T. The independent effects of goal contents and motives on well-being: It's both what you pursue and why you pursue it. *Pers Soc Psychol Bull.* 2004;30:475–486.

14. Kimball LS, Nink CE. How to improve employee motivation, commitment, productivity, well-being and safety. *Corrections Today.* 2006;68:66–74.

15. Baard PP, Deci EL, Ryan RM. Intrinsic need satisfaction: A motivational basis of performance and well-being in two work settings. *J Appl Soc Psychol.* 2004;34:2045–2068.

16. Amabile TM, Hill KG, Hennessey BA, Tighe EM. The work preference inventory: Assessing intrinsic and extrinsic motivational orientations. *J Pers Soc Psychol.* 1994;66:950–967.

17. Sansone C, Thoman DB. Maintaining activity engagement: Individual differences in the process of self-regulating motivation. *J Pers.* 2006;74:1697–1720.

18. Benson SG, Dundis SP. Understanding and motivating health care employees: Integrating Maslow's hierarchy of needs, training and technology. *J Nurs Manag.* 2003;11:315–320.

19. Maurer TJ, Weiss EM, Bareite FG. A model of involvement in work-related learning and development activity: The effects of individual, situational, motivational, and age variables. *J Appl Psychol.* 2003;88: 707–724.

20. Colquitt JA, LePine JA, Noe R. Toward an integrative theory of training motivation: A meta-analytic path analysis of 20 years of research. *J Appl Psychol.* 2000;85:678–707.

21. Webster J, Martocchio JJ. Turning work into play: Implications for microcomputer software training. *Journal of Management.* 1993;19:127–146.

22. Frederick CM, Ryan RM. Self-determination in sport: A review using cognitive evaluation theory. *Int J Sport Psychol.* 1995;26:5–23.

23. Ivengar SS, Lepper MR. Rethinking the value of choice: A cultural perspective on intrinsic motivation. *J Pers Soc Psychol.* 1999;76:349–366.

24. Markus HR, Kityama S. Culture and the self: Implications for cognition, emotion, and motivation. *Psychol Rev.* 1991;98: 224–253.

25. Wagner SL, Lounsbury JW, Fitzgerald LG. Attribute factors associations with work/leisure perception. *Journal of Leisure Research.* 1989;21:155–166.

CHAPTER

7

Group Dynamics

Lana V. Ivanitskaya, Sharon Glazer, and Dmitry A. Erofeev

Learning Objectives

- Explain the difference between a team and a group.
- Define and provide examples of different types of healthcare teams.
- Describe the importance of roles and trust to team functioning.
- Explain socialization and role conflict.
- Analyze how groups are transformed into teams.
- Predict group phenomena that emerge in highly cohesive groups.
- Explain the relevance of CRM style training for tactical teams in healthcare.
- Analyze the present state of knowledge (research methods, findings and limitations) on healthcare team effectiveness.
- Provide recommendations on enhancing team effectiveness.
- Examine how healthcare teams can be affected by new technologies.

■ INTRODUCTION

The ultimate goal of any organization is survival. From the moment of its inception, an organization strives to survive. The most fundamental element of any organization that helps the organization to survive is the individual person. Without a person with a vision and a goal, there is no organization. As Schneider so aptly titles one of his articles, *The People Make the Place,* we find that organizations often forget about this most precious resource.[1] Like one's cultural surroundings, we take the organizational culture for granted, though it was the vision of one that created it, and the efforts of many that made the vision come to life and

109

survive. When people in the workplace fulfill their organizational roles, then the organization thrives.

In the industry of healthcare, people often do not think about the individual who has a vision or the people who keep the organization afloat, because people take for granted that healthcare facilities are readily available, particularly in developed countries. However, there are environmental influences causing healthcare organizations to shut down, mostly due to competition and better service provided by competitors. Healthcare providers can no longer expect that their healthcare facility will survive just by its mere necessity; the business model of the healthcare system has ensured competition for survival of the healthcare organization. Group efforts drive competition. Thus, alone, a single individual cannot create a thriving organizational environment, but instead the organization will survive through group efforts.

In this chapter, we take the readers on a journey toward understanding the basic structure of teams and team processes. We provide definitions for groups and teams, underlying assumptions of each, and explain the role of teams in organizational life. We share a recent strategy for enhancing team efforts, such as that based on aviation's team model of "Crew Resource Management," review common measures of team effectiveness, and discuss factors that predict teamwork success. Finally, we raise awareness of the impact that advanced technologies have on healthcare teams. Although we do our best to tap into the most relevant literature related to groups, teams, and group/team dynamics, we invite readers to learn more about the topic. Throughout this chapter we reference books, articles, and other sources on work teams and groups. You can use these references as a starting point for expanding your knowledge about this topic. They are not, by any means, exhaustive or reflective of all that is available. We admittedly omit numerous excellent resources and by no means intend that this list reflect our favorites. The list is simply a place to start your additional exploration of this topic.

■ GROUPS AND TEAMS

Defining Groups and Teams

A **group** consists of two or more people who interact with each other and share a common purpose. Groups will often identify themselves as distinct from other groups. A **team** is a *type* of group. Therefore, all teams are groups, but not all groups are teams. In order to be a team: (1) individuals' actions must be interdependent and coordinated, (2) each member must have a specified role, and (3) members must share common task goals or objectives. Teams are often depicted as a group of people sharing leadership of and working together on a specific project, whereas a group (but not a team) consists of individuals who work independently and are led by a strong, focused individual. Team members take responsibility collectively, whereas groups that are not teams take individual responsibility. The goals of teams are developed collectively, whereas groups (that are not teams) are mandated their goals. Team meetings tend to be open-ended and members of teams desire to be a part of it. In contrast, non-team group meetings are specific and efficient (e.g., breastfeeding support groups in the hospital often set specific agendas and end at a specific time). Members of groups do not necessarily desire to join, but go because they feel they must (e.g., mothers have found breastfeeding to be extremely challenging and want structured advice).

■ GROUPS AND TEAMS IN HEALTHCARE ORGANIZATIONS

In order to understand the role of teams in healthcare organizations, we need to consider multiple components or levels of organizations. The most basic component of an organization is the individual level, which is sometimes referred to as the micro level of the organization. The organization itself is typically labeled as a part of the macro level. The group level is in the middle and thus referred to as the meso level. Members of an organization are typically associated with at least one meso level. In the healthcare setting, particularly the hospital setting, individual contributors are members of numerous groups. For example, there are profession-based groups (nurses, physicians, or pharmacists) and groups responsible for running different units (neonatal care unit, intensive care unit, or recovery room). There are also different times of day in which members of the different professions and the different units work. Contributors to the organization who work solely night shifts may rarely interact with those who work morning only shifts, but they each play an important part in achieving the goal of maintaining the health and well-being of the clients. The ways in which these contributors interact is virtual and not real-time vis-à-vis clear notes and paper trails for others to follow. Another special team type, a transient team, is composed of health professionals who come together for a short time and disband immediately after the problem is solved (e.g., a pregnant patient with multiple medical allergies, high-risk for blood clotting, and high anxiety would require the efforts of a team of physicians that include hematologist, neonatologist, obstetrician, psychologist, and anesthesiologist).

Limieux-Charles and McQuire provide a typology of healthcare teams based on the team's primary purpose or contribution to healthcare organizations.[2] *Management teams* are responsible for administrative functions. *Quality improvement teams* are dedicated to improving healthcare processes and outcomes. *Teams that deliver care* are defined based on the patient population (e.g., mental health patients), disease type (e.g., stroke), and care delivery setting (e.g., acute or chronic). Inter-professional care delivery teams (such as the transient team described above) have the advantage of drawing upon different, but complementary areas of expertise of their members. This is particularly important for performing tasks that demand highly complex knowledge and skills that are difficult or time consuming to acquire. Compared to individual health professionals, healthcare teams are often considered more capable of providing patient-centered care and responding to challenges of cost containment or reorganization. It is not surprising then that the number of work teams in healthcare organizations is on the rise.[2]

In the healthcare industry, there is also a clear hierarchy of professional groups. Physicians outrank nurses and nurses outrank medical assistants. Although there is a hierarchy of positions, each member needs to communicate effectively with others in order to achieve a common goal. The healthcare industry culture often dictates that team members engage in structured, hierarchical, demanding, and direct communication. These cultural norms emerged in response to the extreme pressures healthcare teams face in crisis situations. However, research evidence suggests that these normative behaviors may be abandoned when certain professional groups possess greater expertise than those who are more influential in the hierarchy, particularly with regard to the use of new technologies.[3,4] We will discuss examples of such changes in the second half of this chapter.

■ ROLES, DIVERSITY, AND TRUST

Each member of an organization holds a role, or set of shared expectations, in the organization. A **role** is the part one plays in a given context. In the organizational context, a person can hold numerous roles, including the roles of supervisor, co-worker, and advisor. The role one plays in any given context serves a specific function. The function include activities or behaviors that the role player believes are expected of him. For example, when one is a nurse-head of shift, then the function served is that of supervisor for nurses in a given unit during a given timeframe. The person in this role (i.e., the focal person) is expected to perform his or her duties that are formally and informally, implicitly and explicitly dictated. Expectations for role behaviors are sent by others who are impacted by the focal person's role. These other stakeholders include the focal person's subordinates, supervisor(s), other administrators, co-workers, clients/patients and patients' families, and others with whom the focal person is in contact and who influence the focal person's role fulfillment. All these people belong in the focal person's **role set**. Thus, the role set includes people who have a stake in the focal person's role fulfillment. Members of one's role set **encode and send** messages (i.e., **role senders**) to the focal person (i.e., **role receiver**) who then **decodes and interprets** the message. The intended message is a derivation of what is sent and received. Various **filters** influence the way we encode and send messages and the way in which we listen or decode and interpret messages. Our filters are shaped over time through personal, observed, or studied experiences. Both **role senders** and **role receivers** are responsible for the way an intended message is interpreted. A key component to healthy group dynamics is communication of role expectations. When roles are poorly or insufficiently communicated, the focal person may perceive that he or she is not fulfilling the role or has been given unclear or conflicting messages so that stressors (i.e., perceived demands) pertaining to the role begin to form.

The filters we develop also impact how we behave in a diverse workforce. In the healthcare industry, populations are diverse in numerous ways, including education, sex, affinity, orientation, ethnicity, and professional background. These elements of differences often creep into communication of expectations and one way of ensuring better communication is overcoming ignorance about differences among co-workers. A meta-analysis on team composition shows that homogenous groups perform better on simple, well-defined, low complexity tasks, whereas heterogeneous groups perform better on more difficult, complex tasks for which there is limited data from which to work.[5] The diversity of heterogeneous teams, therefore, stimulates creativity. Table 7-1 shows that diversity is one of the key ingredients to healthy group dynamics.[6]

Trust is an emotional and logical act that is developed through experiencing seemingly predictable situations, exchanging information about oneself with others, reciprocation of different unspecified deeds when needed, and opening up oneself to vulnerability of being taken advantage of with the expectation that one's vulnerabilities will not be exposed. Groups that forge a sense of trust among its members will be more cohesive and desirable to others. In addition to trust is **respect**. Respect refers to the willingness to listen to the feelings and ideas of others. Trust and respect are essential for successful human relations and, therefore, group functioning. Trust is particularly important when

---

Table 7-1 Healthy Group Dynamics Require Healthy Human Relations

There are four key ingredients to healthy human relations:

1. *People* make the workplace.
2. *Business dealings are personal* dealings tied to conversations and relationships.
3. *Collaborative work* relationships are the key to successful mission accomplishments.
4. *Diversity* breeds innovation, understanding, and creativity.

Adapted from Manning G, Curtis K, McMillen S. (1996). *Building Community: The Human Side of Work.* Cincinnati, OH: Thomson Executive Press.

team members do not meet face to face. In the hospital setting, healthcare providers who work daytime hours trust the evening hour healthcare providers will provide clearly written notes and information so that there will be little confusion about the on-going care of patients. For example, a neonatal care evening shift nurse trusts that the infant's physician, who visited early in the morning, has left explicitly clear instruction for the care of the infant and that if the physician did not, the attending nurse at the time did. If poor instructions were written and something bad happened to the infant, trust in the physician and day shift nurse would be completely destroyed. Therefore, in order to develop a sense of trust, group members must demonstrate:

1. Sensitivity: Demonstrating genuine care of others' ideas, affects, and experiences.
2. Open communication: Informally or formally expressing negative and positive thoughts and feelings.
3. Vulnerability: Self-disclosing honestly without worry of impressing others.
4. Respect for the individual: Regarding others in a positive manner.

■ GROUP PROCESSES

Socialization

Role senders are key players in socializing us. **Socialization** is an important process that helps us internalize the organization's culture. An organization's culture is comprised of values, norms, language (i.e., acronyms), beliefs, symbols, and assumptions that develop over time and begin with the founder of the organization. In the case of hospitals, the culture is established by both the administration and the board of the hospital, as well as the general culture of healthcare.* It is through the process of communication among organizational contributors that people begin to socialize into the organization's culture. Once people are socialized they develop shared mental models of how things will work in the organization. When "things" do not work, conflict arises, because one is unable to fulfill his or her role properly. Thus, **role conflict** arises when a focal person's ideas of his or her requirements are incongruent with expectations from role set members.

---

*This culture has been changing over the past decade from total healthcare to a business model that reduces stays in hospital care to the minimum needed before one might be able to continue care by others outside the hospital setting. This model enables hospitals to continue profiting and surviving.

Role Conflict

There are four types of role conflict.[7–9] *Intrarole* conflict arises when the focal person is conflicted with two different activities to engage in or ways of doing things. The focal person, therefore, violates his or her values or standard ways of doing things. For example, all of a manager's subordinates have been fabulous performers, yet Human Resources requires the manager to down-rate some subordinates in order to (falsely) demonstrate that there are differences in subordinates' performances. *Intrasender* conflict arises when the focal person perceives that a role sender(s) has unrealistic expectations that the focal person believes he or she cannot fulfill. For example, a manager is asked to train his or her subordinates by the end of the month on a new technology that he or she is also unfamiliar with. *Interrole* conflict has to do with the focal person having too many incompatible roles in the organization. For example, a manager sits on a committee to improve work processes, yet until the new process is approved must enforce the current poor process that is in place. Finally, *intersender* conflict arises when the focal person is faced with at least two conflicting requests or incompatible processes. For example, the focal person (e.g., a nurse) may be asked to administer medication to a patient, but the patient adamantly opposes taking the medication, because the dosage is incorrect. The general distinction between these four types of conflict is whether the focal person is perceiving the incongruence with his or her own standards or values (intra-) or whether the focal person recognizes the conflict arising due to incompatibilities among others and/or policies (inter-).

■ GROUP FORMATION

There are four steps in transforming a group into a team. These steps are: (1) forming, (2) storming, (3) norming, and (4) performing. The forming step is the initial encounter in which there is some polite, social discourse. In the storming step, members of the group begin to develop conflict, particularly over position status, power, and influence. By the third step (i.e., norming), members of the group develop and agree upon rules for behaviors and engagement. Finally, in the fourth step, members of the group accept their positions and the rules, and begin to work together as a team. Evidence of team formation is the sense of cohesion and trust.

Group **cohesion** refers to a shared vision, unity of goals and objectives, pride in group membership, and collective group identity. Carron also noted that a clear structure for communication is also evident in cohesive groups.[10] Clear roles would also help groups develop cohesion. High-interaction teams, such as those found in tactical or surgical teams, are likely to require greater cohesion than low-interaction teams. Having a strong sense of purpose and identity in group membership would likely yield greater surgical success than when sense of purpose or identity is low. Thus, being a part of a surgical team in which the head surgeon is highly respected would likely yield greater cooperation among members of the team than when the surgeon is fairly new and not known. When purpose or identity with group goals are low, then mistakes, such as operating on the wrong hand or leaving an instrument in the body, might occur. This example typifies task cohesion, because members of the group are required to cooperate in order to achieve the goal. There is also social cohesion, which is the extent to which group members get along. Five factors influence the extent to which groups are cohesive. These factors are represented in terms of five S's:

- Stability—refers to the duration of the group. Groups that have been around for many years are more attractive to potential new members; knowing that a group is stable perpetuates cohesion.

- Similarity—refers to the extent to which personal characteristics of members are the same. Group members that are similar in age, ethnic background, education level, attitudes, sex, nationality, etc. are likely to be more cohesive.

- Size—refers to the number of members in the group. Group coherence tends to negatively relate with group size.[11,12]

- Support—refers to the instrumental or emotional aid and encouragement supervisors give to subordinates and peers give to one another, the greater the support, the greater the cohesion.

- Satisfaction—refers to members' contentment with other group members, their performance, and socialization into the group's normative practices.

■ GROUP PHENOMENA

Highly cohesive groups are often subject to group phenomenon, such as groupthink or group polarization. This is because in groups, people tend to be more extreme or less argumentative than when asked to make a decision alone. **Groupthink** is the phenomenon in which all members conform and accept the ideas of a strong other.[13,14] This happens when the unity of the group becomes of utmost importance. The desire for unanimity overrides efforts for appropriate decisions. The result of such decision making is usually very bad. The head surgeon may be viewed as the most knowledgeable group member. When faced with a dilemma in the operating room, the surgeon may seek others' advice, but pose his or her own ideas before soliciting others. Members of the team may then offer ideas similar to those the surgeon had originally stated, because something different no longer seems like a plausible solution. Unfortunately, the surgeon was not made aware of some aspect of the patient's bodily function and the decision everyone agreed upon was a bad one. Groupthink typically occurs when members of the group do not question the decision, warnings are rationalized, the group feels invulnerable to error, there is pressure to conform, people self-censor, people desire unanimity, and the group is guarded from contrary viewpoints. **Group polarization** is the exaggeration of group members' positions. Groups tend to polarize when members of the group already have a tendency toward a given position. Polarization of decisions occurs when members fuel the decision with reasons that the decision is correct or downplaying reasons that would negate the decision, without considering reasons why the decision may be *in*correct. Another related concept is **risky shift.**[15] This concept refers to a group's tendencies to make riskier decisions than the average of individual's decisions alone. People feel more comfortable taking risks when all members are responsible for the risk together, as opposed to an individual bearing sole responsibility.

Another phenomenon of groups is social facilitation and social loafing.[16,17] **Social facilitation** occurs when the presence of others serves as a positive stimulus to motivate better performance, particularly on easy or well-rehearsed tasks. Members of a team, for example, may encourage or motivate others to perform beyond what they would normally do otherwise. When the task is difficult or challenging, however, the presence of others can hinder performance. A meta-analysis by Bond and Titus reveals that only 1 to 3% of variance in performance of a complex task is accounted for by the presence of others, whereas presence of others does not particularly help (.3% of variance accounted for in performance) on easy tasks, except to increase the speed in which a task is performed. In a hospital setting, upon starting a new shift, a seasoned nurse may perform the intake of patients more carefully when visitors are with the patient than when the patient is without visitors.

Social loafing is the tendency of others to expend less effort as the size of the group increases. This happens most often on easy tasks. When the task is complex, social loafing is not as likely to occur. Often, mundane tasks that anyone can perform yield social loafing. This is why clear roles are extremely important, particularly when it comes to the safety, health, and well-being of others. The concept of social loafing, however, is not generalized to all contexts, particularly national contexts.[18] In collective nations, social loafing among in-group members (i.e., people who are perceived to be important members of one's group) does not occur. Instead, when there is no accountability or accountability to out-group members, there is individual loafing. Thus, we caution people about the transferability of this and other theories we have discussed to cultures other than the United States.

Groupthink, group polarization, risky shift, and social loafing are examples of undesirable outcomes of group work. We will return to this topic later in the chapter when we discuss group effectiveness.

■ APPLICATION OF CREW RESOURCE MANAGEMENT (CRM) TO HEALTHCARE

In highly tactical groups, where safety, efficiency, morale, and customer satisfaction are of utmost importance, team members must have clearly defined roles, engage in clear communication, and allow each team member to be an equal contributor. One industry that requires high standards for safety is aviation. Until the late 1970s and early 1980s, the captain was the supreme commander and everyone deferred to the captain's decisions. Rarely did flight attendants voice concerns over situations, because it was expected that the captain was aware of every on-going detail of his flight. CRM* was developed in 1979, after human error was identified as the primary cause of many air transport accidents. The purpose of CRM is to promote utilization of human resources on the flight deck.[19] The success of CRM is evident from its popularity as a training program worldwide. The most important ingredient to CRM is communication. Indeed, communication is relevant at every point of group interaction and CRM training focuses on techniques to provide performance feedback.[20] Nearly every major airline implements CRM in training flight crews. Improving safety, efficiency, morale, and customer satisfaction has three training stages:

1. Avoiding error
2. "Trapping" errors before they are committed
3. Mitigating error consequences

These steps are not only essential for air flight, but also for the care of patients, particularly in surgical teams, where the resident surgeon is often perceived as the supreme commander of the operating room. Sexton, Thomas, and Helmreich[21] compared flight cockpit crew members (including captains, first officers, and second officers) with operating room personnel (including surgeons, surgical residents, anesthesiologists, and nurses) on perceptions of teamwork, including measures of hierarchy. Results show that surgical residents and attending surgeons believe there is a high level of teamwork (73% and 64%, respectively) whereas anesthesiologists, surgical nurses, and nurses report lower levels of teamwork (39%, 28%, and 25%, respectively). Just under 55% of attending surgeons believed that junior team members have the right to question decisions of senior team members. In contrast, 94% of airline cockpit members endorsed questioning of senior

---

*When developed in 1979, the term CRM stood for "Cockpit Resource Management," however, to incorporate flight attendants, it was changed to "Crew Resource Management."

crew members. Operating room members were more likely to agree that "even when fatigued, [they] perform effectively well during critical times" (ranging from 47% of attending anesthesiologists to 60% of surgical nurses) than pilots (26%). These results suggest that CRM has been helpful in deterring potentially false self-perceptions of good performance during fatigue and for reinforcing the need to listen and take under advisement all team members equally. Results also suggest that surgeons have a false perception that they create a team atmosphere in the operating room. Junior or hierarchically lower level operating room members do not feel a team atmosphere as much as surgeons do. The results might also be a bit misrepresentative, because they do not include flight attendants' perceptions of teamwork, hierarchy perceptions, and effective performance under fatigue. Moreover, the results are self-reported and not other-reported.

Nonetheless, results generally indicate that CRM style training for tactical teams in healthcare are highly relevant, including operating rooms, emergency rooms, labor and delivery rooms, and cardiac arrest response teams.[21] Indeed, such training programs have been developed for operating rooms and anesthesiologists (Anesthesia Crisis Resource Management).[22–25] It is expected that as barriers of hierarchy begin to break down in critical tactical units in healthcare, there will be fewer errors. CRM fosters open communication, clarity of roles, standardization of routine activities, and checklists to limit complacency.

■ PERFORMANCE AND GROUP EFFECTIVENESS

State of Knowledge about Healthcare Team Effectiveness

Over the past 50 years, researchers studied small groups and teams in the airline industry, sports, human services (e.g., police and firefighting teams), military, manufacturing industry, and more. Most studies on teams were done outside of healthcare settings; therefore, much remains unknown about the effectiveness of healthcare teams. Healthcare managers can gain useful insights from research on non-healthcare teams, yet, they should exercise some caution while applying this knowledge to healthcare organizations. General models of team effectiveness are often based on team characteristics, processes, and outcomes that are not completely relevant to healthcare settings.[2] For example, numerous studies of non-healthcare teams focus on "intellectual teams" that are different from "work teams" in healthcare.[26]

Research on healthcare teams suffers from lack of well-developed measures, such as team effectiveness; therefore, it is hard to evaluate the outcomes of teamwork in healthcare organizations. Team effectiveness measures are broadly divided into two categories: objective and subjective. *Objective outcomes* incorporate data from medical records, administrative databases, and standardized assessments. They are less dependent on respondents' opinions and judgments than *subjective outcomes*. Table 7-2 shows how researchers who studied healthcare teams defined team effectiveness. Healthcare researchers measure outcomes of teamwork in many different ways, therefore, it is challenging to compare and summarize results of different studies.

As can be seen in Table 7-2, some measures used to assess team effectiveness, such as mortality, length of stay, or cost of care might not have a strong direct link to the actual task that a healthcare team is performing. If fluctuations in mortality, length of stay, or cost of care are caused by

Table 7-2 Common Outcome Measures Used in Studies of Team Effectiveness	
Objective Measures	**Subjective Measures**
Patient-centered measures	
Healthcare utilization	Patient/caregiver satisfaction
Medication prescriptions	Patient/caregiver morale
Hospital (re-)admission	Perceived patient post-discharge outcomes
Hospital utilization in last 180 days of life, before and after intervention	
Length of stay	
Re-admission to critical care	
Hospital-acquired complications	
Patient functional status	
Health-related quality of life	
Compliance with recommendation	
Mortality: predicted and actual	
Staff-centered measures	
Nurse retention	Nurses' satisfaction with coordination of care and team performance
Team effectiveness as measured by an external evaluator	Staff members' satisfaction with work quality and environment
	Patient-rated quality of nursing
Organizational measures	
Treatment cost/cost of care	
Diagnostic timeliness	
Time to adopt new procedure (e.g., minimally invasive cardiac surgery)	
Innovativeness of treatments	
Patient flow	
Length of stay	
Patient volume	
Ability to accept admissions	

other factors that are not related to teamwork, then these outcomes will serve as poor indicators of team effectiveness. When evaluating team performance, it is important to ask, "What tasks are team members expected to perform effectively?" and to select outcomes relevant to those tasks.

How Researchers Study Healthcare Team Effectiveness

Given the challenges in evaluating team performance, how do we know which teams are effective and under what conditions are they effective? There is much information available to teach one how to design, train, lead, and manage team performance.[2,27–30] In healthcare research, this evidence comes from three types of studies. One type of study is known as **intervention studies,** which compare teamwork versus non-teamwork. A second type is **team redesign studies** that compare redesigned care delivery teams with usual team care. A third type is **correlational field studies** that examine linkages between team characteristics, processes, and outcomes. Summary literature review and research (i.e., meta-analyses) efforts bring together evidence from numerous team studies and the authors evaluate these studies for strength and consistency. To date, these summary studies have been based on team effectiveness data from different industries and not just healthcare. Findings that are consistent, based on solid theory, and supported with extensive research are ready for application in organizational settings. Table 7-3 shows ready-for-application interventions that can be used to improve team effectiveness in a variety of settings.

In the section that follows, we will review major findings from research on effective healthcare teams.

What Healthcare Research Tells Us about Team Effectiveness

Studies That Compare Team vs. Non-Team Healthcare
In several acute and home care settings, traditional care that is sequential, discipline-based, and delivered by individuals was redesigned to create a multidisciplinary geriatric care team. Researchers who had access to these organizations compared the outcomes of team-based and non-team-based healthcare. One consistent finding was that team-based healthcare was associated with higher patient satisfaction and health-related quality of life. Other findings were mixed. In four studies of geriatric patients in the Veterans Administration (VA) system, patients' functional status, mental health, mortality, and dependence were better in the multidisciplinary team setting than in the traditional, non-team healthcare setting.[31–34] Three other studies conducted outside of the VA system did not replicate this finding.[35–37] In a different study, an implementation of hospital-wide critical care and medical emergency outreach teams led to improvements in patient outcomes, such as higher survival rates, decreased readmission to critical care, and shorter length of stay.[38] Overall,

Table 7-3 Evidence-Based Practice: Interventions That Improve Team Effectiveness

Intervention	Application Examples
Team design	*Selection:* Selecting individuals based on their teamwork competencies, ability to perform the task, cognitive ability, etc. or based on their ability to learn new skills required for teamwork.
Regulation of performance	*Goal setting:* Helping the team to set difficult and specific goals, facilitation of acceptance and commitment to those goals, provision of team feedback, assistance in obtaining knowledge, and strategies necessary for accomplishing the goals *PROMeasure performance management tool:* Assisting teams in understanding their work and its outcomes by identifying effectiveness measures relevant to the team's task (e.g., medication errors), scaling of measures in effectiveness units, and drawing of contingency tables that show a link between the team's inputs and outputs to identify the most valuable strategies for accomplishing team's goals.
Training strategies	*Cross-training:* Helping team members understand each other's jobs. *Simulation-based training:* Using scripted scenarios to allow the team to practice both routine and rare (but potentially life threatening) experiences. *Crew Resource Management (CRM):* Applying a variety of techniques to train teams on competencies related to coordination and skill integration—mutual performance monitoring, backup behavior, feedback, communication, and interpersonal relations.
Leadership	*Task and support behaviors by the team leader:* Structuring team members' task activities and concern with their needs and feelings. *Transformation and transactional leadership:* Facilitating team members' motivation and effort, for example, by providing (a) clear expectations, (b) rewards that are contingent on team performance, (c) appealing vision of the future, (d) meaningful goals, and (e) corrective behavior management. *Leader-member exchange (LMX):* Developing dyadic relationships with team members to yield different roles (trusted members with enlarged roles and leadership latitude vs. members with more prescribed roles subject to supervision).

Adapted from Kozlowski and Ilgen, 2006.

these findings suggest that team care can positively affect outcomes for patients and health organizations.

Care by multidisciplinary healthcare teams, however, tends to be more expensive than non-team care, and some question if the costs outweigh the gains in decreased service utilization.[34] This is particularly the case with home-based primary care teams that offer 24/7 contact for geriatric patients. These teams do pre-approval for hospital readmissions and assist in discharge planning. Additional costs associated with team care include increases in the number of drug prescriptions and service utilization by mental health patients.[39,40] These cost analyses reveal some contradictions. For many patients, especially those from underserved populations, an increased utilization of healthcare services is a desirable outcome because it is likely to improve their health. If these patients are uninsured or underinsured, however, their increased utilization of emergency rooms can become a threat to organizational survival. In other words, increased service consumption can be a positive outcome from a patient's perspective and a negative outcome from the organizational perspective. Despite the fact that many teams are costly to implement, patients who receive team-based care often achieve better clinical outcomes than those treated in a traditional way.

Intervention Studies

An **intervention** is a broad term that includes many strategies for improving situations. With respect to group dynamics, they are efforts toward making teams more effective. An intervention can be a training session on conflict resolution, changes made to team structure, and the development of guidelines outlining team members' roles. Published studies on efforts to design more effective healthcare teams describe interventions to improve team members' autonomy, diversity, and interdependence (e.g., interdisciplinary rounds) training, Continuous Quality Improvement (CQI) training, and goal-setting training. Enhancing autonomy of team members and ensuring team integration leads to improved staff-centered outcomes, such as increased job satisfaction and retention of nurses who worked in inpatient settings and of staff in an inpatient acute care unit.[41,42] In another study, greater autonomy led to improved patient outcomes, specifically, declined hospital readmissions among home care team patients.[43] CQI training is linked to improved patient outcomes in one study but two earlier studies did not find this link.[44–46] Finally, goal setting training leads to greater effectiveness at the individual level and improved team efficacy.[47]

Correlational Studies

Unlike other types of studies described above, field studies are less likely to rely on experimental or quasi-experimental designs. Researchers who conduct field studies examine relationships between a variety of organizational factors and team effectiveness. Table 7-4 shows examples of factors that correlate with team effectiveness (e.g., organizational context in which healthcare teams operate, tasks teams perform, healthcare team design, and processes that take place within teams). In these studies, team effectiveness data (objective and/or subjective) was gathered at the same time as data for other variables included in the study. There were no interventions implemented and no random assignment to team and non-team conditions. Although these studies improve our understanding of the relationships between team effectiveness and other variables, we have to be careful drawing causal conclusions, because they are only correlational studies. For example, Table 7-3 shows that in past studies of healthcare teams, quality improvement (QI) practices were positively associated with team effectiveness. Do QI initiatives (cause) create more effective teams (outcome) or do effective teams (cause) initiate QI activities (outcome)? These questions suggest that team effectiveness may be both the cause and the outcome.

In their comprehensive review of literature that was not limited to healthcare, Campion and colleagues identified several broad categories of factors that relate to team effectiveness.[48,49] These are job design (self-management, participation, task variety, task significance, and task identity), team composition (heterogeneity, flexibility, relative size, and members' preference for teamwork), contextual factors (training, managerial support, inter-team communication, and cooperation), task interdependence (task interdependence, goal interdependence, and interdependent feedback/rewards), and processes (potency, social support, workload sharing, as well as communication, and cooperation within the group). Potency refers to a group's belief that it can be effective. Process factors were found to have the strongest relationships with team effectiveness.[49]

Negative Outcomes of Teamwork

In this chapter, we discussed many reasons for organizing employees into teams and ways in which these teams can make healthcare organizations more effective. Teams must be designed and managed properly in order for them to be effective. If the design of the teams is flawed, then the so-called team may be no better, or may even be worse, than independent individuals working toward a goal. Trying to transition too quickly into a team model might also lead to productivity erosion. Without following the four steps needed for forming a cohesive team, including identifying each contributor's role, some team members may not be team contributors. An example of team erosion is **free riding** by a team member whose contributions to teamwork cannot be singled out. Another is reduction of effort by a high performer who believes that other team members do not do their share of work. Finally, teams may erode when there is reduction of effort by a low performer who feels dispensable and redundant compared to other, highly capable team members. Other negative consequences of poorly designed teams are poor coordination, low job satisfaction of team members, bad decision making, and conflict. These outcomes yield further low efficiency and high costs of teamwork.

To avoid these negative outcomes, healthcare administrators can take steps to design better teams, train team members to work together, man-

Table 7-4 Contextual, Task, Design, and Process Factors Associated with Health Team Effectiveness

Construct	Specific Measure	Relationship with Team Effectiveness Higher Team Effectiveness: ↑ Lower Team Effectiveness: ↓
Organizational context	Primary-case solo practice structure	↑
	Dispersion of service across greater number of hospitals	↓
Task features	Workload (caseload)	↑
	Rules and procedures	↑
	Quality improvement practices	↑
	Clarity of task, goals, leadership	↑
	Interdependence	↑
Team design	Team size	Unclear or ↓
	Years of member experience	↑
	Years of team experience	↓
	Diversity: disciplinary, age, ethnic	↑
	Willingness to learn	↑
Team processes	Interdisciplinary collaboration	↑
	Conflict	↓
	Team climate	↑

Adapted from Limieux-Charles and McQuire, 2006.

age team performance, structure the work performed by the team, and provide support to team members. This chapter describes many of these steps; their summary appears in Table 7-5.

In the next section, we discuss recent technological developments that are affecting teamwork in healthcare.

Technology and Healthcare Teams

Rapidly developing telecommunications lead to a spread of telehealth— new practices of delivering healthcare services over distance. Telehealth may become a practice of choice for specialty services, such as radiology, oncology, cardiology, dermatology, and mental health services. It can serve rural, underserved, and isolated populations, as well as managed care networks in urban settings.[50] Telehealth can increase interactions between patients and providers of clinical services, between specialists and practitioners, and between families and mental health professionals. It presents new challenges for healthcare employees who work together to serve patients over distances. Some of these challenges include, but

Table 7-5 Making Healthcare Teams More Effective: Recommendations for Health Administrators

Strategy	Recommendations for Health Administrators
Select	Select team members who have . . . • Diverse but complementary expertise; and • Skills and knowledge relevant to team's task. Select the fewest possible number of team members. Select employees who prefer working in a team rather than alone.
Train	Train team members on team processes. Cross-train team members on each other's tasks (a scheduled program of rotating assignments).
Manage performance	Manage performance of the *team*, allow the team to manage its members. Set clear and challenging goals that reinforce team members' interdependence. Link interdependent goals to performance of the *entire* team through team feedback and rewards. Promote workload sharing by helping the team identify and reward each team member's individual performance.
Design work	Consider team's tasks and organizational culture to decide how much . . . • Autonomy from management control can be given to the team; • Task variety can be given to each team member; • Team's responsibility can be expanded to a distinct piece of work that is meaningful to team members; and • Team members' interdependence can be enhanced through resource sharing, using each other's inputs, etc. Re-distribute decision-making power: Share power between leaders and team members directly involved in solving operational problems. Empower team members to make their own decisions. Communicate about the importance of the work that the team is doing in terms of its consequences for patients, other employees, organizational mission, etc.
Support teams	Be a coach who promotes a "can do" attitude among team members. Encourage positive interaction and social support, especially when the tasks are mundane, difficult, or stressful. Facilitate communication and cooperation between the team and the rest of the organization (other teams, departments, etc.). Ensure that organizational leaders at all levels support teams.

Campion and Higgs, 2005.

are not limited to, new skill requirements for technology-enabled communication among group members, performance management of groups that operate virtually without face-to-face meetings, coordination of group work over distance, and re-formulation of group members' roles and decision-making power.

Implementation of new technology in healthcare organizations demonstrates a need for substantial changes in team members' work routines. A case study by Harvard University researchers Edmondson, Bohmer, and Pisano illustrates processes that took place in 16 operating room (OR) teams that successfully or unsuccessfully implemented a minimally invasive cardiac surgery.[51] Minimally invasive cardiac surgery requires greatly modified teamwork routines (e.g., greater communication, psychological safety promoted by the leader, new behaviors by team members, and collective learning from past experiences). Unsuccessful OR teams were those assembled based on contributors' seniority or availability, rather than skills. Moreover, leaders of poorly performing teams discouraged or remained neutral to others' input. Like with CRM, group leaders (surgeons) need to empower the team by assuming a role of "a partner, not a dictator."[51] Team members will respond to a leader's signals and attempt new behaviors of information sharing and error correction, which leads to the development of new group work routines. Collective learning was possible when OR teams took time to discuss past and upcoming cases. This study shows that a shift to new technologies may require substantial changes in teamwork. The researchers demonstrated that teamwork routines are hard to change, but execution of old routines with new technology often results in poor outcomes for patients, team members, and healthcare organizations.

Finally, Barley explicates the growing importance of relying on technicians' (e.g., emergency medical technicians, medical technicians, and radiological technologists) interpretations and decisions.[52] Today, healthcare professionals with more years of education than technicians must often depend on technicians' expertise. Although physicians outrank technicians in the organizational hierarchy, power relationships are not always consistent with what may be expected. In fact, it is unclear whether medical technicians are experts or servants to those in their role set, particularly because technicians offer critical healthcare information that physicians and radiologists may not detect. In Barley's study, technicians acknowledge the importance of approaching a higher-ranking group member, such as a radiologist or a physician, without "coming across like . . . a [physician]."[52] At the same time, technicians act as physicians' consultants, advisers, and sometimes even teachers because they possess unique expertise. They have *contextual knowledge*—the ability to make sense of small differences and signs in output that others miss or misinterpret, specialized skills (e.g., inserting an intravenous needle), heuristics (e.g., how to position a patient to detect the presence of a gallstone), etc. Barley's study depicts how hierarchical relationships can be modified when knowledge is re-distributed at a lower level. New clinical technologies, described by Edmondson and colleagues, and re-distribution of technical knowledge, explained by Barley, are transforming healthcare groups. These groups can be better coordinated through collaboration rather than through chain-of-command communication. However, to make it happen, those with expertise must be empowered to make critical care decisions.

■ CHAPTER SUMMARY

Inter-professional teams (rather than groups or individuals) are equipped to deliver the highest quality of care. In a team, individuals' actions are interdependent and coordinated, each member has a specified role, and members share common task goals or objectives. Healthcare organizations have different types of teams—management teams, quality improvement teams, and teams that deliver care. Inter-professional care delivery teams draw upon different, but complementary, areas of expertise of their members.

A team member's role is the part one plays in a given context. A key component to healthy group dynamics is communication of role expectations. Trust is developed when team members experience seemingly predictable situations, exchange information about oneself with others, reciprocate, and open up. People begin to socialize into the organization's culture through the process of communication. Once team members are socialized, they develop shared mental models of how things will work in their team. Role conflict arises when a focal person's ideas of his or her requirements are incongruent with expectations from role set members. Groups transform into teams through forming, storming, norming, and performing. Cohesive groups may develop group phenomena, such as groupthink, that limits their effectiveness.

When evaluating team performance, it is important to ask, "What tasks are team members expected to perform effectively?" and to select outcomes relevant to those tasks. Intervention studies, team redesign studies, and correlational field studies provide evidence on healthcare team effectiveness, which is assessed using both objective and subjective measures. Despite the fact that many teams are costly to implement, patients who receive team-based care often achieve better clinical outcomes than those treated in a traditional way.

Healthcare administrators must take steps to design better teams, train team members to work together, manage team performance, structure the work performed by the team and provide support to team members. Healthcare teams can become more effective through training aimed to enhance their members' autonomy, diversity, and interdependence. CQI training and goal-setting facilitation can also be used to improve team performance. Useful in developing tactical healthcare teams, CRM focuses on avoiding error, "trapping" errors before they are committed, and mitigating error consequences.

Implementation of new technologies impacts healthcare teams: Team members who work at a distance may have limited face-to-face interaction, operation room teams that adopt new technologies must change their work routines, and team members with unique technical expertise must be empowered to share it with others.

Review/Discussion Questions

1. Explain the difference between micro, meso, and macro levels in healthcare organizations. Provide an example of each.
2. What are the characteristics of each type of healthcare group considered in this chapter?
3. Think about a time when you said something that someone has misinterpreted. What was the message and how do you think the person misinterpreted the message? What about your filters shaped the way you molded your message? What might have been the filters acting on the other person's interpretation of the message?
4. Analyze a health team you know. Justify why it is a team and not a group. How are its members socialized? How cohesive is it?
5. Why do healthcare organizations use CRM-style training?
6. Respond to the following questions:
   a. Think of one team of which you are (or were) a member. What makes this team effective? What are the conditions that have influenced the team to be effective?
   b. For the team you identified, list the tasks that this team should be expected to perform effectively. Explain how you understand effective performance in each task. Will your team members agree with this definition?
7. Examine tangible and intangible costs of your recent teamwork experience. List your personal "costs" of being a team member (i.e., costs you would not have incurred if you had worked alone). For example, estimate the cost of your personal time spent attending group meetings and coordinating group members' activities. Did you experience any emotional costs (e.g., costs associated with an interpersonal conflict, elevated strain, or burnout)?
8. Identify at least two other variables from Table 7-1 for which team effectiveness can be both the cause and the effect. In other words, it is possible that these factors (a) are impacted by how effective a healthcare team is and (b) influence team effectiveness. What implications does this lack of causal clarity have on our ability to build effective teams?

Learning Activities

Exercise 1: Characteristics of an Effective Group[53]

Consider each of the following characteristics. Evaluate your group as it is operating now (1 is the lowest rating; 10 is the highest).

1. *Clear mission:* The task or objective of the group is well understood and accepted by all.

   1   2   3   4   5   6   7   8   9   10

2. *Informal atmosphere:* The atmosphere is informal, comfortable, and relaxed. It is a working atmosphere, in which everyone is involved and interested. There are no signs of boredom.

   1   2   3   4   5   6   7   8   9   10

3. *Lots of discussion:* Allow time for discussion in which everyone is encouraged to participate, and discussion remains pertinent to the task of the group.

   1   2   3   4   5   6   7   8   9   10

4. *Active listening:* Members listen to each other. People show respect for one another by listening when others are talking. Give every idea a hearing.

   1   2   3   4   5   6   7   8   9   10

5. *Trust/openness:* Members feel free to express ideas and feelings, both on the issues and on the group's operation. People are not afraid to suggest new and different ideas, even if extreme.

   1   2   3   4   5   6   7   8   9   10

6. *Disagreement is OK:* Do not suppress or override disagreement by premature group action. Examine differences carefully as the group seeks to understand all points of view. Accept conflict and differences of opinion as the price of creativity. Diversity is valued.

   1   2   3   4   5   6   7   8   9   10

7. *Criticism is issue oriented, never personal:* Give and accept constructive criticism. Orient criticism toward solving problems and accomplishing the mission. Personal criticism is neither expressed nor felt.

   1   2   3   4   5   6   7   8   9   10

8. *Consensus is the norm:* Reach decisions by consensus in which it is clear that everyone is in general agreement and willing to go along. Keep formal voting to a minimum.

   1   2   3   4   5   6   7   8   9   10

9. *Effective leadership:* Informal leadership shifts from time to time, depending on circumstances. There is little evidence of a struggle for power as the group operates. The issue is not who controls, but how to get the job done.

   1   2   3   4   5   6   7   8   9   10

10. *Clarity of assignments:* Inform the group of the action plan. When taking action, clear assignments are made and accepted. People know what they are expected to do.

    1   2   3   4   5   6   7   8   9   10

11. *Shared values and norms of behavior:* There is an agreement on core values and norms of behavior that determine the rightness and wrongness of conduct in the group.

    1   2   3   4   5   6   7   8   9   10

12. *Commitment:* People are committed to the goals of the group.

    1   2   3   4   5   6   7   8   9   10

Exercise 2: Group Members' Roles

What is your current **role** in this classroom context? Write the role in the large middle circle in Figure 7-1 and specify the members of your **role set**. Write the names of these people in the small circles stemming from the large one.

1. What do the members of your role set expect of you? Write at least 3–5 expectations.
2. On what information have you based your determination that these are expectations of you (implicit/explicit, formal/informal messages)?
3. Ask a member of your role set if you have clearly understood what you think is expected of you by this particular person. If it is not, ask for clarification.

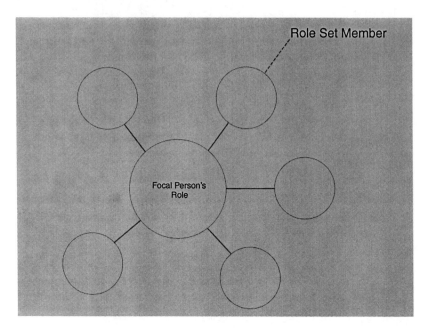

Figure 7-1   Exercise 2: Group Members' Roles.

Exercise 3: Group Polarization[54]

Peter Gray (1993) suggests a simple exercise that readily demonstrates the group polarization effect. Before lecturing on group decision making in Chapter 7, have your students declare on a Likert-type scale how strongly they agree (rated 7) or disagree (rated 1) with some statement or idea. For example, "Senators should have a term limit." Collect the responses and divide students into like-minded groups for a short, 5-minute discussion. After the group discussion, have students rate their agreement with the proposition again on the same Likert-type scale.

Results should be consistent with group polarization; those who initially agreed should agree more strongly after group discussion, and those who initially disagreed should disagree even more strongly after group discussion. According to Gray, asking your students to speculate about the causes of the effect should generate the same explanations generated by psychologists over the years (i.e., that members are exposed to new, persuasive arguments, and that members gradually take a more extreme position in order to be viewed positively by others). An added benefit is that, in addition to learning the group polarization effect in a memorable way, students learn that they can successfully "think like researchers" in generating plausible explanations for observed events.

Case Study[51]

Two surgical teams from different hospitals have a similar composition—nurses, perfusionists, an anesthesiologist, and a surgeon (team leader). Two nurses who are members of different teams provided the following accounts of their teamwork:

> Nurse A: "We all have to share the knowledge. For example, in the last case, we needed to reinsert a guidewire and I grabbed the wrong wire and did not recognize it at first. And my circulating nurse said, 'Sue, you grabbed the wrong wire.' This shows how much different roles don't matter. We all have to know about everything. You have to work as a team."

> Nurse B: "There is a painful process of finding out what didn't work and saying 'We won't do that again.' We are reactive. The nurses have to run for stuff unexpectedly. . . . If you observe something that might be a problem you are obligated to speak up, but you choose your time. I will work around [the surgeon]. I will go to his PA [physician's assistant] if there is a problem. . . . If I see a [surgical] case on the list [for tomorrow] I think, 'Oh! Do we really have to do it! Just get me a fresh blade so I can slash my wrists right now."

Question: Apply your knowledge of teams and team processes to explain possible causes for team members' experiences. What interventions can you recommend to address concerns expressed by Nurse B?

References

1. Schneider B. The people make the place. *Personnel Psychology*. 1987; 40:437–453.
2. Lemieux-Charles L, McGuire WL. What do we know about health care team effectiveness? A review of the literature. *Med Care Res Rev*. 2006; 63:263–300.
3. Barley SR. Technicians in the workplace: Ethnographic evidence for bringing work into organizational studies. *Adm Sci Q*. 1996;41:404–441.
4. Edmondson AC, Bohmer RM, Pisano GP. Disrupted routines: Team learning and new technology implementation in hospitals. *Adm Sci Q*. 2001; 46:685–716.
5. Bowers CA, Pharmer JA, Salas E. When member homogeneity is needed in work teams: A meta-analysis. *Small Group Research*. 2000;31:305–327.
6. Adapted from Manning G, Curtis K, McMillen S. *Building Community: The Human Side of Work*. Cincinnati, OH: Thomson Executive Press; 1996.
7. Kahn RL, Wolf DM, Quinn RR, Snoek DJ, Rosenthal RA. *Organizational Stress: Studies in Role Conflict and Ambiguity*. New York: Wiley; 1964.
8. Rizzo JR, House RJ, Lirtzman SI. Role conflict and ambiguity in complex organizations. *Adm Sci Q*. 1970;15:150–163.

9. Schwab RL, Iwanicki EF, Pierson DA. Assessing role conflict and role ambiguity: A cross validation study. *Educ Psychol Meas*. 1983;43:587–593.

10. Carron AV. *Social Psychology of Sport*. Ithaca, NY: Movement Publications; 1980.

11. Liden RC, Wayne SJ, Jaworski RA, Bennett N. Social loafing: A field investigation. *Journal of Management*. 2004;30:285–304.

12. Shaw ME. *Group Dynamics: The Psychology of Small Group Behavior*. New York: McGraw-Hill; 1981.

13. Janis I. *Victims of Groupthink*. Boston: Houghton-Mifflin; 1972.

14. Janis I. *Groupthink* (2nd ed.). Boston: Houghton-Mifflin; 1982.

15. Stoner JAF. A comparison of individual and group decisions involving risk. Unpublished Master's Thesis, Massachusetts Institute of Technology; 1961.

16. Bond CF, Titus LJ. Social facilitation: A meta-analysis of 241 studies. *Psychol Bull*. 1983;94:265–292.

17. Karau SJ, Williams KD. Social loafing: A meta-analytic review and theoretical integration. *J Pers Soc Psychol*. 1993;65:681–706.

18. Earley PC. East meets West meets Mideast: Further explorations of collectivistic and individualistic work groups. *Acad Manage J*. 1993;36:319–348.

19. Helmreich RL, Merritt AC, Wilhelm JA. The evolution of Crew Resource Management training in commercial aviation. *Int J Aviat Psychol*. 1999; 9:19–32.

20. Kern T. Controlling for Pilot Error: Culture, Environment, and CRM. New York: McGraw-Hill; 2001.

21. Sexton JB, Thomas EJ, Helmreich RL. Error, stress, and teamwork in medicine and aviation: Cross-sectional surveys. *Br Med J*. 2000;320:745–749.

22. Helmreich RL, Schaefer H G. Team performance in the operating room. In MS Bogner (ed.), *Human Error in Medicine*. Hillside, NJ: Erlbaum; 1998.

23. Howard SK, Gaba DM, Fish KJ, Yang G, Sarnquist FH. Anesthesia crisis resource management training: Teaching anesthesiologists to handle critical incidents. *Aviat Space Environ Med*. 1992;63:763–770.

24. Gaba DM, Howard SK, Fish KJ, Smith BE, Sowb YA. Simulation-based training in Anesthesia Crisis Resource Management (ACRM): A decade of experience. *Simul Gaming*. 2001;32:175–193.

25. Gaba DM, Fish KJ, Howard SK. *Crisis Management in Anesthesiology*. Oxford, UK: Churchill Livingstone; 1994.

26. Oandasan I, Baker GR, Barker K, Bosco C, D'Amour D, Jones L, Kimpton S, Lemieux-Charles L, Nasmith L, San Martin Rodriguez L, Tepper J, Way D. *Teamwork in Healthcare: Promoting Effective Teamwork in Healthcare in Canada*. Ottawa: Canadian Health Services Research Foundation; 2006.

27. Doran, D. Teamwork – Nursing and the multidisciplinary team. In L McGinnis Hall (ed.). Quality Work Environments for Nurse and Patient Safety (pp. 39–66). Toronto: Jones and Bartlett Publishers; 2005.

28. Kozlowski SWJ, Ilgen DR. Enhancing the Effectiveness of Work Groups and Teams. *Psychological Science in the Public Interest*. 2006;7:77–124.

29. Ilgen DR, Hollenbeck JR, Johnson M, Jundt D. Teams in Organizations: From Input-Process-Output Models to IMOI Models. *Annu Rev Psychol*. 2005;56:517–543.

30. Stewart GL. A Meta-Analytic Review of Relationships Between Team Design Features and Team Performance. *Journal of Management*. 2006;32:29–55.

31. Caplan GA, Williams AJ, Daly B, Abraham K. A Randomized, Controlled Trial of Comprehensive Geriatric Assessment and Multidisciplinary Intervention After Discharge of Elderly from the Emergency Department—The DEED II Study. *J Am Geriatr Soc.* 2004;52(9):1417–1423.

32. Cohen HJ, Feussner JR, Weinberger M et al. A controlled trial of inpatient and outpatient geriatric evaluation and management. *N Engl J Med.* 2002;346:905–912.

33. Hughes SL, Cummings J, Weaver F, Manheim LM, Conrad KJ, Nash K. A randomized trial of Veterans Administration home care for severely disabled veterans. *Med Care.* 1990;28(2):135–145.

34. Hughes SL, Weaver FM, Giobbie-Hurder A, Manheim L, Henderson W, Kubal JD, Ulasevich A, Cummings J, the Department of Veterans Affairs. Cooperative Effectiveness of Team-Managed Home-Based Primary Care: A Randomized Multicenter Trial. *J Am Med Assoc.* 2000;284(22):2877–2885.

35. Becker PM, McVey LJ, Saltz CC, Feussner JR, Cohen HJ. Hospital-acquired complications in a randomized controlled clinical trial of a geriatric consultation team. *J Am Med Assoc.* 1987;257:2313–2317.

36. Kerski D, Drinka T, Carnes M, Golob K, Craig W. A Post-geriatric evaluation unit follow-up: Team versus nonteam. *J Gerontol.* 1987;42(2):191–195.

37. Zimmer JG, Groth-Juncker A, McCusker J. A randomized controlled study of a home health care team. *Am J Public Health.* 1985;75:134–141.

38. Ball C, Kirkby M, Williams S. Effect of the critical care outreach team on patient survival to discharge from hospital and readmission to critical care: Non-randomized population based study. *Br Med J.* 2003;327:1014–1016.

39. Hedrick SC, Chaney EF, Felker B, Liu CF, Hasenberg N, Heagerty P, Buchanan J, Bagala R, Greenberg D, Paden G, Fihn SD, Katon W. Effectiveness of collaborative care depression treatment in Veterans' Affairs primary care. *J Gen Intern Med.* 2003;18(1):9–16.

40. Liu CF, Hedrick SC, Chaney EF, Heagerty P, Felker B, Hasenberg N, Fihn S, Katon W. Cost-effectiveness of collaborative care for depression in a primary care veteran population. *Psychiatr Serv.* 2003;54(5):698–704.

41. Weisman CS, Gordon DL, Cassard SD, Bergner M, Wong R. The effects of unit self-management on hospital nurses' work process, work satisfaction, and retention. *Med Care.* 1993;31:5

42. Cassard SD, Weisman CS, Gordon DL, Wong R. The impact of unit-based self-management by nurses on patient outcomes. *Health Serv Res.* 1994;29:4.

43. Ling CW. Performance of a self-directed work team in a home healthcare agency. *J Nurs Adm.* 1996;26(9):36–40.

44. Chin MH, Cook S, Drum ML, Jin L, Guillen M, Humikowski CA, Koppert J, Harrison JF, Lippold S, Schaefer CT. Improving diabetes care in midwest community health centers with the health disparities collaborative. *Diabetes Care.* 2004;27(1):2–8.

45. Doran-Irvine DM, Baker GR, Murray M, Bohnen J, Zahn C, Sidani S, Carryer J. Clinical improvement: An interdisciplinary intervention. *Health Care Manage Rev.* 2002;27(4):42–56.

46. Goldberg HI, Wagner EH, Fihn SD, Martin DP, Horowitz CR, Christensen DB, Cheadle AD, Diehr P, Simon G. A randomized controlled trial of CQI teams and academic detailing: Can they alter compliance with guidelines? *Journal of Quality Improvement.* 1998;24:130–142.

47. Gibson CB. Me and us: Differential relationships among goal setting training, efficacy, and effectiveness at the individual and team level. *Journal of Organizational Behavior*. 2001;22(7):789–808.

48. Campion MA, Medsker GJ, Higgs AC. Relations between work group characteristics and effectiveness: Implications for designing effective work groups. *Personnel Psychology*. 1993;46:823–850.

49. Campion MA, Papper EM, Medsker GJ. Relations between work team characteristics and effectiveness: A replication and extension. *Personnel Psychology*. 1996;49:429–452.

50. Jerome L, DeLeon P, James L, Gedney J. The coming of age of telecommunications in psychological research and practice. *Am Psychol*. 2000;55(2).

51. Edmondson AC, Bohmer R, Pisano GP. Disrupted routines: Team learning and new technology adaptation. *Adm Sci Q*. 2001;46:685–716.

52. Barley, SR. Technicians in the workplace: Ethnographic evidence for bringing work into organizational studies. *Adm Sci Q*. 1996;4:404–441.

53. Adapted from: Manning G, Curtis K, McMillen S. Building Community: The Human Side of Work. Cincinnati, OH: Thomson Executive Press; 1996.

54. Gray P. Engaging students' intellects: The immersion approach to critical thinking in psychological instruction. *Teach Psychol*. 1993;20:68–74.

CHAPTER

8

Power and Politics

Lee W. Bewley

Learning Objectives

- Describe the effect of power in a health organization.
- Identify the sources of power for individuals in a health organization.
- Describe how health professionals can achieve power in the health-care setting
- Describe the elements of politics and the association of politics and power in a health organization within Mintzberg's Political Game Playing framework.

■ INTRODUCTION

The modern hospital is manned by hundreds of employees serving multiple departments, services, and clinics, and representing scores of human capital perspectives ranging from health executive to administrative staff. Each of the staff members and the collective groups of staff in various service areas bring unique perspectives, experiences, expectations, and capabilities to the organization; however, the staff, individually and collectively, shares a common, universal element in organizational behavior: the ability to decide whether, and to what degree, to dedicate their efforts toward achieving goals and objectives established by management.

Autonomy of alignment with management direction among staff and work groups is not unique to hospitals among health organizations. Medical group practices, managed care organizations, health plans, and virtually all health organizations face the management problem of shaping and directing the behavior of staff in the workplace. Successful management practices in organizational behavior are positively associated with operational outcomes, higher levels of employee commitment, and greater prevalence of organizational citizenship behaviors. Conversely, management that fails to positively develop staff behaviors is more likely to achieve decremented operational outcomes, lower levels of employee commitment, and higher rates of employee detachment from the organization.

The essential component of management in achieving positive development of organizational behavior among employees is the appropriate utilization of power by an individual in an organizational setting, ranging from a single staff member to the entire enterprise. Power is the ability to stimulate productive action. The key element of this ability in an organization is inherent in the nature of the relationship between an individual and the staff that may be influenced by power. An individual in isolation has no one that he may influence; consequently, his power is effectively benign. On the other hand, an individual who regularly interacts with staff in an organization is clearly more likely to exert or experience influence and, therefore, has the potential to employ power in the course of work. The foundation for power is based on the nature of the interaction between a staff member who seeks to influence another staff member or group. Generally, the level of power and corresponding likelihood of a successful conveyance of influence is based on an evaluation of characteristics or context aligned with the executive, manager, or individual seeking to leverage power to achieve influence. For instance, the higher the level of power a hospital nursing staff perceives the vice president for nursing in a community hospital to possess as a consequence of certain characteristics inherent in the executive and the organization context of the position, the higher level of influence that the executive is likely to be able to achieve in the hospital.

Another important consideration in the interaction of members in an organization relative to power and influence is the practice of organizational politics. Politics in business is usually associated with attempts to influence or to achieve power contrary to or misaligned with the primary design or goals of the organization. There are a number of mechanisms in which individuals or groups in health organizations may seek to employ organizational politics to gain power and exert influence.

■ SOURCES OF POWER

What are the characteristics or organizational contexts that enable a member of a health organization to achieve power in order to positively influence staff in the organization? The two broad domains of power generation include individual-based characteristics and organizational structure. Fellow staff members will assess the level of power an individual possesses based upon characteristics inherent in the individual and the position that the individual holds in the organization. There are several components of both individual- and structural-based power sources.

Individual Based

A seminal writing in organizational behavior by French and Raven outlines five primary sources of power based on individual characteristics evaluated by staff subject to the potential influence of an individual. These individual characteristics include legitimate power, reward power, coercive power, expert power, and referent power.[1,2] Each of these bases of power is neither mutually inclusive nor independently exclusive as a rule of practice. Separate or combinations of each of the sources of individual-based power may be leveraged to achieve influence in an organization.

Legitimate

Legitimate power derives primarily from authority. It is the reflection of an assignment or duty position allocated to an individual in an organization, which is recognized and understood by other staff, particularly by staff members that occupy subordinate positions. Subordination to another individual in an organization facilitates the opportunity to command, direct, or change employee actions by the staff member with authority provided that the subject subordinates fall within the relevant bounds of control available to the senior staff member. For instance, the chief executive officer (CEO) of a hospital possesses legitimate power and practically all of the staff in the hospital exists within the CEO's bounds of authority. However, the vice president for nursing services also holds similar, significant legitimate power in the organization, but staff working in areas other than nursing will likely moderate the level of power perception of the nursing executive.

Reward

Reward power is based in the perception by staff that an individual either possesses something that is desired by individuals or groups in an organization or that the individual can reasonably coordinate to deliver something of value to members of the staff. Examples of rewards that may be conveyed range from simple praise to bonuses or promotions. It is important to note that if a manager or executive is not perceived by staff to be either able or willing to generate rewards, then the ability of an individual to use reward power to influence staff to achieve organization goals will bear no fruit.

Coercive

The contrary power perspective of reward power is coercive power or the perception of members of an organization that an individual has the ability to mete out punishment or sanctions ranging from a mild annoyance to professionally or personally devastating. Similar to reward power, if the organizational staff judge that an individual either does not have the ability or the constitution to adjudicate coercive actions to individuals or groups in the organization, then the executive or manager that attempts to employ this form of power to achieve influence will likely fail in their efforts.

Expert

The individual-based characteristic of expert power is particularly effective and clearly identifiable by attributes specific to an individual. Practically any characteristic, credential, or ability that reflects relatively rare expertise and a unique ability to positively contribute may serve as the basis for expert power. However, the essential element of establishing power, like all forms of potential power, is that staff that may be subject to the attempted influence of an individual seeking to leverage expert power must recognize, understand, and accept the characteristics of the individual who may attempt to establish power. For instance, people unfamiliar with many health professions may equivalently judge the expert power of a physician assistant and an emergency medical technician.

Referent

The final individual-based power source is referent power. As people in an organization positively associate specific personal or behavioral characteristics to an individual that causes them to be inclined to agree with or seek to please another individual that is judged to have charisma, then referent power is developed in an organization by an individual. The enduring essential element of this power generation process is that the members of the organization generate this power by associating favorable personal judgments to a focused individual based on the manner in which that individual interacts with people.

Structural Based

In addition to individual-based sources of power in organizations, there are certain aspects of firms that have the potential to generate power based upon the structural characteristics of the enterprise. These structures include resource power, decision-making power, and information power. Each of these sources of power may be employed individually or in combination to exert influence in organizations to facilitate achievement of organizational goals and objectives.[3,4]

Resources

Perhaps no other aspect of an organization, particularly in a capitalistic society, is emblematic of power than the possession and control of essential resources to achieve some individual or collective end. The breadth and depth of potential resources that may generate power is extensive, but the strength of the power generation is positively associated with the relative scarcity of the resources in the relevant market context and in the strength of being essential or desired. Individuals that have the capacity to direct, divert, withhold, and/or provide resources clearly have the capacity to influence others, potentially in relationships that are lateral or ascendant rather than a traditional subordinate or down-stream perspective.

Decision Making

Individuals that hold a position within the structure of an organization that either make or facilitate decisions clearly have the capacity to be able to influence individuals or groups within the firm. If appropriately utilized, the ability or opportunity to make decisions within an organizational context potentially affect each of the other prime sources of power and, thus, can be a potent source of power if staff influenced by the individual with decision-making authority recognize this power.

Information

The common refrain that "information is power" is generally true. Information that is essential, valued, and/or sought by individuals within an organization serves as the basis for power for key individuals who possess or have access to information that could yield influence. Just as possession and control of resources may generate influence opportunities in ascending or lateral organizational strata, information power may also achieve influence up, across, and down the organizational boundaries depending upon the level of value individuals in the organization place on the information.

Summary of the Sources of Power

The prime use of power in an organization is to influence individuals and/or groups to generate positive actions aligned with the goals and objectives of the firm. Each of the component sources of power with the individual and structural domains of power generation exist as potential levers to generate influence and corresponding action within an organizational context (see Figure 8-1).

Sources of Power for Health Professionals

Health professionals have a number of mechanisms for achieving power within the organizational context, particularly given the degree of specialization among professions that create varying and relative scarcity of human resources. Furthermore, the prevalence of executive positions in organizations, credentialing services, and the asymmetrical access to resources and information yield accessible means for achieving power to generate influence.[5] Table 8-1 outlines some mechanisms that health professionals may use to achieve power in health organizations.

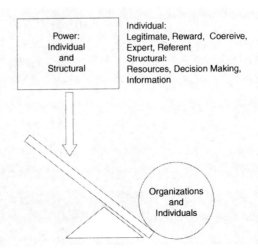

Figure 8-1   The Effect of Power.

Table 8-1 Sources of Power for Health Professionals			
	Physicians/ Dentists	**Nurses**	**Allied Health Providers**	**Health Administrators**
---	---	---	---	---
Legitimate	Owner, Partner, Chief	VP, Head Nurse	Owner, Partner, Chief	CEO, Administrator
Reward	Contingency Based	Contingency Based	Contingency Based	Contingency Based
Coercive	Contingency Based	Contingency Based	Contingency Based	Contingency Based
Expert	MD, DO, DMD	MSN, Ph.D.	M.S., D.PT., Ph.D.	MHA, MSHA, MBA, FACHE, Ph.D.
Referent	Past Actions, Interpersonal Interactions	Past Actions, Interpersonal Interactions	Past Actions, Interpersonal Interactions	Past Actions, Interpersonal Interactions
Resources	Clinical	Nursing	Clinical	Business Processes
Decision Making	Clinical Staff	Nursing Staff	Clinical Staff	Business Processes
Information	Patient Diagnosis	Case Management	Patient Diagnosis	Business Processes

■ POLITICS IN HEALTH ORGANIZATIONS

The development and use of power in organizations to generate influence is generally associated with the primary mission of the organization, which is usually to enable principles and agents to provide an adequate return on investment to the owners of the enterprise in for-profit health organizations or to achieve higher levels of societal benefit in the context of non-profit health organization. Organizational politics exists as another process of shaping power and influence; however, the basis and intent of these processes are not always aligned with organizational goals and objectives and, in fact, may be contrary to the benefit of the firm for the gain of individuals or interest groups.

Elements of Playing Politics

What are the characteristics of organizational politics? Generally, the elements of playing politics include actions taken outside the bounds of established organizational processes, actions taken to benefit individuals or groups often to the detriment of the organization, and intentional, premeditated actions focused solely on the attainment and/or preservation of power. Essentially, playing politics is an individually motivated event undertaken with the principle intent to improve one's own personal benefit.[6,7]

Mintzberg's Political Games

Mintzberg articulated a model of organizational interaction focused on the development, maintenance, and employment of influence in firms among employees that often exists outside the established bounds of the enterprise, but intermittently achieves outcomes that align with the interests of the organization. Mintzberg's model of political games outlines the players, conditions, and power/influence relationships in an organization context along with the primary reasons for playing each of the games. The following depictions illustrate how health professionals may play these games in health organizations.[8,9]

Insurgency

This game involves individuals or small groups that resist authority or some legitimate power. If the CEO of a community hospital was considering an unpopular closure of the Neo-Natal Intensive Care Unit (NICU), then the staff may leak details of the plan to the local newspaper or to board members in an attempt to have the plans derailed.

Counter-Insurgency

This game involves senior leaders, executives, and/or individuals with legitimate power countering the political insurgency efforts of subordinate staff. In the NICU scenario, the CEO could censure discussion of hospital plans outside of the hospital or take actions to punish staff that leaked information.

Sponsorship

This game involves subordinate or junior staffs that seek to improve their power position in the organization by seeking patronage and sponsorship from more senior and powerful staff members. An example of this might be represented by the actions of a junior actuary in a health insurance company that are directed to gaining valuable developmental time with the chief executive of the firm.

Alliance-Building

This game involves line leaders with legitimate power coordinating across operational lines to solidify their power base. Each of the respective head nurses in a hospital may develop relationships across wards to enhance their power base.

Empire-Building

This game involves line leaders with legitimate power angling to attain and accumulate key, essential resources within the organization to bolster their power base. A partner in a group practice management could play this game by seeking to concentrate the most productive providers in his clinic at the expense of the other partner clinics.

Budgeting

This game is similar to empire-building game; however, focus of line leaders is solely on attaining a greater portion of the operational budget and effectively crowding out other aspects of the firm. The emergency services director that seeks to upgrade his facilities by allocating 90% of the annual capital budget would be playing this game.

Expertise

This game is played by employing expert power in a manner that is oriented exclusively to improving the power base on the individual. A highly regarded physician that practices pediatric neurosurgery demands specific facilities, equipment, and support staff with the prime rationale being that no one else in the hospital understands what is required to do his or her work.

Lording

This game is played by staff members with potentially excess legitimate power who overly leverage their power to firmly establish their own power base and diminish the power of other staff. The president of the medical staff, who perpetually reminds the administrator that he or she is the medically trained professional in public and private forums, may be playing the lording game.

Line vs. Staff

This game is played between staff members with alternatively legitimate and expert powers generally intended to diminish the power standing of one individual or group. Staff conflicts between administrators and clinicians may often resort to these political games.

Rival Camps

This game is played when multiple groups aggregate around polarizing issues and seek a "winner takes all" outcome to completely establish power by dashing the power and standing of the other group. A division between the medical staff and nursing staff relative to operational procedures could develop into this game.

Strategic Candidates

This game is played by individuals or groups with legitimate power to change the fundamental framework or direction of the organization. Individuals seeking to become the CEO, who advocate different views of the future in terms of mergers or alliances versus remaining a stand-alone facility, may play this game.

Whistle-Blowing

This game is played by levering information power to stop or inhibit action within the organization. An example of this game would involve staff coming forward to the press or the board of directors with information to prevent the firing of a popular staff member.

Young Turks

This game is played with the most aggressive political goals intended, which result in a revolutionary change in the process or content of leadership and power in the organization. Employees or junior leaders of a healthcare system seek to buy the system.

Figure 8-2 depicts the various political games that members of a health organization may play in the development of personal power to achieve influence.

■ CHAPTER SUMMARY

Power facilitates influence in health organizations and is derived from individuals and structure. Health professionals may develop power from several perspectives and sources. Some of this is resource dependent and some is based on individual choices. Power provides the basis for political games and competition. Organizational politics are played to advance the power and influence of individuals. Individuals and subgroups may play a number of political games in a health organization.

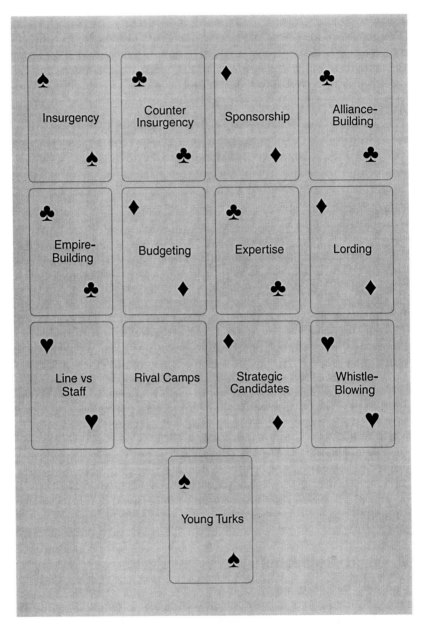

Figure 8-2 Mintzberg's Organizational Political Game.

Review/Discussion Questions

1. What are the two prime sources of power in health organizations?
2. What are specific determinants of power for individuals in health organizations?
3. How does power vary among health professionals?
4. What is the prime motive for playing organizational politics in health organizations?
5. What are the various political games that health professionals may pursue in health organizations?

Learning Activities

1. Evaluate members of an organization to determine their respective bases of power.
2. Scan *New York Times* and *Wall Street Journal* articles for health organizations that are in distress, and evaluate the content and process of any relevant political game playing in those organizations.

References

1. French J, Raven B. The Basis of Social Power. *Studies in Social Power*. Ann Arbor, MI: Institute for Social Research. 150–167; 1959.
2. Ivancevich J, Matteson M. *Organizational Behavior and Management* (4th ed.). Chicago: Irwin, 361–376; 1996.
3. Bass D, Burkhardt M. Potential power and power use: An investigation of structure and behavior. *Acad Manage J*. 1993;June:441–470.
4. Pfeffer J. *Understanding Power in Organizations*. Marshfield, MA: Pitman Publishing, 104–122; 1981.
5. Shi L, Singh D. *Health Services Professionals*. *Delivering Health Care in America: A Systems Approach*. Sudbury, MA: Jones and Bartlett, 117–148; 2004.
6. Velasquez M, Moberg D, Cavanagh G. Organizational statesmanship and dirty politics: Ethical guidelines for the organizational politician. *Organ Dyn*. 1983;Autumn:65–79.
7. Yoffie D, Bergenstein S. Creating Political Advantage: The Rise of Corporate Entrepreneurs. *Calif Manage Rev*. 1985;Fall:124–129.
8. Mintzberg, H. *Power In and Around Organizations*. Englewood Cliffs, NJ: Prentice Hall, 171–271; 1983.
9. Mintzberg, H. The organization as political arena. *Journal of Management Studies*. 1985;22:133–154.

CHAPTER

9

Conflict and Interpersonal Relationships

Gerald R. Ledlow

Learning Objectives

- Define conflict and give examples of real and potential conflict situations.
- List and describe the different conflict management styles.
- Apply the conflict management style decision tree to real or hypothetical conflict situations.
- Develop a practical model of conflict management in healthcare organizations.
- Describe four factors in building professional and positive interpersonal relationships.
- Explain how trust and disclosure work together in building relationships.
- Explain how quality communication leads to better conflict management and conflict outcomes as well as better interpersonal relationships.

■ INTRODUCTION

Conflict is inevitable. Interpersonal relationships are required to lead and manage a successful healthcare organization. Conflict occurs when interdependent people have different goals amid an environment of scarce resources.[1] Assumed in that definition, interpersonal relationships must exist. March suggests that each individual in an organization has different goals; even if the goals are slightly different, conflict can occur. [2] There are conflict situations across the continuum of contexts and there are countless types of interpersonal relationships. This chapter will focus on healthcare organizations as the context, and the intent is to provide you knowledge, skills, and abilities to lead and manage healthcare organizations with the understanding that conflict is inevitable, necessary, and can produce positive quality outcomes. Also, positive and mutually beneficial interpersonal relationships with all healthcare organization stakeholders, physicians, surgeons, nurses, administrators, housekeeping staff, volunteer staff, and community leaders to name only a very few, are tightly tied to leadership and management success in healthcare operations.

Healthcare organizations are complex and usually large entities. "The theories of Maslow, McGregor, and Argyris suggest that conflict between individuals and individuals and the organization would get worse as organizations became larger (with greater impersonality, longer chains of command, and more complex rules and control systems). As society becomes better educated and more affluent (producing more people whose higher-level needs are salient) more conflict will occur."[3] Communication, knowledge, and situational assessment are keys to successful conflict management and building solid interpersonal relationships. Communication that contains information that is timely, accurate, useful, and frequent (without being annoying) nurtures trust; trust creates an environment for interactive, inclusive, and open communication, an essential element for successful conflict management and in developing quality relationships.

Leading change management experts recommend using conflict in your organization to "stir the pot" to create change. Conflict creates change; the question is, "is the change positive?" If you train your organization to manage conflict where internal and external relationships are treated with respect, then you are much more able to use conflict to positively change your organization rather than destroy it. It starts with communication, knowledge, and skills; it starts with you as the leader and manager. It is recommended that the reader review the chapters in this text on leadership, decision making, and communication to broaden understanding of conflict and interpersonal relationships. This chapter will be different in that the case study will be presented early in the chapter as a context to think about and reflect on conflict management and interpersonal relationships as you read about the topic areas.

Case Study

A CEO of a major healthcare organization planned a major push to earn internal provider and staff support and community/customer/patient brand identity for a new patient service where additional emphasis would be on customer satisfaction. The leader's vision was communicated frequently to the organization's stakeholders. Everyone rallied around the new vision and began to get involved with the planning of the programs. Everything seemed liked it was working; the plan to communicate a new vision started to get people working, but very soon thereafter, problems arose. Providers began to battle with administration, customers began to demand access to the new services, and different staff sections began to argue over trivial issues concerning the programs. What proved to be a catalyst to conflict, the new programs, was eventually put on the "back-burner." What happened? The CEO reflected on this, and the conclusions were

1. The new programs made staff insecure about their jobs. The staff felt they needed to be a "part" of the new vision/new programs but were not given a forum to be "officially" included.
2. A vision may not be enough. A clear objective plan with clear lines of authority of who does what for the new programs should have been communicated "up front." The staff was not guided/focused on the tasks at hand.
3. The staff may not have been sufficiently trained to meet the new expectations the CEO set with the vision.
4. Stakeholders (internal and external) were jockeying for "position" to gain the CEO's favor rather than concentrating on the new programs.
5. There was no constructive way to handle the conflict situations that occurred. Training was clearly needed.

Has this happened to your organization? Maybe this story was about your organization.

■ CONFLICT MANAGEMENT

Conflict connotes negative thoughts, such as in metaphors of "battle," "war," "aggression," and "violence." However, conflict is inevitable and necessary for a vibrant organization. Five basic frameworks form the basis of modern conflict management theory and application: psychodynamic theory, field theory, experimental gaming theory, human relations theory, and inter-group conflict theory. Conflict that is channeled and managed is a rational route to change, improvement, thought creation, and organizational longevity if not survival. The existence of conflict means there are opportunities to find improved alternative solutions to the current state of affairs. Of course, conflict can negatively impact the organization, but pessimism should not be the overriding default of leadership, management, or human existence for that matter. Leaders and managers can manage conflict and train others to apply skills and tools of conflict to achieve successful and improved outcomes in their professional lives. Leaders communicate meaning in everything they do. If messages are incongruent, goal conflicts and inconsistencies soon become part of the organizational culture.[4–6]

Hand-in-hand with conflict management is interpersonal relationships; factors of interpersonal relationships are overviewed in the last half of this chapter. Learning, as an organization, to constructively manage and succeed in conflict situations is a foundational construct of leadership and management.

Conflict occurs wherever interdependent people or groups (that means they depend on each other in some fashion for some need) have different goals or aspirations of achievement amid an environment of scarce resources.[7] Simply, people, individually or in groups, working together with other individuals or groups who have different goals, needs, or desires where a full complement of resources are not available to satisfy those goals, needs, or desires, will have conflict. We all live, work, and socialize with other people and share the limited resources available (rarely, if ever are resources not limited), so conflict will happen and does happen to varying degrees of intensity. At one end of the spectrum, conflict can be a situation identified by two parties and those parties identify the problem and work together to solve it (problem-solving style) and at the other end is violence (competing style) with bodily harm, such as a war, which is the failure of conflict management.

Conflict is both an individual and group phenomenon. Western society tends to teach children to "smooth over" conflict; do you remember a parent saying to "play nice" or "you have to learn to share"? Fairness, morals, social norms and mores, along with the application of any of the multiple distributive justice methods, contribute to conflict situations when one party feels less than an equitable distribution of resources has occurred. Quality conflict management should produce the following outcomes:

- A wise agreement if an agreement is possible
- An efficient solution
  - An innovative solution, potentially
  - Movement toward positive change in the organization
- A better relationship between the conflicting parties (or at least not damage the relationship)

So with all these expectations, how can you manage conflict? Basically, different situations require different styles; training organizational stakeholders on the effective use of conflict styles is also imperative.

Conflict Styles

There are six basic conflict management styles. Each person has a dominant or primary style and secondary style that are relatively stable (like personality style) but all six styles can be learned, applied, and mastered. Conflict styles are a learning skill set. The more you learn and master, the more flexible you are in conflict situations. Later a decision tree is shown that can help you select which conflict style to use based on the situation (answering several yes or no questions); it is imperative to understand and be able to apply different conflict styles since situations will differ daily. The six styles presented are shown as an amalgam of multiple scholars' work for purposes of expanding your knowledge; the styles are:[1,8-12]

1. Accommodating
2. Avoiding
3. Collaborating
4. Competing
5. Compromising
6. Problem Solving

The basic styles are chosen based on the situation. It is important to note that during conflict situations, one party can select (knowingly or unknowingly) one style and the other party can select a different style. Only in problem solving do both parties knowingly choose that style and work together. In order to understand the situational context, and what style to select, each style is presented with its associated situational context below:

Accommodating

- When you find you are wrong; to allow a better position to be heard, to learn, and to show your reasonableness.
- When issues are more important to others than to you; to satisfy others and maintain cooperation.
- To build social capital for later issues.
- To minimize loss when you are outmatched and losing the conflict.
- When harmony and stability are especially important.
- To allow subordinates to develop by learning from their mistakes.

Avoiding

- When an issue is trivial or more important issues are pressing.
- When you perceive no chance of satisfying your needs.

- When potential disruption outweighs the benefits of resolution.
- To let people cool down and regain perspective.
- When gathering information supersedes immediate decision making.
- When others can resolve the conflict more effectively.
- When issues seem a result of other issues.

Collaborating

- To find an integrative solution when both sets of concerns are too important to be compromised.
- When your objective is to learn.
- To merge insights from people with different perspectives.
- To gain commitment by incorporating concerns into a consensus.
- To work through feelings that has harmed an interpersonal relationship.

Competing

- When quick, decisive action is vital (e.g., emergency situations such as a disaster or terrorism incident or accident).
- On important issues where unpopular actions need implementing (e.g., cost cutting, enforcing unpopular rules, discipline).
- On issues vital to company welfare and survival when you know you are right.
- Against people who take advantage of noncompetitive behavior.

Compromising

- When goals are important, but not worth the effort or potential disruption of competing.
- When opponents with equal power are committed to mutually exclusive goals.
- To achieve temporary settlements to complex issues.
- To arrive at expedient solutions under time pressure.
- As a backup when collaboration or competition is unsuccessful.

Problem Solving

- May not always work (takes two to make this style work).
- Requires the identification of a broader range of strategies.
- Points for problem solving
  - Both parties must have a vested interest in the outcome (the resolution).
  - Both parties feel a better solution can be achieved through problem-based collaboration.

- Both parties recognize the problem is caused by the relationship, not the people involved.
- Focus is on solving the problem, not on accommodating differing views.
- Both parties are flexible.
- Understanding that all solutions have positive and negative aspects.
- Both parties understand each other's issues.
- Problem is looked at objectively, not personally.
- Both parties are knowledgeable about conflict management.
- Allow everyone to "save face."
- Celebrate successful outcomes openly.

Clearly, the styles are different and, thus, should be used contingently based on the situation that presents itself in conflict environments. The dynamic nature of healthcare organizations requires leaders and managers to become competent with each conflict style. Again, training organizational stakeholders is also critically important. To show the contingent nature of conflict styles, a merging with a well-known leadership model is highlighted. From a leadership contingency perspective, review the Ohio State and Michigan Leadership studies. Conflict management styles can be arrayed graphically as shown in Figure 9-1, similar to leadership styles.

Before discussing the decision tree, additional factors should be considered for the successful leader and manager of healthcare organizations.

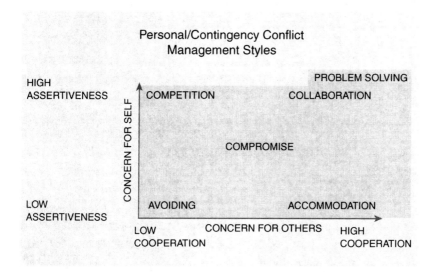

Figure 9-1 Conflict Styles Regarding Concern for Self and Others.[13]

Essential steps for leaders and managers in conflict management when in the early stages of conflict are to:

- Stay calm and rational.
- Use facts (do your homework).
- Understand the resource implications and limitations surrounding the conflict.
- Listen to how you feel and know what you want or need.
- Try to imagine what the other(s) feel, want, and need.
- Use a process to select a strategy such as the decision tree method.
- Rehearse your strategy.
- Be prepared to modify your approach if necessary.

When you are in the midst of conflict, it is important to keep these tenets in mind:

- Separate the people from the problem or conflict as much as possible.
- Focus on interests, not positions.
- Avoid always having a "bottom line."
- Think about the worst and best solutions and know what you can "live with."
- Generate several possibilities before deciding what to do.
- Insist that the result (resolution) be based on some objective standard.

Negotiation is similar to conflict resolution. There are several important points from Fisher, Ury, and Patton's 1991 work, *Getting to Yes: Negotiating Agreement Without Giving In* (2nd ed.), that are salient for conflict management. These recommendations reinforce previous points already presented and lean toward the problem-solving style of conflict:[14]

- Do not bargain over positions.
- Separate the people from the problem.
- Focus on interests, not positions.
- Invent options for mutual gain.
- Insist on using objective criteria to resolve the issue.
- Use your "best alternative to a negotiated agreement" (BATNA; this means, what is the worst case scenario if nothing is resolved?).
- Get the other party to negotiate.

Now, we will turn our attention to selecting a conflict style based on the situation. With six styles to select from, it is important to study each style and become familiar with the styles so that the selection method, a decision tree, becomes understandable. Remember that five styles are at your "control" while the sixth style, problem solving, requires that both parties consciously and upon agreement select that style.

Conflict Style Selection

Selecting a conflict style depends on several factors. These factors rest in the interpersonal relationship with others (that is those in the conflict against you), resources available (like time), resources not available, importance of the issues at hand, and other associated elements. Taking these factors from the decision tree model, the factors consist of the following in the form of high/yes or low/no answer to questions:

1. Is/are the issue(s) important to you?
2. Is/are the issue(s) important to the other party?
3. Is the relationship with the other party important to you?
4. How much time is available and how much pressure/stress is there to come to a resolution? *Of note, an answer of "High" means High Pressure.*
5. How much do you trust the other party?

Review Figure 9-2 noting the questions at the top and the associated high/yes and low/no answers to each of these questions. Follow the path until you come to the conflict management style that is recommended to employ given the conflict situation. An example will be provided following your review of the figure.

The following is an example illustrating two points, how to use the decision tree and the caution associated with using the avoiding style:

You are in a conflict situation with another employee at the hospital. You have prepared yourself by reviewing all the points made

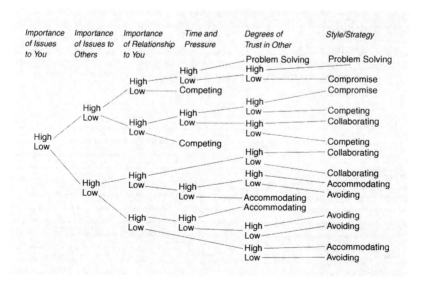

Figure 9-2 Conflict Management Style Decision Tree (Modified).[1]

previously in this chapter. Now answer the questions based on the decision tree model:

1. Is the issue important to you? *You determine the answer is low.*
2. Is the issue important to the other party? *You determine the answer is high. (Why else would this person make such a big deal out of it?)*
3. Is the relationship with the other party important to you? *You determine the answer is low. (This is the caution: how does this equate to using the avoiding style?) Eventually, the avoiding style will deteriorate the relationship with the other person or party.*
4. How much time is available and how much pressure/stress is there to come to resolution? *You determine there is high pressure to come to a resolution.*
5. How much do you trust the other party? *You determine you do not really trust the other person, so the answer is low.*
6. OUTCOME: *The style recommended is the Avoiding Style.*

Conflict management is a critical and necessary skill with both technical (styles and decision tree) and relationship (communication and trust building) components. Conflict as a state of nature, situational framework, conflict styles, and the application of conflict styles with a recommendation selection method has been presented. See the overview of interpersonal relationships in the next section.

■ INTERPERSONAL RELATIONSHIPS

In organizational life, interpersonal relationships are required, beneficial, and enhance our daily professional lives. There are key elements or factors that facilitate improved, positive, and mutually beneficial relationships. Yukl in 1989 proposed a taxonomy of managerial behaviors in which one of the four major domains of managerial life was "Building Relationships"; in this domain, managing conflict and teambuilding, networking, supporting and developing, and mentoring were the actual behaviors and activities managers (and leaders) were recommended to engage in to strengthen relationships.[15] A healthcare organization leader and manager, as mentioned before, must establish, enhance, and grow relationships with a myriad of organizational stakeholders both internal and external to the organization. There is no better method to build relationships than going to visit people in their environment or location; many know this as "management by walking around," but it is a powerful approach. This section will provide an overview of those factors that will enhance relationships. Each factor presented has monumental importance; there are many factors in relationships, however, four key factors constitute the remainder of the chapter.

Factors to Strengthen Relationships

Relationships refer to the feelings, roles, norms, status, and trust that both affect and reflect the quality of communication between members of a group.[16]

Relational communication theorists assert that every message has both a *content* and *relationship* dimension, where:

- Content contains specific information conveyed to someone, and
- Relationship messages that cue or provides hints about whether the sender/receiver likes or dislikes the other person(s).

Communicating with someone that provides both content and positive relationship information is important. The reader is recommended to read the decision-making and communication chapter for information on confirming and disconfirming communication and evaluative and descriptive communication. Confirming and descriptive communication lends itself to positive and enhanced relationships while disconfirming and evaluative communication lends itself to a reduction in the relationship bond. Language, tone, and nonverbal communication work together to provide meaning that comes from you and is interpreted by another person. Some important information regarding nonverbal communication is:[16,17]

- Nonverbal communication is more prevalent than verbal communication.
  - Eye contact
  - Facial expressions
  - Body posture
  - Movement

- People believe nonverbal communication more than verbal communication.
  - 65% of meaning is derived from nonverbal communication

- People communicate emotions primarily through nonverbal communication.
  - 93% of emotions are communicated nonverbally

Consider frequency of communication that is timely, useful, accurate, and in reasonable quantity to reinforce and validate the relationship. As for factors, one important factor is *quality communication of sufficient and desired frequency.*

The next factor, *disclosure,* relates to the type of information you and the other person in the relationship share with each other; disclosure is one factor that can help you "measure" or evaluate the depth and breadth of a relationship. The "deeper" the information disclosed, the closer the bond of the relationship. Also, the broader the topics of information and experience sharing—family, work, fishing together, or playing golf—suggests a closer bond for the relationship as well. Self-disclosure can be categorized and actually measured. In the model below, level 5 illustrates a weak relationship bond whereas level 1 shows a strong relationship bond. Disclosure or self-disclosure is strongly and positively correlated (or connected to where more trust means more disclosure) to trust. Again, trust starts with quality communication. Shown, are Powell's self-disclosure levels:[16]

- Level 5: Cliché communication
- Level 4: Facts and biographical information
- Level 3: Personal attitudes and ideas
- Level 2: Personal feelings
- Level 1: Peak communication (rare; usually with family or close friends)

For a better understanding of self-disclosure, this concept is:[16]

- A function of ongoing relationships
- Reciprocal
- Timed to what is happening in the relationship (contextual/ situational/relational)
- Should be relevant to what is happening among people present, and
- Usually moves by small increments

Factor three is *trust*. Build and earn trust over time through honest interaction (communication and experiences). Honesty, inclusion, and sincerity directly link to building trust. Trust is an essential component of a quality, positive relationship. Honesty is being truthful and open concerning important pieces of information that you share with another person. Inclusion is about including the other person in the relationship in activities and experiences that are important to them, you, and both of you. Inclusion is also about making sure the other person is part of the "group" in the organization. Sincerity is meaning what you say, meaning what you do, and not keeping a record or account of the relationship (not keeping score). Over time, if honesty, inclusion and sincerity are the basis of your interaction with others, positive and quality relationships will begin to grow.

The fourth factor is *cultural competence*. This factor is not only based on ethnical or national dimensions but socio-economic factors as well. For instance, consider the cultural differences in surgeons as opposed to nurses as opposed to facility technicians or linen staff or consultants. Every stakeholder group, every individual has a varying culture of uniqueness. Understanding those cultural issues, walking a mile in someone else's shoes, is a factor important to building solid interpersonal relationships. Understanding and modifying your approach to relationship building and enhancement based on cultural differences will serve you well in leadership and management positions. Some elements of importance concerning cultural competence follow.

Culture is a learned system of knowledge, behavior, attitudes, beliefs, values, and norms that a group of people shares.[16,18] Culture is a difference that makes a difference.[16] Cultural differences have been categorized, initially from the work of Hofstede, into the following (four are presented here, there are several more):

* Language
* High vs. low context
* High vs. low contact
* Time (mono-chronic vs. poly-chronic)

First, language is the structure, rules, and annunciation of symbols; Spanish, English, Mandarin Chinese, German, and Flemish are examples of language. High-context cultures place more emphasis on nonverbal communication; physical context is important in interpreting the message and the stress is on the receiver of a message to understand the intended meaning. Low-context cultures places more emphasis on verbal expression; the sender is responsible for relaying meaning to the receiver verbally. Sometimes, people from a high-context culture will find those from a low-context culture less credible or trustworthy. Someone from a low-context culture may be more likely to make explicit requests for information ("talk to me," "do you know what I mean?"). In contrast, a person from a high-context culture expects communication to be more indirect and relies on cues that are more implicit.[16] People from high-context cultures may consider a low-context person overbearing, dominant, and talkative.

High-contact and low-contact cultures differ as well. People from some cultures are more comfortable being touched or being in close proximity to others (high-contact) whereas some people want more personal space, typically have less eye contact, and are uncomfortable with being touched by others. This is similar to personal and social space. Some people want larger areas of "space," while others are comfortable with less "space." Mono-chronic and poly-chronic cultures differ with perceptions and use of time. Mono-chronic cultures are precise; time is to be used and manipulated. Poly-chronic cultures are not as precise on time; time is what it is, events flow in their intended pattern as they happen. It is not unusual to have a mono-chronic culture person arrive at a scheduled meeting 5 minutes early, only to be irritated and mad by the time a poly-chronic culture person arrives 30 minutes past the scheduled time. Although organizational rules such as adherence to schedules are important, some understanding of time perception differences can reduce potential "anger" when both cultures understand the perceptions of each other.

Four factors have been presented in order to assist in interpersonal relationship building. These factors, coupled with a review of the decision-making and communication chapter of this text, will greatly assist in building relationships with all healthcare organization stakeholders. It is recommended that the reader, considering limited space in this chapter and volume, further study communication, disclosure, trust, and cultural competence within the context of interpersonal relationships using the modern literature on the topic. Additionally, seeking out and getting a mentor who clearly has earned the respect of others by establishing many quality relationships will serve you well for many years; learn from your mentor in both relationship building and conflict management.

Leadership and Management Roles

Building relationships while being in a leadership or management role is not always easy. However, you can build relationships, professionally, while maintaining your position, power, and authority. If honesty, inclusion, and sincerity (building blocks of trust) are the basis of your quality communication that is culturally competent, then you can maintain your role while building relationships. You can gauge the relationship by disclosure levels; disclosure is where leaders and managers must consciously draw the line for their personal level of disclosure. Disclosing too much or too much too soon or too often can reduce your position, power, and authority; being personally "disclosure conservative" is a good initial approach when building new relationships. To conclude this section on interpersonal relationships, Yukl recommends the following based on leader and manager behaviors and activities to promote relationship building:[19]

GUIDELINES: For Supportive Leadership:
- Show acceptance and positive regard.
- Be polite and diplomatic, not arrogant and rude.
- Bolster the person's self-esteem.
- Provide assistance with the work when needed.
- Be willing to help with personal problems.
- Be a great listener.

GUIDELINES: For Integrative Problem Solving:
- Foster mutual trust.
- Identify shared objectives and beliefs.
- Identify specific reasons (not personalities) for the conflict.
- Consider a range of acceptable solutions.
- Try to find an optimal solution.

GUIDELINES: For Team Building:

- Emphasize common interests.
- Use ceremonies and rituals.
- Use symbols to develop identification with the work unit.
- Encourage and facilitate satisfying social interaction.
- Hold team-building sessions.
  - Involve frank and open discussion of interpersonal relationships.
  - Involve yourself in group processes in an effort to improve them.
- Use process consultants when and where appropriate.

■ CHAPTER SUMMARY

This chapter has provided an overview of conflict management and interpersonal relationships from a "knowledge to skills to application" perspective. Clearly, it is recommended that the reader pursue additional study in the topical areas of conflict management, problem solving, decision making, team building, relationship building, networking, communication, and mentoring (including being mentored).

Conflict is inevitable, necessary, and exists when interdependent parties have different goals amid scarce resources. Conflict styles can be learned, mastered, and selected given the situation. A conflict management decision tree can aid in style selection. Interpersonal relationships are vital for leaders and managers in healthcare organizations, while communication, along with other factors, serves as a foundation for relationships. Given this, there is a need to periodically train organizational stakeholders in conflict management and in developing positive professional interpersonal relationships.

Review/Discussion Questions

1. What is conflict and can it be avoided?
2. Can conflict be managed throughout the organization and how?
3. What are the styles of conflict management and what is important about each style?
4. The case study in this chapter presented a conflict situation. What organizational strategy can the CEO use to get the organization back on track considering conflict management?
5. What factors impact interpersonal relationships? What factors outside of the presented factors in this chapter are important to your relationships?
6. What things destroy relationships? What builds relationships?

7. What items in the lists of recommendations (guidelines) did you find most important to relationship building?

8. Based on the case study of this chapter, are there relationship-building strategies that could be used to improve the situation?

References

1. Folger JP, Poole MS, Stutman RK. *Working Through Conflict: Strategies for Relationships, Groups, and Organizations,* (3rd ed.). NY: Longman; 1997.

2. March JG, Weisinger-Baylon R. *Ambiguity and Command: Organizational Perspectives on Military Decision Making.* Marshfield, MA: Pitman Publishing; 1986.

3. Bolman LG, Deal TE. *Reframing Organizations: Artistry, Choice, and Leadership.* San Francisco, CA: Jossey-Bass Publishers, 152–153; 1991.

4. Ledlow GR, Bradshaw DM, Shockley C. Primary care access improvement: An empowerment–interaction model. *Mil Med.* 2000;165(2);390–395.

5. Ledlow G, Cwiek M, Johnson J. Dynamic culture leadership: Effective leader as both scientist and artist. Global Business and Technology Association International Conference. In N. Delener, C. Chao (eds.). *Beyond Boundaries: Challenges of Leadership, Innovation, Integration and Technology.* 694–740; 2002.

6. Schein EH. *The Corporate Culture Survival Guide: Sense and Nonsense About Culture Change.* San Francisco, CA: Jossey-Bass; 1999.

7. Folger JP, Poole MS, Stutman RK. *Working Through Conflict: Strategies for Relationships, Groups, and Organizations,* (3rd ed.). New York: Longman; 1997.

8. Burton J. *Conflict: Resolution and Prevention.* New York: St. Martin's Press; 1990.

9. Cahn D. (ed.). *Intimates in Conflict: A Communication Perspective.* Hillsdale NJ: Lawrence Erlbaum; 1990.

10. Canary DJ, Cupach WR, Messman SJ. *Relationship Conflict.* New York: Sage; 1995.

11. Cupach WR, Canary DJ. *Competence in Interpersonal Conflict.* New York: McGraw-Hill; 1997.

12. Hocker JL, Wilmot WW. *Interpersonal Conflict.* (4th ed.). Madison, WI: WCB Brown & Benchmark; 1995.

13. Note: This is an aggregation of multiple scholars' work as referenced in endnotes 5–10 above and a modification of the leadership studies at Ohio State and Michigan University accredited to Stogdill and Likert; as for the leadership component, "Concern for Task" was substituted with "Concern for Others."

14. Fisher R, Ury W, Patton B. *Getting to Yes: Negotiating Agreement Without Giving In* (2nd ed.). New York: Penguin Books; 1991.

15. Yukl G. *Leadership in Organizations* (3rd ed.). Englewood Cliffs, NJ: Prentice Hall; 1994.

16. Beebe SA, Masterson JT. *Communicating in Small Groups: Principles and Practices* (5th ed.). New York: Addison-Wesley Educational Publishers Inc.; 1997.

17. O'Hair D, Friedrich GW, Wiemann JM, Wiemann MO. *Competent Communication* (2nd ed.). New York: St. Martin's Press; 1997.
18. Schein EH. *The Corporate Culture Survival Guide: Sense and Nonsense About Culture Change*. San Francisco, CA: Jossey-Bass; 1999.
19. Yukl G. *Leadership in Organizations* (3rd ed.). Englewood Cliffs, NJ: Prentice Hall, 191–218; 1994.

CHAPTER

10

Leadership Theory and Influence

Gerald R. Ledlow and M. Nicholas Coppola

Learning Objectives

- Discuss and explain the foundations of leadership theory as theory and models are developed and evolve.
- Discuss and compare different leadership perspectives and theories.
- Develop a personal leadership definition.
- Describe how individuals are motivated to perform effectively and develop motivational plans with which to lead people.
- List and define factors or components of leadership and how those factors contribute to leadership.
- Describe behaviors, actions and processes that foster quality leadership of individuals and groups.

■ INTRODUCTION

This chapter provides an overview of the complex and exciting topic of leadership. Within the study of graduate education, business practice, and organizational analysis, there is no topic more important than the study of leadership. The study of leadership is a relatively recent niche within the realm of organizational behavior and analysis; however, fewer topics promote more interest and have more stakeholder consequences. Furthermore, no great leaders of our time have become successful and prosperous without first understanding the principles of leadership; this applies to both famous and infamous leaders. Some leaders are born with charismatic and instinctive leadership skills. However, all great leaders must devote time, energy, and study to various aspects of leadership in order to master the discipline while mastering competencies in situational assessment, motivation, communication, and understanding dynamic group behavior. Whatever the case, students of leadership should consider this discipline one of the more important aspects of personal and professional education.

This text emphasizes leadership in organizations by contributing two chapters for study: (1) Leadership Theory and Influence and (2) Leadership and Transformation. The chapter, Leadership Theory and Influence, is presented first, followed by the next chapter, Leadership and Transformation. These chapters focus on the essentials of leadership, noting that not all theories can be presented in two chapters, and bring many theories together from a wide range of disciplines.

Why is leadership important to the study of healthcare?

History has recorded leaders' exploits for thousands of years. Anthropology, archeology, social anthropology, political science, business, communication, health administration, and other disciplines have contributed to the foundations of leadership theory and practice. Many studies of great leaders and leadership have been centered on the United States or "Western" based models. However, as we have begun to enter a more global community without barriers and walls, more effort has been focused on international applications of leadership. This "globalism" of leadership study and practice has forced the study of leadership to look outside traditional boundaries for better ways to train, teach, and evaluate leaders.

Regardless of cultural identity, all healthcare executives lead people and manage resources. This involves focusing the collective energy of both managing people and resources toward meeting the needs of the external environment (that is, focusing on the mission of the organization).

It is important for leaders to understand that the individuals that make up this human resource component are comprised of people with vastly different education, training, and experience. These same individuals also have vastly different roles within the organization—and no leader can understand the complexity of all aspects of jobs within the system. As a result, a good leader's job is to successfully motivate individuals within the organization toward goal-directed behavior that supports the leader's vision and the organization's mission. Finally, the last important job of leaders is the management of non-human resources in the system. The role of a healthcare administrator, healthcare executive, or healthcare manager is to merge the complexity of leading people and the complexity of managing resources into a culture that serves communities by maintaining and improving the health of individuals in those communities. This is done by influencing the people and resources under their stewardship to serve those individuals that come to healthcare organizations for assistance, to build strong and effective relationships with their communities, and, especially, to build working relationships with the public health infrastructure in their communities. Learning about the various descriptive theories in this chapter will assist the burgeoning student of leadership in assessing his or her own personal penchants for managing human and non-human resources.

■ DEFINING LEADERSHIP

Conservative leadership scholars, who embrace the empiricists' view, suggest that the understanding of leadership is founded in traditional research methods. In this view, concepts of leadership may be discerned through the development of testable hypotheses and the operationalization of demonstrable unit variables derived from latent constructs. Liberal leadership enthusiasts advocate that leadership is an art and, like beauty itself, may lie in the eye of the beholder. Compounding this debate is the fact that framing leadership is not culture free. Techniques and activities developed in one society may need to be altered in order to be effective in another. For example, American society recognizes leadership regardless of age or gender. However, Asian and Middle Eastern societies place heavy emphasis on gender and age as precursors to leader recognition.

Regardless of art or science, the discussion of leadership is ancient. Researchers can find numerous scriptural writings predating modern times that describe the exploits and qualities of leaders. Much of this early spiritual teaching suggested great leaders should be beneficent and altruistic. However, a millennium and a half later in 1530, Machiavelli suggested one of the qualities of a good leader was to be malevolent and feared. Since these times, there have been as many methods to define leadership as there are ways to measure the phenomenon. Leadership is (perhaps) one of the most widely debated and broadly defined domains within the realm of organization behavior. For example, when the famed American Indian and Cavalry fighter Geronimo was asked what made him a good leader, he replied, "The ability to ride a strong horse."[1]

The lack of a clear and accepted definition and model of leadership theory is a fundamental challenge within the literature. For example, the definition of leadership in Webster's dictionary is somewhat tautological. The first two entries state that, "leadership is the position of office of the leader," and/or "leadership is the capacity or ability to lead." Further review of the term "leader" in Webster's dictionary is similarly tautological with definitions stating a leader is "one who leads." With such a nebulous definition on which to base research, it is no wonder that researcher's continue to debate on various models and methods to study leadership.

Strong partisan opinions on differentiating the study of leadership from other disciplines have occupied volumes of text and decades of debate within the literature. For example, a review of searchable databases onsite at the Library of Congress in Washington, DC, employing a series of partially overlapping searches using the words leader, leadership, manager, executive, supervisor, and director covering printed material from 1945–2005 suggested the common media (comprising television, radio, and newspapers) has popularized the term "leader" making these words synonyms with other descriptive terms in the English language. For example, the discussion of leadership and leaders has transcended traditional boundaries and is often used to describe phenomena associated with celebrities, pop culture icons, inspirational personnel, and sports figures, to name a few. Despite well-respected literature that distinctly separates leadership from other descriptive identifiers, leadership continues to be used to describe a plethora of activity in society.

Regardless of definition, due to this metastasized creep in cultural application through the decades, the terms leader and leadership have dominated fashionable connotations associated with non-equivalent positions resulting in a popularly accepted hierarchy. Being a leader is better than being a manager, supervisor, or subject matter expert. Being designated a leader rather than a manager (or something else) results in an artificial perception of status, which translates to a "feel good" perception for the individual. Perhaps this is in part associated with the competition associated with competing for the best employees—as well as other cultural challenges. For example, a review of want ads in several professional organizations lists few vacancies for industry managers; however, the want ads do list several positions for industry leaders. This ongoing debate on the differentiation of management versus leadership continues to occupy a great deal of the literature. However, large and respected organizations such as the American College of Healthcare Executives and a majority of the Masters of Business Administration schools clearly separate the two disciplines.[2] Management enthusiasts may recognize the war has long since been lost and that management represents a cluster of variables under the umbrella of leadership theory.

As stated earlier, within the referred literature, leadership is said to be as much an art as a science.[3] Furthermore, the study of leadership suggests that no one model guides the process of leadership study. As a result, the study of leadership has focused on distinct niches and amorphous constructs rather than any one general model. This different approach to leadership theory sets it apart from the study of other disciplines such as the study of vertebrate evolution or astronomy. Both these disciplines have popularly accepted theories that help explain phenomena. The study of leadership is quite different and still vehemently debated among organization behavior scholars. With so many available and partisan positions on leadership, it is easy to understand why there continues to be vehement debate on defining, testing, framing, and understanding the concept of leadership. As for an overarching definition, leadership is best described as the *ability to assess, develop, maintain, and change the organizational culture to optimally meet the needs and expectations of the external environment.* Needless to say, there are many components, elements, behaviors, knowledge, skills, and abilities that a leader needs to master to meet the expectations of this definition. The following sections build on the foundation of leadership and influence in the hope that the definition of leadership written above becomes salient.

■ A CHRONOLOGICAL REVIEW OF LEADERSHIP THEORY

1840–1880

The Great Man Theories
The urge to study leadership as a scientific property of human behavior is a relatively modern discipline. Machiavelli may have written one of the first recognized treatises on leadership in 1530; however, the first relevant scientific theories were not posited until the mid-1800s. From approximately 1840 to 1880, great man theorists Carlyle, Galton, and James studied great men from history who exhibited certain behavior characteristics and had documented successful outcomes, such as prosperity, political standing, or affluence. Based on the study of these characteristics the authors suggested that in order to be a good leader, one would have to emulate the characteristics of these men. Such characteristics often also centered on an individual's race and gender. Not surprisingly, many of the great men from the early chronicles were Anglican, male, and Caucasian.

Some authors combine great man and trait theories into a common field of study, while others do not. In the early study of great man theories, an inordinate amount of weight was placed on certain immutable variables such as gender, race, height, and oration. Mutable variables, such as social class, education, and religion, also has factored heavily into the early great man theories. As the study of historical figures evolved, scholars began to exam commonalities among great historical figures and developed a finite list of traits. The primary focus on traits eventually evolved into a distinct discipline called, "trait theory." This niche concept suggested that leaders are defined by various characteristics, such as intelligence, extraversion, experience, education, confidence, and initiative. It was said that possession of these traits distinguished a leader from a follower in early trait-based theories.

1938

Trait Theory

The re-emphasis on traits was solidified as an acceptable practice in 1938 and 1939 when authors Lewin, Lippitt, and White's research became the benchmark studies of their time.[4,5] These scholars studied the leadership styles of two groups of 10 and 11 year-olds in mask-making clubs. During the experiment, they noted that the two groups demonstrated two distinct behavior types—authoritarian or democratic. The study led to the subsequent examination of the impacts on production, group tension, cooperation, and feelings of "we'ness" versus "I'ness." These early studies have become some of the more often cited and highly quoted leadership and social psychology studies of the modern era. Accordingly, much of the modern research in leadership theory today may trace its roots back to these earlier studies. Unfortunately, the failure of the theory to attribute any single trait, or set of traits, that could systematically explain leadership success across various situations promoted a paradigm shift in leadership study to analyze the effects of situations on leader behavior.

1950

Postmodern Trait Phase

As the original study of trait-based theories developed, some have characterized the phenomena as the postmodern trait-based phase. The postmodern trait phase of leadership suggests that the study of leadership can be evaluated based on certain successful and admired personality and social traits. The underlying assumption is that some people have traits and skills that make them more likely to seek and attain leadership positions. In the first half of the 20th century, over 100 studies sought to find causal influence from traits such as intelligence, personal adjustment, originality, enthusiasm, and persistence (among others) to successful outcomes. However, a major limitation is that traits associated with one leadership situation may not predict leadership ability or outcome in another situation. Stogdill conducted several reviews of research in the trait arena (Table 10-1). He concluded that recognition of the relevance of leader traits is not a return to the original trait approach (more system oriented/interrelated research today).[6] The trait theory of leadership eventually evolved into the study of leadership behaviors.

Late 1950s

Theory X and Theory Y[6]

Between the trait and the behavior phase of leadership research, the concept of Theory X and Theory Y emerged. In the late 1950s, McGregor hy-

Table 10-1 Stogdill's Successful Leader Traits and Skills

Traits	Skills
Adaptable to situations	Clever (intelligent)
Alert to social environment	Conceptually skilled
Ambitious and achievement oriented	Creative
Assertive	Diplomatic & tactful
Cooperative	Fluent in speaking
Decisive	Knowledgeable about group tasks
Dependable	Organized
Dominant	Persuasive
Energetic	Socially skilled
Persistent	
Self-confident	
Willing to assume responsibility	
Tolerant of stress	

Yukl G. (1994). *Leadership in Organizations* (3rd ed.)., Englewood Cliffs, NJ: Prentice Hall.

pothesized that leaders generally hold one of two contrasting sets of assumptions about people. He additionally suggested that these two dichotomous sets of assumptions would influence leadership behavior. For example, if managers/leaders assumed that their followers were lazy, indifferent, and uncooperative, then they would be treated accordingly. Conversely, if they viewed their subordinates as energetic, bright, and friendly, they would treat them quite differently. These leadership attitudes toward followers would soon condition the leader to behave in a certain manner. In essence, this theory exemplifies a self-fulfilling prophecy.

Those who hold Theory X assumptions would be autocratic and those who hold Theory Y assumptions would be democratic. A Theory X leader would view a subordinate who was late as irresponsible and would require stricter control, while a Theory Y leader might speculate that this same subordinate may find his or her job boring and may need additional opportunities to stimulate them and improve performance (and behavior). The real contribution of McGregor's work was the suggestion that a manager/leader influenced a leadership situation by these two dichotomous assumptions about people.[7]

- Theory X: People are lazy, extrinsically motivated, incapable of self-discipline, and want security and no responsibility in their jobs.
- Theory Y: People, who do not inherently dislike work, are intrinsically motivated, exert self-control, and seek responsibility.

Theory Y leaders assess themselves (internal modifiers) in areas such as preferred leadership style, motives and limitations, past experiences, and external modifiers such as characteristics of the task, time constraints, organizational norms, structure and climate, past history with group, economic and legal limits, and degree of stability of the organization. Once the assessment is complete, the Theory Y leader chooses a leadership style (which does not mean they will not select an autocratic style depending on the situation). A Theory X leader has one leadership style, autocratic, and has a limited view of the world and does not consider internal and external modifiers.

■ LEADERSHIP PHASE EVOLUTION

Behavior Phase

All phases of leadership research build on each other and interweave into various models of leadership (see Table 10-2). The great man theories and the study of traits eventually evolved into a study of leadership behaviors. Behavior theory gained acceptance in the 1940s and grew substantially into the 1950s. The behavior research phase focused on what styles or behaviors leaders utilized, and how those styles contributed to subordinate satisfaction, performance, and quality. The behavior research first acknowledged that leadership and leading could be a learned skill. Recently, since the 1960s and 1970s, situational leadership (also known as contingency leadership) has gained favor. This research phase suggests that successful leaders must assess the situation and then choose the appropriate leadership style to make the greatest positive impact on subordinate effort.

1947

The Ohio State Leadership Studies[8]
In 1947 under the direction of Stogdill, the Ohio State leadership studies were conducted. The goal of these studies was to determine if there was a relationship between effective leader behavior and subordinates' satisfaction and performance. Two dimensions of leader behavior that emerged were consideration and initiating structure (see Table 10-3). The consid-

Table 10-2 Research Phase Time Line			
Great Man Phase (ca. 450 B.C.–1900)	Trait Phase (450 B.C.–1940s)	Behavior Phase (1940s–1970s)	Situational or Contingency Phase (Present)
Attempts to suggest that modeling the characteristics of successful leaders made one successful	Attempts to determine what specific traits make a person an effective leader	Attempts to determine what particular behaviors leaders utilize to cause others to follow them	Attempts to explain effective leadership within the context of the larger work situation

Table 10-3 Initiating Structure and Consideration

	Manager's Initiating Structure	
	High	**Low**
Manager's Consideration		
High	High performance Low grievance rate Low turnover	Low performance Low grievance rate Low turnover
Low	High performance High grievance rate High turnover	Low performance High grievance rate High turnover

eration structure focused on psychological closeness between the leader and followers while the initiating structure dealt with concern for actively directing subordinates toward job completion or goal attainment.

Surprisingly those who were marked high on both consideration and initiating structure were not always the most effective leaders. Further research along these lines indicated that both of these dimensions were needed for effective leadership. It was more important for a leader to strike a balance between what is appropriate for the situation rather than consistently displaying high consideration and high structure at all times. The following comments delineate the summary of conclusions of how effective leader behavior relates to follower satisfaction and performance:[9]

Consideration

1. Employee satisfaction with a leader is dependent on the degree of consideration displayed by the leader.
2. Leader consideration affects employee satisfaction more when jobs are unpleasant and stressful than when they are pleasant and have low stress.
3. A leader who is high on consideration can exercise more initiating structure without a decline in employee satisfaction.
4. Consideration given in response to good performance will increase the likelihood of future good performance.

Initiating Structure

1. Initiating structure by a leader that adds to role clarity will increase employee satisfaction.
2. Initiating structure by a leader will decrease employee satisfaction when structure is already adequate.

3. Initiating structure by a leader will increase performance when a task is unclear.

4. Initiating structure by a leader will not affect performance when a task is clear.

The major drawback to the Ohio State leadership studies was the limited consideration given to situational differences that may influence leader effectiveness. From this you can see the development of research (future studies) leaning toward situational leadership.

1950

University of Michigan Studies

Conducted around the same time as the Ohio State leadership studies, the University of Michigan leadership studies sought answers to many of the same research questions as their Ohio State colleagues. Not surprisingly, the Michigan study results were similar to those conducted at Ohio State, thus supporting some convergent validity assumptions. As with the Ohio State studies, the Michigan studies suggested grouping leaders into one of two classifications; employee orientated or production orientated. The research suggested that highly productive supervisors spent more time planning departmental work and in supervising their employees. The same supervisors spent less time working alongside and performing the same tasks as subordinates. They, the successful supervisors, accorded their subordinates more freedom in specific task performance and tended to be employee oriented. In contrast, the employee-focused leader focuses his or her time on forging relationships and in maintaining harmony in the work environment. This type of leader is less interested in written policies and formalized delegation of responsibilities.

1955

Skills Perspective

A less discussed and accepted model of leadership is Katz's 1955 skills perspective of leadership. Katz posited that effective leadership is based upon possessing and developing three core skills of technical, conceptual, and human abilities. Technical proficiencies are associated with the work required to transform inputs into outputs. Conceptual proficiencies relate to abstract ideas in the environment that have an effect on ongoing projects. For example, someone with high conceptual properties might be said to "get the big picture." Human proficiencies centered on the employees doing the work within the organization. Within this construct, high emphasis is placed on securing and maintaining relationships within the organization. Katz suggested that if a leader possessed all these skills, he or she would be a successful leader. The skills perspective of leadership is an evolutionary derivative of the early trait theories. While similar in many respects to trait theories, the skills perspective actually identified specific skills and suggested that leadership development and attainment were improbable outside the possession of all three suggested skill constructs.

1964

The Managerial Grid

In 1964, Blake and Mouton posited that a leader with high concern for people and a high concern for production are the best leaders.[6] The "high-high" leader facilitates more "team management" which is evident when the leader shares participation in goal setting, problem solving, and decision making. These "high-high" leaders modeled the behaviors by engaging fully in open confrontation and resolutions of differences, demonstrated initiative, explored fully into the background of problems and projects, engaged in constructive conflict-resolution behavior, made decisions, and engaged in the evaluation of work. This helps to produce quality performance. Much of this research has been accepted by the greater organizational industry at large and has been adopted into many organizational training programs. This theory also supported the proposition that leaders were being developed (behavior leadership phase theories) not just made (trait leadership phase theories). As a result of this

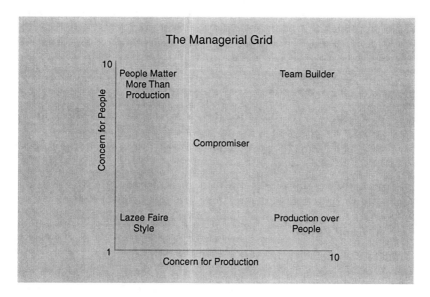

Figure 10-1 The Managerial Grid.

early work, researchers began to recognize that the context or situation played a major role in successful leadership (see Figure 10-1).

1964

Contingency Leadership Phase

Also developed in 1964, Fiedler's contingency model may be the first leadership theory to posit contingency relationships in the field of leadership. This model posits that the performance of groups is based on the interaction between the leader and situation favorableness. The fundamental leadership style ultimately is based on the least preferred co-worker (LPC).[10] The leader's style of managing personnel can then be geared toward micromanagement (structured) or autonomous management (unstructured). Additionally, this model evaluates the interaction between leader traits and situations. The basic premise of the model is that effectiveness is contingent on having a match between leader and follower styles.[10] Fiedler identified the degree of cooperation offered by followers (commitment), clarity of the group's task (structure), and the leader's formal authority to direct and reward followers (power). He referred to those factors collectively as the degree of situational control or favorableness on a preferred co-worker scale. The contingency model of leadership assumes that the style of a leader is fixed and that a leader cannot be sensitive to tasks and followers concurrently.

Fiedler argues that changing an individual's leadership style is difficult. He proposes that, instead, organizations should "engineer the job to fit the leader" or place individuals in situations that fit their style. A "backdoor" approach to situational leadership is offered here. Fiedler specifically identified three situational factors that are present in any situation where a task-oriented style, as opposed to relationship-oriented leadership, is more likely to be effective: (1) leader-member relations, (2) task structure, and (3) position power of the leader.[6]

- Leader-member relations: the extent to which the group trusts and respects the leader and is willing to follow his or her directions
- Task structure: the degree to which the task is clearly specified and defined or structured
- Position power: the extent to which the leader has official power, that is, the potential or actual ability to influence others due to their position in the organization (also known as legitimate power by French and Raven)

This theory defines leadership effectiveness in terms of work group performance. It postulates that work group performance is contingent upon the match between: (1) a person's leadership style, and (2) the "favorableness" of the leadership situation. In essence: Work Group Performance

= Leadership Style + Situational Favorableness. According to Fiedler, the term leadership style is a leader's manner of acting in a work situation, which depends upon his or her personality, and therefore is relatively fixed. Two key factors are important to understand in this theory or model of leadership:

- *Leadership style:* To determine a person's leadership style, Fiedler developed a measure called the least preferred co-worker (LPC) scale. This instrument describes the one person with whom he or she worked least well with among all the workers they have ever supervised.

- *Situational favorableness:* This refers to the degree a situation enables a person to exert influence over a work group. Three factors are used to measure this component: (1) Leader-member relations, which is the quality of the relationship between the leader and followers. (According to Fiedler, this is the most important determinant because it directly contributes to the influence the leader will have over his or her followers.) (2) Task structure is the degree to which a group's assignment can be spelled out in a step-by-step fashion; the higher the degree of task structure the more influence the leader will be given. (3) Position power is the authority to reward and punish followers, hire and promote them, and receive the backing in their decisions.

There are several important issues regarding Fielder's model of leadership: (1) Evidence suggests other situational variables, such as training and experience, contribute to leader effectiveness. (2) There is some doubt whether the LPC scale is a true measurement of leadership style; critics contend its interpretation is speculative and inadequately supported. Critics question the reliability of the measurement of leadership style and the range and appropriateness of the three situational components. The other significant element in situational leadership is organizational culture. Simply, culture is a group's unique view of the world. Every organization, from a family to a conglomerate, has an overriding organizational culture and various sets of sub-cultures. Leaders must attend to cultural issues to be successful.[11] Some researchers have suggested that leadership strategies in any setting have strong underlying similarities but must change as the setting changes over time. Even though the organization is essentially the same, change in the environment, such as continuous changes in healthcare organizations (regulations, technology, socio-economic, and demographic), may require leaders to change their strategy/style to be effective.

Because of this groundbreaking development in leadership research, a training program was developed in order for leaders to learn how to adapt their circumstances to fit their set leadership styles, but it was found to have questionable success.[12] However, the contingency model does not explain why leader-situation matches or mismatches occur.[13] To help bridge the gap-filled reality constructed by Fiedler, other theories contend the personalities of leaders are not as pertinent as the awareness of their leadership styles in addition to how they use their self-awareness or self-knowledge to adapt to situations, instead of attempting to change the situation to reflect their style.[13]

1971

House's Path-Goal Theory

Developed in 1971, House's path-goal model is based on expectancy motivation theory (that is, people are motivated by an expectation of a reward, in simple terms). In this theory, leaders make paths to goals as clear as possible based on the current situation, environment, and personnel surrounding and competing with the goal. The premise of the theory is that the leader will have a positive impact on the follower's motivation toward the goal. It is coined a path-goal approach because leader behavior is expressed in terms of a leader's influence in clarifying the paths followers travel toward work and personal goal attainment.[14] An important proposition of path-goal theory suggests that when task demands are unclear or ambiguous, decreased employee satisfaction and unlikely accomplishment of the goal happen.[15] To be effective, the leader must adapt behavior to the task at hand, subordinate's needs, and how his or her efforts will be perceived by subordinates.[16] Leadership training could then focus on matching the appropriate behavior to the situation, and leaders would know when to choose between leadership structure and follower consideration.

As Yukl suggests, this theory attempts to combine basic elements of Vroom's expectancy theory of motivation with a situational perspective.[6] According to the expectancy theory, motivation depends on a person's belief that effort will lead to performance, and that performance will lead to rewards that are valued. If any one of these three variables (expectancy, instrumentality, and valence) drops in value, then motivation decreases. The path-goal theory describes how leader behavior affects these expectancies. The leader's task contains two elements: (1) goal element—increase the number and kinds of rewards that the followers would receive for performance outcome (social exchange theory), and (2) path element—make the path easier by removing the obstacles that inhibit goal accomplishment.

The basic premise is that leader behavior and situational variables influence subordinate outcome. There are four types of leader behavior: (1) directive leadership (provides specific guidelines and "expectancies" to subordinates), (2) supportive leadership (friendly and approachable, demonstrating concern for the well-being and personal needs of subordinates), (3) achievement-oriented leadership (leaders who set challenging goals, expect best performances, and show confidence in subordinates' performance), and (4) participative leadership (leaders who consult with subordinates and elicit their suggestions before making a decision).

Situational variables play a major role in this theory such as: (1) subordinate characteristics (ability, need for self-esteem and self-actualization, and personality traits such as rigidity, authoritarianism, and closed-mindedness) and (2) task characteristics (ambiguous to non-ambiguous, simple versus difficult, stressful versus non-stressful, dull versus interesting, and safe versus dangerous). These variables, coupled with leader style, assist in work outcomes.

1973

Normative Decision Theory

Vroom-Yetton-Jago's normative decision-making model was originally developed in 1973 and subsequently modified in 1988.[17] The model assumes that no one decision-making model is appropriate. However, the theory postulates that there are two types of decision-making styles adopted by leaders: group decisions and individual decisions. These decisions are then defined based on personnel resources and the situation. Additionally, the normative decision theory proposed that the effectiveness of a leader's decision-making style is contingent on situational factors.[18] For example, the authors suggest that the effectiveness of a decision is a function of three classes of outcomes, each of which may be affected by the decision process used. These are the quality or rationality of the decision, the acceptance or commitment on the part of subordinates to execute the decision effectively, and the amount of time required to make the decision. The authors state that when the task is familiar and followers supportive, then it is appropriate for a leader to adopt an autocratic style. When the task is ambiguous, then the leader should use consultative strategies, and when follower support is in question, then the leader should use a participative strategy. The shortcoming of this theory is that it is mainly prescriptive and does not address what leaders actually do when faced with a particular situation. The theory is also limited to decision making and neglects other important leadership elements such as motivation and the development of followers. The normative decision theory provided a foundation for subsequent leadership theories, such as the situational leadership theory. Although updated since 1973, the model continues to be little empirical support for the model within the literature.

1975

Leader-Member Exchange Theory

Graen and Cashman posited the leader member exchange theory (LMX) in 1975.[19] This model suggests that leaders accomplish work through various personal relationships with different members of the group. Leaders give tasks that are more positive to members who they feel support them. LMX suggests behavior is not consistent across subordinates. As a result, leaders classify subordinates into two groups, an in-group and an out-group. Subsequently, the leader adapts to individual needs for direction, contact, and supervision on a follower basis. This creates a unique relationship with every different member of the group, called a "dyadic." Graen and Cashman later coined the term vertical dyad linkage (VDL), where leaders and members of each dyad form leader-group interactions, judgments, and opinions. The key with this theoretical model of leader behavior is that the emphasis is on the interaction of the leader with the supervised group. For example, the leader exchanges resources, such as increased job latitude, influence on decision making, and open communication, for members' commitment to higher involvement in organizational functioning. This research embraces the social exchange theory that suggests that leaders must offer an exchange (bonus, increased status, etc.) for improved or additional performance by subordinates. This approach has been criticized because it does not study the organizational outcomes associated with the exchange relationship and links exchanges in diverse and inconsistent ways. However, the obvious reality of many leaders treating employees differently based on personal relationships is a common reality in the workforce that merits additional attention.

1977

Situational Leadership Theory

From 1969 through 1977, Hersey and Blanchard developed the situational leadership theory.[20] Situational leadership theory (SLT) is defined as a leadership style driven by the situation at hand. This model specified the readiness of followers, defined as the ability and willingness to accomplish a specific task, as the major contingency that influences appropriate leadership style. Situational leadership theory is based on the relationship of three components: (1) directive behavior (task behavior) the leader provides followers; (2) the amount of supportive behavior (relational behavior) a leader provides; and (3) the development level (maturity) of the follower, which is derived from the amount of competence and commitment demonstrated while performing a specific task. Competence is the degree of knowledge or skills gained from education, training, and/or experience needed to do the task, and commitment is defined as the combination of confidence and motivation displayed by the follower to do the task. A follower can be competent but not committed to do a task, consequently needing support to regain the devotion to accomplish the task.

SLT also suggests that individual leadership style should be matched to the maturity of the subordinates.[21] Situational leadership theory demonstrates that there is no one best style of leadership. People in leadership and management positions become more effective when they use a leadership style that is appropriate to the development level of the individual or group they want to influence. Maturity is assessed in relation to a specific task, and the psychological maturity and job experience of the follower. The leader may then exercise various levels of delegating, participating, selling, and telling in completing assigned tasks and goals. Application of the correct leadership style based on the developmental level of the follower or group is the key ingredient in this model; however, sometimes there are situational variables that may affect the leadership style. Some situational variables are time constraints, supervisory demands, and job demands. Each style varies the leadership approach based on the aforementioned situational factors. Most recent leadership approaches include additional dimensions of leadership, whether or not the leader utilizes a transactional or transformational style.

While contingency and normative decision approaches are both types of situational theory, Hersey-Blanchard's approach is more centric as it depends on the amount of tasks and people that the leader adopts in reference to the level of subordinates' commitment and competence. The greater the subordinates' level of commitment and competence, the less the leader has to provide task-based and relation-based leadership. The situational leadership theory holds that successful leadership is achieved by selecting the correct leadership style depending upon the readiness of the followers.

1978

Transformational Leadership
Burns introduced the transformational leadership model into literature in 1978.[22] Transformational leadership is a process where leaders and followers raise one another to higher levels of motivation. This model borrows from earlier trait theories developed earlier in the decade. In the transformational model, the leader motivates followers through internal rewards. Leader motivation techniques include emphasis on personal charisma, individual attention to the follower and intellectual stimulation of the task. Transformational leaders motivate followers through appealing to strong emotions within the group.

Within the study of transformational leaders, Burns posited two types of leaders, transactional and transformational.[22] Transactional leadership attempts to preserve and adhere to existing work constraints, while transformational leadership seeks to upset and alter norms. Transactional leaders exchange rewards and promises for their team members' efforts. Transformational leaders are visionaries who seek to raise the level of consciousness in their followers and promote the goals of the organization, not individuals.

Burns has suggested that transactional leadership involves values, but they are values relevant to the exchange process. These values include honesty, fairness, responsibility, and reciprocity. Furthermore, the theory suggests that bureaucratic organizations enforce the use of legitimate power and respect for rules and tradition rather than influence based on inspiration. For Burns, leadership is a process, not a set of discrete acts. Burns described leadership as "a stream of evolving interrelationships in which leaders are continuously evoking motivational responses from followers and modifying their behavior as they meet responsiveness or resistance, in a ceaseless process of flow and counterflow. At the macro level of analysis, transformational leadership involves shaping, expressing, and mediating conflict among groups of people in addition to motivating individuals."[6]

In 1985, Bass built on Burns' work and proposed a theory of transformational leadership that is measured primarily in terms of the leader's effect on followers.[6] Followers of a transformational leader feel:

- trust
- admiration
- loyalty
- respect

And they are motivated by the leader to do more than the original expectation:

- By making followers more aware of the importance of task outcomes
- By inducing them to transcend their own self-interest for the sake of the team
- By activating their higher-order needs

Bass's original theory included three behaviors of transformational leaders; the fourth was added later to transformational behaviors:

- **Charisma:** leader influences followers by arousing strong emotions and identification with the leader
- **Intellectual Stimulation:** leaders increase follower awareness of problems and influence followers' view as problems from a new perspective

- **Individualized Consideration:** providing support, encouragement, and developmental experiences for followers
- **Inspirational Motivation:** extent that the leader communicates an appealing vision using symbols to focus subordinate effort and model (role modeling; Bandera's social learning theory) appropriate behavior

Like Burns (1978), Bass viewed transactional leadership as an exchange of rewards for compliance; transactional behaviors are:[22]

- **Contingent Reward:** clarification of work required to obtain rewards
- **Active Management by Exception:** monitoring subordinates and corrective action to ensure that the work is effectively accomplished
- **Passive Management by Exception:** use of contingent punishments and other corrective action in response to obvious deviations from acceptable performance standards

■ CHAPTER SUMMARY

This chapter has presented a chronological overview of leadership and leadership theories as a manner to present information and ideas that have formed the foundation to modern leadership thought. The progression from great man, to trait, to behavior, to situational or contingency leadership theories has been presented. The theories of leadership presented here are the major works that have influenced the study of leadership for the past few decades. Unfortunately, not all leadership theories can be listed in this chapter. However, the key and seminal leadership theories presented here have formed the lineage and foundation to modern leadership study. Table 10-4 provides an overview of the theories presented and assists in understanding the niche-specific goals of each theoretical leadership theory.

In summary, the study of leadership is complex, interconnects with all aspects of organizational life, and is essential to the success of an organization. This chapter set the foundation of leadership study over the past century and establishes the basis for the next chapter, Leadership and Transformations. The importance of understanding the concept of "leading people and managing resources" is critical in that situational assessment, motivation, and communication are key skills of successful leaders. The following table serves as the chapter summary for the leadership models presented.

Table 10-4 Model Overview (illustrates the aforementioned models in a grid for visual inspection and comparison)

Theory	Goal	Antecedent Framework	Constructs	Variables	Relationship	Utility for Greater Understanding in the Fields
Carlyle, Galton, and James Great Man (early to mid 1840–1880)	Identify immutable traits of past leaders so that future leaders could be identified	Perhaps Machiavelli	Physical characteristics	Immutable physical characteristics	Possession of characteristics is leadership	Evolved into trait theory over time
Lewin, Lippitt, and White's Trait Theory (1938–1939)	Identify mutable traits of past leaders so that future leaders could be identified	Great man theory	Intelligence, extraversion, physical stature	Outcomes of intelligence, extraversion, physical stature	Those with "leadership" traits should be good leaders	Incorporated into broader leadership studies such as behavioral and situational theories
McGregor Theory X and Theory Y (1950)	Identify lazy and self-motivating personnel	Early trait theories	Laziness and motivation	Various	Laziness equals failure and motivation equals success	Suggests motivated leaders can achieve more than lazy leaders
Stodgill and Coons Ohio Leadership Studies (1950)	Identify individual dimensions of behavior	Early trait theories	Initiating structure and consideration	Work-related variables and satisfaction	Leaders who set high standards while respecting employees achieve high outcomes	Organization management design
Michigan Leadership Studies (1950)	Identified leader objectives associated with performance effectiveness	Early trait theories	Employee-oriented and production oriented	Satisfaction and goal attainment	Focus is on employee task performance	Task organization and employee workload

Table 10-4 Model Overview (illustrates the aforementioned models in a grid for visual inspection and comparison)

Theory	Goal	Antecedent Framework	Constructs	Variables	Relationship	Utility for Greater Understanding in the Fields
Katz's Skills Theory (1955)	Identify individual dimensions of behavior	Early trait theories	Technical, conceptual, and human abilities	Various traits and outcomes	Must have all three to be successful	Production outcomes
Blake and Mouton Managerial Grid (1964)	Focus is on attitudes	Early trait theories, motivation, and management	Concern for results and concerns for people	Satisfaction, outcomes, and productivity	Those with both high centers for people and results are most effective	Team building and consensus making
Fiedler's Contingency Model (1964)	Discern variables affecting group performance	Motivation and management	Situation favorableness-preferred co-worker scale	Task and relationship orientation	The more favorable the relationship (or perceived relationship) between the leader and follower, the higher degree of task orientation is accomplished	Psychology, management teams
House's Path Goal Model (1971)	Predict leadership effectiveness based on communication of leader intent; expectancy motivation theory	Earlier works in expectancy, motivation, and satisfaction; Vroom's expectancy theory	Perception of: work, self-development and path to goals; communications: directive, supportive, participative, and achievement	Rewards, goals, accomplishment, personal characteristics, environment	Leader behavior; will be motivational to the extent it assists subordinates to accomplish assigned goals	Management communication

(continues)

Table 10-4 Model Overview (illustrates the aforementioned models in a grid for visual inspection and comparison) (continued)

Theory	Goal	Antecedent Framework	Constructs	Variables	Relationship	Utility for Greater Understanding in the Fields
Vroom-Yetton-Jago's Normative Decision Making (1973)	Model assumes that no one decision-making model is appropriate	Earlier works	Quality or rationality of the decision, the acceptance or commitment on the part of subordinates to execute the decision effectively, and the amount of time required to make the decision	Various	Better decision making achieved through balancing construct dimensions	Decision making
Graen's Leader-Member Exchange and Vertical Dyad Linkage (1975)	Tasks are accomplished based on personal relationships	Katz and Kahn (1966) motivation, equity, and organizational citizenship behavior	Vertical dyad linkage	In-group and out-group	Satisfaction will be higher with the in-group leading toward goal attainment	Motivation, satisfaction, delegation

Table 10-4 Model Overview (illustrates the aforementioned models in a grid for visual inspection and comparison)

Theory	Goal	Antecedent Framework	Constructs	Variables	Relationship	Utility for Greater Understanding in the Fields
Hersey-Blanchard's Situational Leadership (SLT) (1977)	The four leader choices are to tell, sell, participate, or delegate	Graen's (1975) LMX and VDL and other antecedent theories	Directive behavior, supportive behavior, development level	Structure variables of time, supervisory, and job demands	Optimizing four leadership choices to environment constraints maximizes outcomes	Delegation and decision making
Burns Transformational Leadership (1978)	Leaders and followers raise one another to higher levels of motivation	Max Weber's charismatic leadership (1947)	Charisma, intellectual stimulation, environment	Rewards	Followers of a transformational leader feel: • trust • admiration • loyalty • respect	Motivation and satisfaction

Review/Discussion Questions

1. What traits, behaviors, and situational factors can you list of a leader you admire, and what makes you admire them?
2. How would you define leadership, and what would your leadership model look like?
3. What three critical factors would make you a good leader and why?
4. What does it mean to "Lead People and Manage Resources" within the healthcare organization context?
5. Why do you want to be a leader and what is your "vision" of leadership?
6. Explain the progression of leadership theories and models through time and how models are "built" upon each other?
7. Are the models presented descriptive or prescriptive? Explain.
8. To serve as the case study discussion question, without using names, what person in your experience was a great leader and who was a poor leader? What attributes of leadership were most profound in both cases and what context did you observe in those leaders?

References

1. Wintle J. The Dictionary of War Quotations. New York: Free Press; 1989.
2. Aldag R, Buck J. The New York Times Pocket MBA Series: Leadership & Vision. *The New York Times*, Mighty Words, Inc. and the American College of Health Care Executives. Directory of search firms, Vol. 16; 2001.
3. Hughes RL, Ginnett RC, Curphy GJ. *Leadership—Enhancing the Lessons of Experience* (3rd ed.). New York: Irwin/McGraw Hill; 1999.
4. Lewin K, Lippitt R. An experimental approach to the study of autocracy and democracy: A preliminary note. *Sociometry*. 1938;1:292–300.
5. Lewin K, Lippitt R, White R. Patterns of aggressive behavior in experimentally created social climates. *J Soc Psychol*. 1939;10:271–301.
6. Yukl G. *Leadership in Organizations* (3rd ed.). Englewood Cliffs, NJ: Prentice Hall; 1994.
7. Bedeian AG. *Management, Effective Leadership*. New York: Dryden Press; 1986.
8. Gordon J. *A Diagnostic Approach to Organizational Behavior* (3rd ed.). Englewood Cliffs, NJ: Prentice Hall; 1991.
9. Filley AC. *The Complete Manager.* Champaign, IL: Research Press, 57–60; 1978.
10. Fiedler FE. *A Theory of Leadership Effectiveness.* New York: McGraw-Hill; 1967.
11. Schein EH. *The Corporate Culture Survival Guide: Sense and Nonsense About Culture Change.* San Francisco, CA: Jossey-Bass; 1999.
12. Jago AG. Leadership: Perspectives in theory and research. *Manage Sci.* 1982;28:315–336.
13. Northouse PG. *Leadership Theory and Practice.* Thousand Oaks, CA: Sage Publications; 2001.
14. Mawhinney TC, Ford JD. The path goal theory of leader effectiveness: An operant Interpretation. *Acad Manage Rev.* 1977;2:398–411.

15. Greene CN. Questions of causation in the path-goal theory of leadership. *Acad Manage J*. 1979;22:22–41.
16. Schriesheim C, Glinow M. The path-goal theory of leadership: A theoretical and empirical analysis. *Acad Manage J*. 1977;20:398–405.
17. Vroom VP, Jago A. *The New Leadership: Managing Participation in Organizations*. Englewood Cliffs, NJ: Pretence Hall; 1988.
18. Vroom VH, Yetton PW. *Leadership and Decision-Making*. Pittsburgh, PA: University of Pittsburgh Press; 1973.
19. Graen GB, Cashman JF. A role making model in formal organizations: A developmental approach. In JG Hunt, LL Larson (eds.). *Leadership Frontiers*. Kent, OH: Kent State University Press, 143–165; 1975.
20. Hersey P, Blanchard K. (1969). *Management of Organizational Behavior: Utilizing Human Resources*. Englewood Cliffs, NJ: Prentice-Hall; 1969.
21. Hersey P, Blanchard K. *Management of Organizational Behavior: Utilizing Human Resources* (2nd ed.). Englewood Cliffs, NJ: Prentice-Hall; 1977.
22. Burns J. *Leadership*. New York: Harper Row; 1978.

11

Leadership and Transformation

Gerald R. Ledlow, M. Nicholas Coppola, and Mark A. Cwiek

Learning Objectives

- Discuss the process of leadership based on the models presented in this chapter.
- Explain and list factors where leaders influence organizational culture.
- Describe, compare, and contrast organizational culture from organizational leadership, based on the definition of leadership from the previous chapter.
- Describe the strategies and discuss the applications of the dynamic culture leadership model.
- Describe the strategies and discuss the applications of the omnibus leadership model.

■ INTRODUCTION

As we learned in the previous chapter, leadership is a complex field of study. Mature and experienced leaders acknowledge having to adjust their personal leadership style based on the organization that they work in, the types of employees they are leading, and who is available for the tasks that need to be performed. Practiced leaders often will conduct a 360-degree self-assessment of their personal leadership ability once every 2 or 3 years and make adjustments to their behaviors, foci, and training. Some leaders may find they have slowly allowed themselves a dictating rather than delegating mode of leadership, and be unaware that decisiveness on their part can be interpreted at times as an uncaring attitude. Other leaders may find that a desire to be consensus-driven and collaborative has crept into a pattern of protracted group discussions and decision-making avoidance. Change creates the necessity to master ambiguous situations and to provide structure and meaning to complex organizations. This requires continuous leadership growth and development for those that lead in dynamic organizations. Thus, the dynamic culture leadership model prescribes a sequence of leadership-based activities and processes essential to steer the organization well. Lastly, some leaders may have become so comfortable with their "inner circles" of senior level vice presidents and department heads that the collective wisdom of the group is no longer heard or encouraged. In this regard, the charismatic qualities that may have led the CEO to his or her position of eminence may not be relative to maintaining effectiveness in the long run.

This chapter presents several aids for both students of leadership and mature practitioners of the art and science of leadership to learn from. In this chapter, we present two evolving models of leadership that should assist young leaders in honing their personal leadership practice. The expectation is that these models will invoke thought, reflection, and discussion. These models are the dynamic culture leadership model and the omnibus leadership model. Both of these models are prescriptive in that they provide a strategy for success and a model for implementation. Also, this chapter presents a list of recommended leadership measurement tools to conduct personal and organizational evaluations.

■ PRESCRIPTION ONE: THE DYNAMIC CULTURE LEADERSHIP MODEL

Superb leadership is required at all levels of the healthcare organization, due to the increasingly dynamic nature of the healthcare environment. This reality was the catalyst for the development of the dynamic culture leadership (DCL) model, a model that is still in development. Leadership in this model is recognized at three levels as the critical ingredient in the recipe for overall business success: at the personal level, at the team level, and certainly at the organizational level. The challenge is to focus the knowledge and skills of organizational leaders and to empower the total organization to complete its mission, to reach its vision, and to compete successfully in an environment that constantly changes. The DCL model is presented here in overview form and is intended to fit within the transformational leadership paradigm.

The dynamic culture leadership model provides both a descriptive and high-level prescriptive process model of leadership.[1] The model emphasizes a sense of balance that needs to be maintained in order to achieve a sustainable and continuing level of *optimized* leadership. "Optimized leadership," like the concept "high quality," is not necessarily a norm to be achieved at all times. Rather, it is a worthy goal, an ideal state. No individual (and certainly no organization) can in all situations and at all times enjoy a steady state of higher-level leadership. There are, however, many individuals—and organizations—that continuously optimize their ability to function at high leadership levels by consciously (and even unconsciously) cultivating the various elements of the model.

Optimized leadership is certainly attainable for any person and any organization, but it usually requires concentrated effort to overcome past habits, ideas, and tendencies. Ultimately, *individual* leaders comprise a leadership team. The team, therefore, must be diverse in style and competencies while being anchored to a set of values and operating principles of the organization. The assessment instrument for individuals and teams for this model is based on a leadership-management continuum and an art-science continuum.

The following table describes the characteristics of "leadership" as compared to "management," and "science" as compared to "art." It is important to note that organizations need leaders, managers, scientists, and artists working together to achieve success over the long term. Figure 11-1 illustrates the macro descriptive model while Figure 11-2 shows the prescription (or processes) associated with the model.

Table 11-1 shows the differences in *leadership* versus *management*. Table 11-2 shows the differences in *science* versus *art*. It is important to keep in mind that organizations need a leadership as well as a management mentality/capabilities, as well as a science and an art mentality/capabilities, in order to survive and thrive in its external environment.

Table 11-1 Explanation of the Leadership-Management Continuum (DCL)	
Leadership	**Management**
Longer time horizon	Shorter time horizon
Vision then mission oriented	Mission oriented
Organizational validity (Are we doing the right things?)—environmental scanning and intuition	Organizational reliability (Are we doing things correctly and consistently?) Compliance to rules and policies and rule development
Does the organization have the correct components (people, resources, expertise) to meet future as well as current needs?	How can current components work best now?
Developing and refining organizational culture to meet external environment needs	Maintaining organizational climate to ensure performance
Timing and tempo of initiatives and projects	Scheduling of initiatives and projects

Table provided by New Visions Network, LLC, © 2007, all rights reserved.

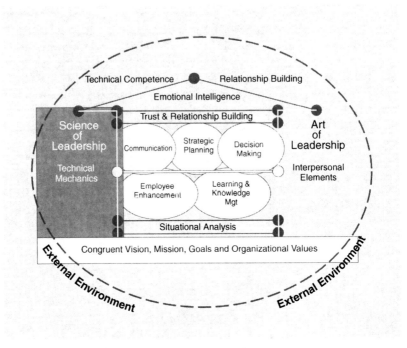

Figure 11-1 The Dynamic Culture Leadership (DCL) Model.

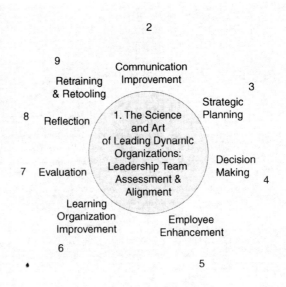

Figure 11-2 The Leadership Process (DCL) Model.

Table 11-2 Explanation of the Science-Art Continuum (DCL)

Science	Art
Technical skills orientation— forecasting, budgeting, etc. . . .	Relationship oriented—networking, interpersonal relationships
Decisions based more on analysis	Decisions based more on perceptions of people
Developing systems— important to organizations	Developing relationships and networks— important to organizations
Expert systems	Experts as people
Cost control and evaluation of value important	Image and customer relationships important

Table provided by New Visions Network, LLC, © 2007, all rights reserved

The dynamic culture leader model entails a leadership process, as shown in Figure 11-2, emphasizing leadership team assessment, communication improvement, strategic planning, decision-making alignment, employee enhancement, and learning organization improvement. Leaders who follow the sequence shown in Figure 11-2 on a regular cycle have the best potential to deal with change in their environment, while building a culture that is effective even during times of change. Figure 11-3 illustrates the leadership team assessment (this is Step 1 as shown in Figure 11-2) for ten members of a hospital leadership team as it compares to the current operational environment and the demands of the external environment. As shown, there is a tension between what the leadership team tends to be (more *leadership* oriented with a reasonable *science* and *art* balance) versus a more *management* and *science* emphasis of leadership demanded by the external environment; the operating environment can be found within that tension. The external environment requirements, as perceived by the leadership team, are skewed toward *management* and *science* (the analytical manager quadrant). The perception of leadership would lead one to believe that the external environment requires greater cost control, accountability, and adherence to policies and rules, although relationships are still important, as is some leadership focus.

Assessing an organization's leadership team is essential. Aligning the team to bring diversity of style, skills, experience, and abilities is essential for organizations to maintain a robust, resilient, and even opportunistic, personality. In this model and assessment, cultural and individual diversity is valued so as to better respond to dynamic organizational and external environments. Diversity of focus and organizational goals are not advantageous; a diverse leadership team brings robustness to solving organizational problems as long as focus on the vision, mission, and goals are similar across the leadership team. An assessment that looks at leadership as a team, across organizational levels, operating environments, and external environment needs, is far better than simply relying on only individual leader assessments.[2]

Figure 11-3 shows the results of a leadership team-style assessment, including operating style and external environment expectations. Note that there is a considerable disconnect between leadership style and external environment requirements. The organizational operating style is *balanced* whereas the leadership style composite is *analytical leader* (skewed toward *science* and *leadership*) and the external environment is *analytical manager* (skewed toward *science* and *management*). This is hypothesized to represent a leadership coping strategy. Aligning additional leadership team members to bring in more *management* and *science* oriented members may be an appropriate strategy. Alternatives to adding team members would be to "buy" or have consultations with those that add *management* and *science* abilities to the organization. However, this can cause a problem in the long term since institutional knowledge could be more easily lost. When leadership style by organizational level is compared, there is much more propensity for *leadership* than *management,* as one looks down the organizational hierarchy, than an organization may be able to tolerate over the long term. In essence, it is important to understand and know the leadership team's style and "personality" as it compares to operating style (how business gets done), as well as the expectations of the external environment.

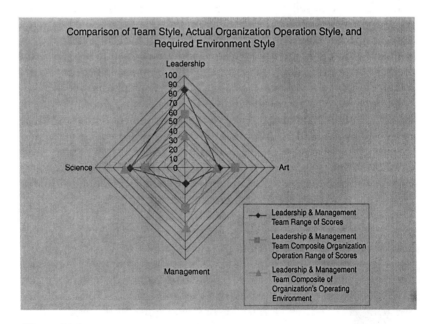

Figure 11-3 Omnibus Leadership Model.

Leaders are gifted in different ways, with different personalities and varying skill sets. All leaders can grow, become more balanced, and achieve greater effectiveness. There are common factors found in those who succeed in becoming dynamic culture leaders, including the desire to learn more about themselves, the motivation to learn and practice new skill sets, and the need to grow and become more tomorrow than what they are today. This is not the easiest path to be taken, but it is the path that optimizes the likelihood of leadership effectiveness and success.

Organizations are more dynamic today than ever before. With the advent of the information age, the fluidity of professional and family life, and the competitive nature of the global marketplace, there exists today more of an entrepreneurial environment in organizations. "Entrepreneurial organizations reflect a different set of underlying assumptions principally because they shift the focus away from producing specific, predetermined behavior by means of direction and formal controls. Instead, they encourage coordination through the shared understanding that will enable individuals to choose effective actions themselves. Organization structure and control systems can no longer be depicted as tools that mechanically determine members' behaviors. We, too, must shift our thinking about organizations away from the organization as an entity, to members' choice and understanding."[3] Leaders in this environment cannot rest on the laurels of "cookie-cutter" methods, but must learn and become effective in developing teams of professionals within dynamic cultures. If one questions the reality of the dynamic nature of organizations today, one need simply consider the realities of human diversity, information overload, the evolution of technology, the sophistication of the consumer, and e-commerce.

Leaders need to have a firm grasp of how to develop an organizational culture that creates a thriving environment for their organization. Schein in 1999 defined "culture" as the basic assumptions and beliefs shared by members of a group or organization.[4] "A major function of culture is to help us understand the environment and determine how to respond to it, thereby reducing anxiety, uncertainty, and confusion."[5] The key question becomes "how do leaders shape culture?" Schein suggests that leaders have the greatest potential for embedding and reinforcing aspects of culture with the following five primary mechanisms:[6]

- **Attention:** leaders communicate their priorities, values, and concerns by their choice of things to ask about, measure, comment on, praise, and criticize.
- **Reaction to Crisis:** increases potential for learning about values and assumptions.
- **Role Modeling**
- **Allocation of Resources**

- **Criteria for Selection and Dismissal:** leaders can influence culture by recruiting people who have particular values, skills, traits, and by promoting them . . . likewise for firing them.

Schein also described five secondary mechanisms:[6]

- **Design of Organizational Structure:** centralized structure reflects that only the leader can determine what is important; decentralized structure reinforces individual initiative and sharing.
- **Design of Systems and Procedures:** where emphasis is placed shows concern and ambiguity reduction issues.
- **Design of Facilities**
- **Stories, Legends, and Myths**
- **Formal Statements**

It is imperative that healthcare leaders understand the factors that influence culture. Culture is more stable and harder to change than "climate," since climate usually is not stable over time. Whether employees are "happy" today (a climate indicator) is only of temporal importance, while culture indicators (such as processes, incentive systems, communication environment, understanding of goals and how they fit into the work to attain goals), are much more meaningful and important.

The dynamic culture leadership model is a set of constructs with the goal of helping unify the various leadership theories that previously have received attention. Further, the DCL model can be studied immediately and utilized by leaders and organizational scholars intent on developing highly effective leadership. In their book *The Success Paradigm*, Mike Friesen and James Johnson discuss the importance of leadership in the integration of quality and strategy to achieve organizational success.[7]

In this book, leadership *process* was described as critical for success. The dynamic culture leadership model is presented as an application of theory to advance existing contingency leadership theories, and coupling all of this with a strategic process. This is therefore presented as a prescriptive model.

Today's complex, ever-changing organizations are experiencing a shortage in leadership effectiveness, not because of the lack of talent or good will, but because of the tremendous balancing act needed for success. This balance of *scientist* attributes and *artist* attributes defined in the dynamic culture leadership model provides the pathway for success. Experts (such as Friesen and Johnson, as well as the authors of this chapter) assert, *leadership* is the pivotal issue in success. The dynamic culture leadership model is intended to become central to the understanding of leadership in organizations and the people who lead them.

The DCL model, in its current state of development, is being tested in both theoretical and practical ways. It provides today a conceptual framework for the better understanding of complex organizations and as a model for advancing leader effectiveness. Further, tools for leadership assessment and direct application are being refined to advance the practical utility of the model in all organizational settings. In summary, the dynamic culture leadership model recommends:

- An assessment of the organization's leadership team and ultimately the development of a team that is diverse in terms of the *leadership, management, art,* and *science* attributes, all while securing itself in the values, beliefs, and mission of the organization.
- An organization's leadership should focus on communication improvement, strategic planning, decision-making alignment, employee enhancement, and learning organization improvement in a regular, cyclical sequence.
- The sequence should be repeated based on the tempo of change in the environment; rapid change creates a need to work through the sequence at a faster pace. It is estimated that in healthcare today, this sequence should be planned for every 3 to 4 years.

■ PRESCRIPTION TWO: THE OMNIBUS LEADERSHIP MODEL

In 1905, the world famous Carnegie Museum of Natural History placed the bones of a prized Apatosaurus on review. The bones remained on display until 1992, when a different team of paleontologists reexamined the fossil. They noticed that incorrect kinesiology had been displayed, and the wrong head had been placed on the dinosaur almost 90 years earlier.[8] However, during those years, hundreds, perhaps thousands of scholars and academics viewed the bones and admired the symmetry and perfection of the fossil—never noticing the 90-year-old error the original paleontologists had made. Is it possible that the study of leadership is likewise suffering from an ancient error in construction? Has the study of leadership become a calculus formula that has become memorized, but never derived? It has been suggested that there are as many methods to define leadership as there are ways to measure it. From a research perspective, this is often very beneficial, as the purpose of research is to look at things in increasing levels of complexity and with the ultimate goal of discerning intricate parts of the puzzle. Is it possible, however, that in the complex study of leadership theory the level of complexities are so intricate that the larger picture is no longer visible? A review of leadership theory suggests the possibility that the answer to this question is "yes."

Furthermore, is it possible that the study of leadership has suffered from *theory creep?* The original concept of *creep,* coined by Casper Weinberger, suggested that *creep* is the absence of a uniform vision, and that this condition results in constant change.[9] The end product of *creep* results in solving problems that have no relationship to the original project or process at all. In other words, the wrong fight is fought.

The study of leadership theory may have suffered from *theoretical creep*. A review of leadership theories in the 20th century suggests leadership studies have crept from the broad- and wide-ranging trait and great man theories to discriminate research efforts that reflect more of an application of unit models of decision making or satisfaction, rather than theory. Supporting this premise, some authors have suggested the problem with organizational theories is that the wrong unit of analysis is applied to inappropriate situations. Furthermore, many authors suggest previous studies may not be looking at leadership issues, but rather evaluating supervisory and interpersonal characteristics.[10–15]

Constructs of the Omnibus Leadership Model

Traditional models of leadership focus on outcomes and trace those outcomes back to specific leadership traits, characteristics, or behaviors, with little emphasis placed on the values associated with intrinsic goal-directed behavior. The "nature versus nurture" debate has long existed within the study of leadership. Are leaders born, or can they be made? The environment certainly plays a role in fostering goal-directed behavior, as do family values, available resources, and education (including both didactic and spiritual education). However, these constructs are often viewed as confounding variables rather than leadership progenitors in traditional leadership models. This is a weakness within traditional leadership study.

Furthermore, traditional leader theories fail to fully integrate the various aspects of confounding variables into one multi-faceted model that allows for a wider range and utility of leadership study. Specifically, constructs such as cultural distinctiveness, higher power influences, and environmental pressures are often disregarded as antecedent constructs for forecasting leader outcomes or explaining past leader behavior. However, these constructs are excellent theoretical examples for forecasting leader outcomes under appropriate conditions.

For example, in the current environment of the *War on Terror*, some leaders feel driven to goal-directed behavior through a higher power mandate. Separate from that which is considered religion or spirituality in its common understanding, a higher power is often classified as a greater belief in a mantra, or distinctive icon, which guides and directs leader behavior and followership in a predictable manner. Rarely however does the discussion of how higher powers impact on the values and goal-directed behavior of leaders take place. In fact, many leadership scholars completely ignore altogether the construct of a higher power influence when examining leadership. Some suggest it is politically incorrect to consider this, while others posit that it is too hard to measure and evaluate. Regardless, the study of higher power influence on leadership is a burgeoning field of interest in the scholarly community.[16–18]

As previously discussed, the preponderance of traditional leadership models focus on outcomes, using indicators of satisfaction and productivity as indices of success. However, many established models also fail to incorporate the aspects of environment and individual culture. Clearly, culture and the environment have a profound impact on the study of leadership theory. As a result, an integrated theoretical model developed by Coppola[19] suggests a solution to this problem. The omnibus leadership model (OLM) borrows from previous literature in the field and provides a different aperture for evaluating leaders and leadership theory. The model offers spatial dimensional constructs of higher order, individual culture, and environment as signposts for other variables or constructs. Furthermore, from these spatial dimensions, the constructs of beneficence, character traits, and resources may be derived.

Higher Order Construct

Higher order principles guide the construct of beneficence, or the practice of "doing good" against the construct of malevolence, or the practice of "doing bad." Higher order principles are themselves derived from family values, spiritual teachings, education, "herd mentalities" in the community, and individual interpretation of the aforementioned spatial dimensions—whether they be consistent or inconsistent with practices or norms of behavior. Certainly, higher order principles guide the development of many leaders. It is a construct that should not be overlooked in future leadership studies.

For example, when applying traditional leadership models, Adolf Hitler might be described as an effective leader, or at least as someone who demonstrated leadership skills, through the example of the successful rebuilding of Germany after WWI. A retrospective application of path-goal leadership theory may justify this proposition. Additionally, it is unquestionable that Adolf Hitler initially inspired hundreds of thousands of followers toward his fascist movement in both Europe and the United States in the late 1930s. A retrospective application of transformational leadership theory may help explain Hitler's retrospective success in this regard. However, to refer to Adolf Hitler as a leader is insulting to the profession of leadership. Adolf Hitler is not thought of as a highly regarded leader in the study of leadership theory today. He is considered, at best, to have been a despot and a dictator. Certainly, a model must be created that allows for the differentiation of leadership and dictatorship.

Individual Culture Construct

The construct of character traits may be derived from the individual cultural spatial dimension. Trait theory itself has dominated the bulk of traditional leadership methodology over the previous century and little additional discussion seemed to have been warranted. However, as mentioned in the previous chapter, cultural distinctiveness clearly acts as an immutable object in the study of leadership theory. Some Asian and

Middle Eastern societies clearly favor gender in the practice of leadership hierarchy, while other societies are more gender neutral. Age is likewise a factor in many Asian societies and is often used as a proxy that suggests experience equates with competence. As a result, it would be inappropriate to apply a transformational leadership model to the evaluation of some societies due to the hierarchal gender- and age-based traits associated with those cultures. For example, in traditional Chinese and North Korean cultures, inquisitiveness and outspokenness may be perceived in a negative light, as opposed the western sense of it showing a search for understanding and an extroverted approach.

Environmental Construct

Leaders cannot execute their vision, inspire followership, and demonstrate legitimate and charismatic attributes unless there are appropriate resources in the environment to assist in the communication of the leader's message. If the environment lacks appropriate resources to assist in the transfer and the communication of the leaders' intent, the leader may not affect significant followership to lead anything. For this reason, we posit that the environmental construct is a necessary precursor to resource availability. Furthermore, leader recognition is not possible without appropriate resources to deliver the leader's message.

Resources have likewise attained a reasonable amount of focus in traditional leadership study; however, resources are generally used as variables unto themselves and not as constructs for measurement.[20] In the OLM, resources may be assessed through both human followership and logistical availability. For example, in the modern study of leadership, vehicles for message delivery have exponentially been available to small groups of individuals who may have been hermetically sealed from the preponderance of the world culture in the past. The advent of the Internet has allowed small fringe groups of previously marginalized peoples to gain standing and respect in the greater world community. If an individual with a provocative website has a message that inspires followership, a lone marginalized individual may find standing and prominence on the world stage. Clearly environmental resources have gained prominence as vehicles for leadership followership.

The Model

The omnibus leadership model meets the needs of future leadership researchers by including the spatial dimensions of higher order and individual culture and environment. Table 11-3 provides a template for this model. Figure 11-4 illustrates Table 11-3 as a conceptual model of the omnibus leadership theory. The benefit of this theory is in capturing constructs that assist in explaining why certain leaders are driven to leadership decisions. For example, many leader decisions are based on values learned from childhood relating to cultural and spiritual teachings that can be acted upon in favorable environments. In understanding and applying this model, it becomes clear on what some leaders base their decisions on, and why some leaders have widespread followership. In fact, followership based on cultural and higher order issues cannot be overlooked in this modern era of the War on Terror and the increasingly globalized society.

Table 11-3 Omnibus Leadership Model

Spatial Dimension	Construct	Description	Variables
Higher order	Beneficence or Malevolence	Altruism or Sadism	Actions Self-serving vs. serving Teamwork: Glory me vs. glory we
Individual (culture)	Character	Extraversion or Introversion Type A or B personality archetypes	Traits, ability & skills
Environment	Resources Stability Turbidity Dynamic	Human followership and logistical availability	Outcomes Action vs. reaction Flight vs. fight

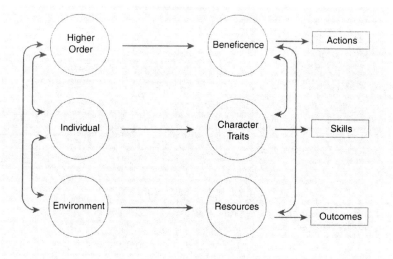

Figure 11-4 Conceptual Model of Omnibus Leadership.

Methods for measuring the omnibus leadership model in the near term may rely on observational and non-experimental studies. Donabedian proposed a similar observational methodology with the now renowned structure-process-outcome quality model in 1966. Donabedian's original article contained few insights for empirical measurement other than to qualify review actions as having merit based on *normative and accepted practices* in the field. Donabedian suggested subject matter experts and panels are required to evaluate his new model.[21] Similar methodologies are necessary for the evaluation of the omnibus leadership model.

Traditional leadership models have previously employed true experimental and non-experimental methods within traditional leadership frameworks. This would continue to be applicable with the omnibus leadership model. Subjects and data may continue to be collected and analyzed utilizing traditional practices and procedures. However, the omnibus leadership model will help guide the researcher toward qualifying specific constructs of leadership for discerning certain phenomena.

In closing, perhaps the Latin term *res ipsa loquitu,* or "the thing speaks for itself," may suggest additional structure to the omnibus leadership model. Leadership is action oriented—"one knows it when he sees it." As a result, leadership theory may continue to confound research efforts. Perhaps leadership scholars must be satisfied with the appreciation of leadership as an art more than a science after all.

Traditional Tools for Measuring Leadership

Much of the leadership research has been descriptive and qualitative. There appears to be less quantitative data. As a result, qualitative research has centered on a "theory building" methodology that uses such methods as biographies, observation activities, informal interviews, and the like. On the other hand, quantitative research is a "theory testing" methodology that tries to prove causality. That is, one thing causes another thing to happen. This is normally associated with statistical applications like the general linear model (t tests, ANOVA, ANCOVA, Regression) or relationships (such as correlations). The theories highlighted in this chapter and the previous one are but a small reflection of the myriad leadership models that have been researched throughout the history of leadership research. Truly, most leadership research has been conducted using surveys, observation, and factor analysis of experts. Rarely have leadership models that link leader styles, situational variables, and outcomes (performance) been evaluated. However, the models summarized in this chapter form the basis of much "cutting edge" leadership thinking today.

A review of the literature suggests that there are a plethora of descriptive tools on the market to measure or evaluate a leader's style or success. Many of these tests use self-report scales. As a result, they introduce and maintain method bias. However, it is possible to control for bias by taking the test multiple times over time. In this manner, a true response score might be found. Table 11-4 profiles these various test tools. All have been widely used in the literature with varying degrees of utility. While our list is certainly not an all-inclusive list of leadership tools on the market, it is felt that a balanced approach to the tools on the market is presented, that are readily available and cost efficient. The authors recommend that readers of this book acquire one or more of the measurement tools listed below and use them as companion guides to this text, in accord with course goals and objectives.

Table 11-4 Leadership Tests and Measures

Test	Measures
Multifactor Leadership Questionnaire	MLQ is designed to measure different characteristics associated with transformational leadership. Three subscales pertaining to transformational leadership include charisma, individualized consideration, and intellectual stimulation.
Leadership Competency Inventory	Developed for individual use, the LCI measures and identifies four competencies essential to effective leadership: information seeking, conceptual thinking, strategic orientation, and customer service orientation.
Leadership Skills Inventory	Developed for individual use, the LSI evaluates and measures competency in: planning and organizational skills, oral and written communication skills, decision-making skills, financial management skills, problem-solving skills, ethics and tolerance, personal/professional balance skills, and total inventory score.
Leadership Practices Inventory, Individual Contributor	Developed for individual use, the LPI assesses five leadership practices: challenging the process, inspiring a shared vision, enabling others to act, modeling the way, and encouraging the heart.
Leadership Practices Inventory	The third edition of this instrument package approaches leadership as a measurable, learnable, and teachable set of behaviors. This 360-degree leadership assessment tool helps individuals and organizations measure their leadership competencies, while guiding them through the process of applying leadership to real-life organizational challenges.

(continues)

Table 11-4 Leadership Tests and Measures (continued)

Test	Measures
Leader Behavior Questionnaire	Developed for individual use, it helps leaders to determine what changes or further skill development are required for them to make full use of their capabilities for visionary leadership: The questionnaire is made up of 50 items measuring ten key leadership scales: focus, respect for self and others, communication, bottom line orientation, trust, length of vision span, risk, organizational leadership, empowerment, and cultural leadership.
Leader Behavior Analysis II, Revised	Developed for individual use, this self scored questionnaire measures team leadership style flexibility, primary and secondary style, effectiveness in matching leadership behaviors to the group situation, and tendencies to misuse or overuse various styles.
Leadership Team Alignment Assessment, Dynamic Culture Leadership	Developed to assess individual and group leadership versus management and science versus art "personalities" in comparison to organizational operating culture and external environment expectations. This assessment incorporates the dynamic culture leadership process of: (1) communication improvement; (2) strategic and operational planning; (3) decision-making alignment; (4) employee enhancement; (5) knowledge management; and (6) repeat. A key premise is that a leadership team that is diverse (in leadership personalities) yet focused on organizational goals is better situated for internal and external changes, thus, dynamic culture leadership.
Leadership Skills Inventory	Developed for individual use, the LSI is a condensed, streamlined version of the self-assessment section in Transforming Leadership. Provides the leader with a tool for assessing his or her effectiveness in self-management, communications, counseling, problem-management skills, consulting, and style shifting. Identifies areas for development of behavioral change to produce maximum results: self-administered, self-scored and self-interpreted.

■ CONCLUSION

The topic of leadership is complex and ever changing. However, as organizations transition, leaders must study and understand the strategic imperative to guide their organizations and to develop a culture that can thrive in the dynamic external environment. Leaders are needed because organizations, the external environment, technology, and people change. The descriptive and prescriptive models overviewed in this chapter were discussed with the intention of facilitating thought, reflection, and discussion of quality leadership practices and outcomes. The ultimate leadership outcomes are organizational survival, longevity, and matching purpose with external needs. In healthcare, these outcomes can be translated into stronger, more productive, healthier, and symbiotic organizations poised to meet change successfully.

Another aspect of leadership neglected in the literature relates to scope and scale of success. For example, a hospital leader, whose organization is very successful financially, may be considered a "good leader," yet if the community is not becoming healthier and more productive, can that person truly be considered a good leader? Leadership ought to be considered in the light of morality and good conscience, and one should understand what successful outcomes are in terms of the greater community served. In addition to studying the models presented in this chapter, it is recommended that the reader review and consider the selections found in the reference section of this chapter.

■ CHAPTER SUMMARY

Two prescriptive leadership models with associated processes were presented, the dynamic culture leadership model and the omnibus leadership model, both of which focus on organizational culture. The understanding of organizational culture is of critical importance, and the development and maintenance of a thriving culture is essential to the long-term survival and success of the organization. Primary embedding and secondary reinforcement mechanisms were presented to guide development and refinement of organizational culture. The healthcare industry, more than many other sectors, needs and requires good leaders.

Review/Discussion Questions

1. How would you apply the dynamic culture leadership model in healthcare organizations?
2. How would you apply the omnibus leadership model in healthcare organizations?
3. Compare and contrast the dynamic culture leadership model with the omnibus leadership model.
4. How do organizational culture and leadership work together?
5. What would you prescribe as a leadership model for healthcare organizations?

References

1. Ledlow G, Cwiek M, Johnson J. Dynamic culture leadership: Effective leader as both scientist and artist. *Global Business and Technology Association (GBATA) International Conference*. In Delener N, Chao C (eds.), *Beyond Boundaries: Challenges of Leadership, Innovation, Integration and Technology*, 694–740; 2002. As first reported in the GBATA publication and provided again herein with permission by New Visions Network, LLC.

2. Conger J, Toegel G. A Story of Missed Opportunities: Qualitative Methods for Leadership Research and Practice. In Parry KW, Meindl JR (eds.), *Grounding Leadership Theory and Research: Issues, Perspectives and Methods*. Greenwich, CT: Information Age Publishing, Inc, 75–197; 2002.

3. Jelinek M, Litterer JA. Toward entrepreneurial organizations: Meeting ambiguity with engagement. *Entrepreneurship: Theory and Practice*. 1995; 19(3):137–169.

4. Schein EH. *The Corporate Culture Survival Guide: Sense and Nonsense About Culture Change*. San Francisco, CA: Jossey-Bass;1999.

5. Yukl G. *Leadership in Organizations* (3rd ed.). Englewood Cliffs, NJ: Prentice Hall; 1994.

6. Schein EH. *The Corporate Culture Survival Guide: Sense and Nonsense About Culture Change*. San Francisco, CA: Jossey-Bass; 1999.

7. Friesen M, Johnson J. *The Success Paradigm*. London: Quorum Books; 1995.

8. American Museum of Natural History. (2007). *Apatosaurus*. Accessed March 2007 from http://www.amnh.org/exhibitions/expeditions/treasure_fossil/Fossils/Specimens/apatosaurus.html

9. Crocker C. The lessons of Somalia. *Foreign Aff*. 1995;74:2–8.

10. Mowday RT, Sutton RI. Organizational behavior: Linking individuals and groups to organizational contexts. *Annu Rev Psychol*. 1993;4:195–229.

11. Antoinette SP, Bedeian A. Leader-follower exchange quality. The role of personnel and interpersonal attributes. *Acad Manage J*. 1994;37:990–1001.

12. Norris WR, Vecchio RP. Situation leadership theory: A replication. *Group and Organizational Management*. 1992;17:331–343.

13. Weick KE. What theory is not, theorizing is. *Adm Sci Q*. 1995;40:385–390.

14. Roberts KH, Glick W. The job characteristics approach to task design: A critical review of the literature. *J Appl Psychol*. 1981;66:193–217.

15. Lowe KB, Gardner WL. Ten years of The Leadership Quarterly: Contributions and challenges for the future. *The Leadership Quarterly*. 2001;11:459–514.

16. Jordan S. *The Effects of Religious Preference and the Frequency of Spirituality on the Retention and Attrition Rates Among Soldiers*. Dissertation Project Submitted to the Faculty of the School of Human Services, Healthcare Administration Program, in partial Fulfillment of the Requirements for the Degree of Doctoral of Philosophy, Capella University, Minnesota; 2006.

17. Fry LW. Toward a theory of spiritual leadership. *The Leadership Quarterly*. 2003;14:693–727.

18. Russell RF, Stone AG. A Review of Servant Leadership Attributes: Developing a Practical Model. *Leadership and Organizational Development Journal*. 2002;23(3):145–157.

19. Coppola MN. A Propositional Perspective of Leadership: Is the Wrong Head on the Model? *Journal of International Research in Business Disciplines*, Business Research Yearbook, International Academy of Business Disciplines. 2004;Vol 11:620–625.
20. Goodman RM et al. Identifying and Defining the Dimensions of Community Capacity to Provide a Basis for Measurement. *Health Educ Behav.* 1998; 25(3):258–278.
21. Donabedian A. *Evaluating the quality of medical care.* Millbank Memorial Federation of Quality. 1966;44:166–203.

12

Decision Making and Communication

Gerald R. Ledlow and James Stephens

Learning Objectives

- Describe and categorize the major domains of applied decision-making theory.
- List and apply the elements of the willful choice or rational decision-making model.
- List and describe the application of a reality-based decision-making model.
- Understand the most used tools of decision making within the methodologies of quantitative, qualitative, and triangulated decision making for individuals, groups, and organizations.
- Define communication and describe the factors of quality communication.
- Describe and apply models for effective leadership and management regarding media richness theory, listening, and culturally competent communication.
- Describe how decision making and communication contribute to effective leadership and management.

■ INTRODUCTION

Competent decision making and communication are essential for successful individuals, groups, and organizations. For decades, communication (consistently the most noted) and decision making have been listed as areas needing significant improvement across all industries and organizational types (for-profit, non-profit, governmental, etc.); this is especially true in public health and health-related organizations including hospitals, clinics, community health departments, and group practices where broad diversity and deep complexity are inherent. A process or prescriptive model of leadership, as compared to descriptive models, suggests that communication improvement and decision-making alignment are vital components to successfully guide organizations to best meet the needs of the external environment, and thus achieve longevity in the marketplace.[1,2]

Easily, volumes of texts could be written and have been written for the topics of decision making and communication. The emphasis in this chapter will be to provide a general overview of decision making and communication and to focus on applications most applicable to entry- and middle-level public health and health organization leaders and managers.

■ DECISION MAKING

Decision making occurs in all organizations. The decision-making process begins with identifying a question, problem, or area needing improvement, or an operational issue. Problems, issues, questions, and operational challenges come to leaders and managers from many different people both within and outside the health organization. Leaders and managers usually are taught to utilize the rational decision-making model using analytical (quantitative) methods and when necessary, couple with group methods (qualitative) such as normative group technique (brainstorming, alternative categorization, prioritizing alternatives, and selecting an alternative based on group consensus) to triangulate (using both quantitative and qualitative methods) on an effective decision. In reality, decision making is not as sterile and ordered as most have been taught. Both willful choice or rational decision-making models, and reality-based or garbage can models, are used in organizations amid a myriad of tools and techniques. The major domains of decision making are:

- Willful choice or rational models
- Reality-based or garbage can models
- Combinations of willful choice and reality-based models

Methods of decision making are:

- Quantitative methods that use tools such as multiple attribute value, probability-based decision trees, analytical mathematical models, linear programming, and similar tools
- Qualitative methods that use tools such as focus groups, interviews (formal and informal), normative group techniques, and similar tools
- Triangulation methods that combine both quantitative and qualitative methods where, classically, qualitative methods are "theory building" and quantitative methods are "theory testing, validating, or confirming"

Next, a review of willful choice and reality-based decision-making models are presented; more time is spent on reality-based models, since this method is the least represented but may be the most applicable to health organizational leaders and managers.

Willful Choice Decision-Making Models

Decision-making models and current understanding implies that decisions are made by rational, intentional, and willful choice. Choice is guided by four basic principles: (1) unambiguous (you know what questions to ask) knowledge of alternatives, (2) probability and knowledge of consequences, (3) a rational and consistent priority system for alternative ordering, and (4) heuristics or decision rules to choose an alternative.[3] These models assume that alternatives are selected based on greatest utility (cost-benefit analysis for example), given the environmental situation (such as a strength, weaknesses, opportunities, and threats [SWOT] analysis), for the organization in line with organizational objectives, goals, and mission. Decision making in engineering, operations analysis and research, management science, and decision theory are variations on the rational and willful choice model.[3] As ascribed in practical application of business practice, the six-step model of decision making puts into application the analytic willful choice model prescribed to today:[4]

1. Identify the problem.
2. Collect data.
3. List all possible solutions.
4. Test possible solutions.
5. Select the best course of action.
6. Implement the solution based on the decision made.

The practical model assumes time and information are abundant, energy is available, and goal congruence of participants (everyone is focused on the same set of goals) has been achieved.

Criticism of Willful Choice Models

Well-known leadership management concepts consider pre-planning (short and long-term) as the method to solve ambiguity (not knowing what to do) in business, but as task complexity increases and time availability decreases, the ability to plan increasingly becomes more difficult.[5] The rapid pace of operations and change in healthcare today makes traditionally based organizations less adaptive and flexible in complex environments.[5] Information and time are assumed to be abundant and relatively free resources in rational and willful choice models, as well as organizational participants in the decision-making process are assumed to have similar (if not the same) goals.[3] These issues are the basis of willful choice model criticisms. Theories of agency (for conflict management) and economics (scarce resources—namely time and information) have attempted to resolve contradictory issues associated with willful choice as an explanatory model. Both the theories of agency and economics depend on rational participants to validate the models.[6] The reality of the health organization world suggests that individual and group preferences change as underlying variables associated with the decision vary, environmental factors evolve, and other organizational decisions are made.[3,7] Reality suggests that preferences of participants in the decision-making process often vary in illogical and emotionally dependent ways. Although considered in the willful choice models, time and information are not considered as valuable or scarce as reality actually suggests.

Neoclassical economic theory suggests that the greatest good occurs when individuals are free to pursue self-serving interests.[6] This further confounds the willful choice decision-making models' underlying assumptions. It is unreasonable to assume that each participant in a decision-making process will have similar self-serving goals and similar joint organizational goals most of the time. These contradictions add further credence that willful choice models should be used when participants' goals are similar, time and information is available in sufficient quantity to use the willful choice model, and participants are well-trained in the use of the model. What is provided here is not a suggestion that one should not use willful choice models, but albeit, use the model in appropriate situations. This leaves the leader and manager in a tough situation; what model should be used when the willful choice model conditions cannot be met? In the discussion that follows, the garbage can model—a reality-based model—is highlighted as an extension of rational decision-making models and adds to the available methods of decision making for the leader and manager in health organizations.

Reality-Based Models: Garbage Can Model Overview

Reality-based models, such as the garbage can model, are intended to extend the understanding of organizational decision-making by emphasizing a temporal context (the situation at one point in time) and accepting chaos as reality. Rational (willful choice) decision-making models are a subset of reality-based models. In ambiguous (do not know what to ask or do) situations where time and information are limited or constrained and "perfect information" impossible to acquire, where organization structure/hierarchy is loosely coupled, and organized anarchy (chaos) seems to embody the organizational persona, analytical decision-making models do not fit reality. The garbage can model, originally designed to reflect decision making in universities, has been used to explain decision-making processes in various organizations and situations. Also, garbage can models have been introduced as possible methods to understand processes such as how an organization learns.[8] For the past two decades, researchers have observed that willful choice models of decision making underestimate the chaotic nature and complexity regarding actual decision-making situations; a large percentage of decisions are made by default where decision-making processes are worked without actually solving anything.[3]

Garbage Can Model Concepts
Organized anarchy, chaos, and bedlam are terms that describe organizational decision making. "Garbage can decisions can occur in any organization but are more likely to be found in 'organized anarchies' where decisions are made under ambiguity and fluid involvement of participants."[3] Garbage can models are attempts at finding logic and order in the mist of decision-making chaos. Garbage, defined as sets of problems, solutions, energy, and participants, is dumped into a can as they are produced (streams of "garbage" in time) and when the can is full, a decision is made and removed from the scenario.[9] "Numerous empirical observations of organizations have confirmed a relatively confusing picture of decision making. Many things seem to be happening at once; technologies are changing and poorly understood; alliances, preferences, and perceptions are changing; solutions, opportunities, ideas, people, and outcomes are mixed together in ways that make interpretation uncertain and leave connections unclear."[3] In management arenas, specifically acquisition decisions, decision-making load, speed required in decision-making, uncertainty, and equivocality (equivocality is another word for ambiguity: not knowing what questions to ask or what to do) are commonplace.[10] Thus the temporal nature of decision-making processes, if taken as "snapshots" in time, would show sequential arrival of problems, solutions, and information in a complex mix of participants, environmental factors, and consequences of prior decisions as reality in the "organized chaos" of decision making in organizations. Since time is not static and multidimensionality is reality, the garbage can model depicts the chaotic nature of decision making.

Concepts are grounded in the ambiguous and uncertain states of nature for the garbage can model. Originally, three states of nature contributed to the model. All three states are immersed in ambiguity and, to a lesser degree, uncertainty; the greater the ambiguity of technology, preferences of participants (the less preferences are known the greater the level of uncertainty) and of the organization, and participation (in more specific terms, attention of participants), the greater the prevalence of garbage can processes in organizational decision making. Ambiguity is defined as ignorance. Not only does this imply lack of knowledge, but a lack of understanding of what questions to ask, what information is available, and what connectivity exists between problem and solution sets and the consequences of implementing solutions. Ambiguity of participation exists when participants in the decision-making process have time demands that compete for attention necessary to solve a problem (make a decision). Since measurement of participation ambiguity depends on many extraneous variables in a sea of limitless situational factors, it is hard to quantify. Yet, attention and energy variations among participants are considered a "given" phenomenon in decision-making processes. Extending original concepts, Takahashi (1997) proposed three additional states of nature ambiguities to the model: (1) fluid participation, (2) divorce of solutions from discussion, and (3) job performance rather than subjective assessments.[9] Regarding individual preference, Pablo and Sitkin suggest that the more risk adverse a decision maker is, the less tolerant they are to ambiguity.[10]

Loose coupling in organizations fosters a garbage can decision-making approach. Loose coupling in an organization is defined as more informal and differentiated with less focus on following the rules but still maintaining structured connectivity of intra-organizational entities. Loose coupling tends to allow a more flexible organization.[11] Organizations that are loosely coupled, in the traditional sense, are more adaptive to change and environmental factors.[3,5,10] The strength of feedback loops determines organizational coupling; stronger feedback loops imply tighter coupling, whereas weaker loops suggest looser coupling.[12] Four criteria for determining the coupling status in organizations are: (1) formal rules where the closer the rules are followed the more tightly coupled (in entrepreneurial organizations, formal rules are not as important); (2) agreement on rules where the greater the employee congruence, the tighter the coupling (entrepreneurial firms agree on social norms rather than formal rules); (3) feedback where the closer the feedback, in time, the tighter the coupling; and (4) attention where empowered individuals allocate energy and time to prioritized areas in their "area" (participation, competence, and empowerment foster focused attention to areas of responsibility). In the garbage can model, the concept of loose coupling is required to understand decision making.[5]

Temporal order replaces sequential order. Time is spatial in that a multitude of issues, problems, information flows, and sensing mechanisms can bombard decision makers in short or long time blocks. How problems and information to resolve the problems arrives in time has relatively equal priority as the evaluation of their importance. Arrival time and sequence in the current context influences decision makers' attention to the situation. "The process is thoroughly and generally sensitive to load. An increase in the number of problems, relative to the energy available to work on them, makes problems less likely to be solved, decision makers more likely to shift from one arena to another more frequently, and choices longer to make and less likely to resolve problems."[3] Individuals in the decision-making process, directly and indirectly, are interconnected and influence the context of the decision at hand.

Attention demands influence decision making. Time and energy must be allocated to understand, evaluate, and formulate a problem, then synthesize relevant information, evaluate options, and finally choose an alternative to counter or terminate the problem. Individuals focus on some things and do not attend to others in the same space of time. Corporate actions, outcomes, and responsiveness are the results of dynamic organizational processes, not heuristics of individual choice.[7] Time and energy combine to form "attention." Attention is a dynamic concept that is highly dependent on load (that is the number of decisions that need to be made).

Lending support to the garbage can concept, rational choice in organizational decision making can be skewed by rituals and symbolism. Symbolic rituals of decision making skew rational attempts to understand the process. Decision making is a process that reassures the organization that values, norms, and logic are upheld; in this light, decision making is a ritual. Lastly, decision making as a process is about showing control and logic in a world of complexity and rapid change. "We made a decision" and "we own the process" implies control of human existence by logical choice. However the choice ritual makes one feel, decision making is not rational, but depictions of organized chaos rationalized by imperfect participants among a myriad of complex and synergized variables.

Decision possibilities in the garbage can model form the spectrum from willful choice models to garbage can–based models. Decisions by "flight," "resolution," and "oversight" are prominent categories in the model. "Flight" is defined as a decision maker's intentional movement (attention shift) to another area of concern (problem). "Resolution" is defined as a decision that uses classical decision-making processes such as willful choice models.[9] "Oversight" is defined as decision makers activating a process or procedure before a problem becomes apparent such as a standing operating procedure or using an established and documented process. Much of the research shows that "flight" was a significant result of much decision making; that means decisions were "overcome by events" or were not made but let to resolve or escalate themselves. So, what does a leader or manager do to deal with the reality of decision making?

Optimization of Decision Making

If a health organization has decision-making processes that resemble the garbage can environment, understanding the issues and proactively creating an environment that improves decision making can benefit the organization. Simulation results of garbage can studies revealed that decision making by resolution was not the prominent result of decision-making processes unless "flight" results are greatly constrained or decision load is light. The prominent results of decision making are "flight" and "oversight"; that means that either decisions were not made or pre-determined and established processes (like standing operating procedures) were used to a greater degree than willful choice models.[9] So why not re-engineer organizations to foster decision making based on goals of the organization, where clearly defined yet challenging goals are set and managers direct subordinates to focus, persist, and provide effort in achieving the goals, comprehend technology, and logically apply rational decision-making processes?[13] The answer is simple: Organizations do not exist to make decisions but to serve the external environment. An organization structured to make decisions will not serve its customers well and eventually will be removed from the marketplace.

Imperfect decision making can be expected. In light of the ambiguous reality of information, preference, differences, and incongruent goals and the problem and information bombardment of the temporally "exposed" decision maker, the garbage can model is a reasonable extension of willful choice theories. Humans strive for processes of willful choice, yet, as the garbage can model proposes, fail to achieve rationality in decision making due to time, energy, attention, uncertainty, ambiguous information, and decision-making load issues. Leaders who can grasp the dynamics of the garbage can are better enabled to promote and foster situations that can position their organizations to make good decisions amid organized chaos and competition. Leaders and managers in health organizations should develop an organizationally sensitive *system of decision making* with the understanding that decision making is not always orderly by:

1. Evaluating the situation and decisions that need to be made across the organization (or within your area of responsibility) and categorizing decisions by quantity, urgency, information needed to make the decision, and variance in decision outcomes

2. Developing readily available information concerning core business functions

3. Standardizing, documenting, and training team members on decisions that need to be made routinely where the same or similar decision outcome is required and by "pushing" those decisions to the lowest levels of the organization as possible but requiring feedback loops

4. Determining decision-making load (quantity in a set time frame) and information available to make decisions for the existing decisions (those not standardized)

5. Determining the importance of a decision to the organization by creating a system of risk determination, urgency, and technological requirements for non-standardized decisions, and

6. Training team members on the decision-making system and processes.

When a decision or decisions need to be made, a health organization leader and manager should:

1. Evaluate the priority and risk of the decision to be made, and determine if this is a standardized decision or a decision that needs to be worked through.

2. Evaluate time available, resources available, participant attention, goals, and incentives.

3. Determine what decision-making method to use, oversight based on established documented processes such as standing operating procedures, resolution using a willful choice model, or by pushing the decision to the appropriate level, individual, or group. It is also important to know when you do not need to make a decision (flight, based on the importance and risk level of the decision at hand).

Understanding that decision making is not a sterile and orderly process in most cases is the essential knowledge required for a leader and manager to develop a reality-based decision-making system. Importantly, organizational decision making *should be aligned* (decisions should be in accordance) with the *organization's mission and vision* statements and *strategic planning–based goals and objectives*. Next, a summary of decision-making tools are presented.

■ TOOLS OF DECISION MAKING

As a summary, tools of decision making vary but are important to be aware of for future study and practice. Study, taking a course, and practice of both quantitative and qualitative decision-making tools are highly recommended. Quantitative methods and qualitative methods will be highlighted while triangulation is a combination of both quantitative and qualitative methods. Considering the next three paragraphs, it is recommended that each tool mentioned (and those not mentioned) be searched, maybe using an Internet search, and discussed, practiced, and role-played with others in the class, group, or organization. Facilitating the decision-making process in a group or organization is an essential skill of leaders and managers and a working competence of decision-making tools is a pre-requisite to such a skill.

Quantitative Methods Summary

Quantitative methods include mathematical and computational analytical models to help us understand the decision-making situation (data turned to information to knowledge) and produce mathematical outcomes of solutions. Some models are rather simple while others can be very complex. Quantitative models assist in putting a "number" on uncertainty. Models include multiple attribute value and multiple utility methods, linear programming, probability, and decision trees based on Bayes' Theorem, and can be as complex as discrete and dynamic simulation. In general, simulation uses theoretical distributions and probabilities to "model" the real-world situation on the computer. From the computer model, response variables produce "outcomes" that can be evaluated. Quantitative models take time and understanding of the important elements (also known as factors or variables) associated with the decision that needs to be made. In most health organizations, quantitative models are gaining momentum but qualified (trained and well-practiced) analysts that understand health processes, and can perform a range of quantitative analyses, are still difficult to find and hire. Even with quantitative analyses in hand, many times leaders and managers skew decisions toward the qualitative side of decision making.

Qualitative Methods Summary

Qualitative methods include a variety of tools from personal intuition, discussions with team members, informal interviews, formal interviews, focus groups, nominal group techniques, and even voting. Qualitative methods are very useful since experience, intuition, and common sense are used to aid decision making by individuals as well as groups. Study and practice of qualitative methods are essential for leaders and managers to facilitate decision making for themselves, groups, and organizations. When quantitative and qualitative methods are combined, it is called triangulation.

Triangulation Summary

Triangulation is a more thorough method to make decisions. Although triangulation takes time, it brings both quantitative and qualitative approaches into the decision-making process. It is common for a group to use nominal group techniques to come to a small set of possible solutions and then for each solution to be analyzed quantitatively. From there the leader or manager can make a decision. Training the group or organization to use triangulation is a good practice for resolving (resolution in reality-based models) decisions. Triangulation can also be used to develop standard operating procedures (known as oversight in reality-based models). Lastly, triangulation can be used to make improvements to processes within the organization.

Summary

Decision making is an integrated process that is embedded in health organizations. Leaders and managers can consciously make decision making better, more efficient, effective, and efficacious while reducing organizational stress. Understanding the nature of decision making and becoming competent as a decision maker, facilitator, analyst, or decision-making assistant (those that help those making the decision) are critical for success as a leader and manager; they are also necessary for success as a team member not in a leadership or management role. Developing a system of decision making within the organizational context and constraints, training others in that system, and becoming a competent user of the system are vital to creating and maintaining excellence in health organizations. Another salient topic, communication, is presented next.

■ COMMUNICATION

Communication is continuous. Communication is necessary. Communication is learned. Communication needs to be improved considering individuals, groups, and organizations. Communication, considering dyadic group and organization, is one of the weakest links in healthcare organizations; there is a plethora of evidence (patient safety, efficiency, morale, etc.) that suggests communication must be improved across the health industry. The rest of this chapter will discuss communication and provide a few vital communication essentials for leaders and managers in health organizations. The essence of communication, media richness, listening, confirmatory language, and basics of culturally competent communication will be the tenets of the rest of this chapter. Again, volumes of texts have been and can be written on each of these topics so more intense study in each of these areas is recommended.

Communication Is Transfer of Meaning

Simply, communication is using symbols, gestures, body movements, and context to transfer meaning to someone else, to groups, and to organizations. Everything you do communicates something to someone. What you do not say or do not do still communicates meaning. Several communication scholars and researchers have stated that, "One *cannot not* communicate!" Being keenly aware of this reality, leaders and managers need to be careful in what they say and do but also in what they do not say or do not do. For example, if a large medical center hospital chief executive officer is seen walking over a crumpled piece of paper laying on the floor of a heavily used hallway in the hospital (not picking the trash up and throwing it away), this sends a message that cleanliness is not important; a "dirty" hospital can be the result in a very short time.

Communication uses verbal (talking), nonverbal (writing such as this sentence), paralanguage (such as tone of voice), body language (such as a shrug of the shoulders), and context (public versus private) to transfer meaning from one person to others. What is communicated from the sender of the message is taken in by the receivers of the message and filtered through their own experiences, knowledge, and assessment of the context of the communication environment. What this means is what is communicated by the sender, with the sender's intended message, must be received and processed by the receiver, given that the receiver will process the message through their own set of filters. In essence, the receiver may process and translate a message with a different meaning than what the sender intended the message to be. Given this reality, leaders and managers must carefully craft messages and then be consistent in their actions (to match their words), paralanguage, and body language and select the proper context with which to communicate their intended message.

Communication, from a macro-perspective, is determined to be "quality" when accuracy, usefulness, timeliness, and quantity are in optimal ranges for the intended audience. Always assess your audience when communicating and use messages consistent with actions, paralanguage, body language, and context that your intended audience will receive, so your audience can process/translate the message to best understand your intended message. When assessing an audience, use the least common denominator approach; that is, craft your message for everyone to understand. If you are talking to a group of physicians, nurses, and non-healthcare community members about a medical situation, use language that a non-healthcare person can understand; the physicians and nurses will also understand what you are discussing. In crafting messages, media richness, confirmatory language, and culturally competent communication are important factors in quality communication. Lastly, listening is of paramount importance for leaders and managers in health organizations.

Media Richness

Communication is critical for successful health outcomes; communication is the vital process that links consumers of care and providers of care.[14] The accurate gathering, documenting, and passing of information that allow high-quality decisions to be made, or for instructions to be followed, are at the crux of what is required to communicate effectively within health organizations. The value of communication in an organization equates directly to how much communication assists the organization in reaching its goals; goals must be clear, measurable, and set within a reasonable time frame.[15] Media richness theory[16,17] offers research and application potential for successful leader and manager communication.

Daft and Lengel (1986) state that organizations process information to reduce uncertainty (the absence of information) and equivocality (ambiguity).[16] Information is processed and communication occurs to accomplish internal tasks of the organization, to coordinate activities, and evaluate external environments.[16] "Uncertainty is a measure of the organization's ignorance of a value for a variable in the (information) space; equivocality is a measure of the organization's ignorance of whether a variable exists in the (information) space."[16] More information reduces uncertainty.[17] Basically, low uncertainty about an issue or problem means an organization has data or information in sufficient quantity to make decisions about the problem, whereas low equivocality means an organization has defined what questions or what data is needed to attempt to solve the problem. Equivocality means that multiple and contradictory interpretations exist about an organizational issue or problem.[17] Leaders and managers differ in information processing response when confronted with uncertainty as opposed to equivocality. Uncertainty causes managers to acquire data, whereas, equivocality prompts the exchange of subjective views among leaders and managers to define problems and resolve conflicts.

Information richness is defined as the ability of information to change understanding within a time interval.[16] The longer the time interval to exchange understanding, the less rich the information. Consequently, the less time required the more rich the information is to the communicators (sender and receiver). The media (such as email, the telephone, or face-to-face conversation) that carries information to intended audiences also has a richness associated with it. A continuum of media richness has been established based on the medium's capacity for immediate feedback, the number of cues and channels utilized, personalization, and language variety.[16,18] In decreasing media richness, the continuum of richness consists of: "1) face-to-face, 2) telephone, 3) personal documents such as letters, memos, and emails, 4) impersonal written documents, and 5) numeric documents."[16] The richer the media, the better equivocality can be reduced; *media low in richness is best used when communicating messages that are understood well and possess standard information.*[16] Simply put, face-to-face interaction works best and bulletin board flyers work the worst in transferring meaning. Leaders and managers must consider what media with which to communicate to ensure the highest probability to transfer meaning to their intended audience.

Confirmatory Language and Culturally Competent Communication

Confirmatory language should be the goal of leaders and managers' communication in health organizations. Confirming language causes people to value themselves more while disconfirming language causes people to value themselves less. Both positive (you are doing great) and negative (your work is not meeting standards) messages can be conveyed using confirming language. The following items are provided by Gibb and provide the basis for developing a confirming communication environment:[19]

- Evaluation vs. Description: evaluation is "you" language; description is "I" language; descriptive language leads to more trust and group cohesiveness. Use descriptive language. Whenever you talk to someone and say "you" or feel you need to point your finger at them, it is probably evaluation language.

- Controlling vs. Problem Orientation: problem orientation is more effective than controlling communication in reducing defensiveness. Focus on a problem and communicate together; do not control communication with your personal issues; find a problem to discuss together.

- Strategy vs. Spontaneity: strategy (like controlling) suggests manipulation so be spontaneous (or at least communicate as such) in communicating with someone; do not take out a list and say, "I have three things to talk with you about."

- Superiority vs. Equality: supportive climates occur under participation and equality. Communicate as equals rather than as supervisor and subordinate; talk as if you were equals even though you may not be equal in organizational status.

- Certainty vs. Provisionalism: flexible, open, and genuine thinking fosters a supportive climate; do not be a "know it all."

Being culturally competent in communication is important as well. Below are some considerations a leader and manager should attend to when crafting messages and communicating with others (these concepts were originally the work of Hofstede in his cultural studies as cited from Beebe and Masterson in 1997 [see Table 12-7]).[19]

- **Individualism:** Individualistic cultures value individual recognition, self-actualization, rights, and freedoms over collectivistic achievement (the United States, Great Britain, and Australia are examples).

- **Collectivistic:** Cultures where the group or team achievement is valued more than individual achievement (Japan, China, Taiwan, Venezuela, Columbia, and Pakistan are examples of countries who score high on collective approaches to work methods).

- **Conversational Style:**
  - Western cultures: control is exerted through speaking.
  - Eastern cultures: control is expressed through silence and an outward show of reticence.

Table 12-1 Individualistic vs. Collectivistic Assumptions from Beebe and Masterson

Individualistic Assumptions	Collectivistic Assumptions
Most effective decisions made by individual	Most effective decisions made by group
Planning is centralized	Planning is done by all concerned
Individuals should be rewarded	Group or team should be rewarded
Individuals primarily work for themselves	Individuals primarily work for the team
Healthy competition important	Teamwork is important
Meetings are for sharing information	Meetings are for team decision making
Key objective: advance your own ideas	Key objective: group consensus

Beebe SA, Masterson JT. (1997). *Communicating in Small Groups: Principles and Practices*, (5th ed.). New York, NY: Addison-Wesley Educational Publishers Inc.

- Time:
  - Mono-chronic: time is linear and segmented, precision is valued (North America and Europe).
  - Poly-chronic: laissez-faire attitude of time, human existence does not proceed by clockwork (Africa and South America).

- Status and Power:
  - High-status group members:
    - talk more
    - communicate more often with other higher status individuals
    - have more influence
    - are less likely to be ignored
    - are less likely to complain about their responsibilities
    - talk to entire group
    - are likely to serve in leadership roles
  - Low-status group members:
    - direct conversation to high-status individuals
    - communicate more positive messages to higher status people
    - are more likely to be ignored
    - communicate more irrelevant information

Understanding the cultural considerations of your audience will assist in crafting messages and consistent behaviors.

Listening

Lastly, leaders and managers in health organizations must be good listeners. Listening not only helps gather vital information but also shows empathy and trust. Empathy and trust are essential to building relationships with others. The better your relationship with others the better communication and decision making will become. Below is a simple yet effective listening model from Beebe and Masterson:[19]

- Hearing: receiving the message as sent

- Analyzing: discerning the speaker's purpose and using critical/ creative judgments

- Empathizing: see and understand the speaker's viewpoint

    "People seen as good leaders are also seen as good listeners."[19]

Guide to Effective Listening or Listening Model:

1. Stop
2. Look
3. Listen
4. Ask questions
5. Paraphrase content
6. Paraphrase feelings

One of the most significant differences in listening for those in healthcare is to who we are willing to listen. Because of advancement in new technology and changes in business practices, we have changed who we listen to, what we are listening for, when we listen to them, and how we listen to them.[20] In addition to various complications of listening to knowledge, and the issue we are listening to people from a variety of cultures—the stage may be designed for more changes in our listening behaviors.

Active listening becomes extremely important when we interact with individuals from different cultures. Listening to someone requires individuals to be focused on more than what has been said, but we must also observe the behavior of the individual. People who are active listeners are more aware of nonverbal messages and more able to communicate effectively with people in their own culture and other cultures.[21] There is an African custom when one person greets another person by saying "I see you." The other person then responds by saying "I see you too." Both individuals have said, by this verbal communication and their nonverbal behavior of eye contact, that they respect each other's presence. They now have become more sensitive to each other's needs to communicate.

How we listen can vary by age of the listener. Younger workers prefer to use electronic tools and older workers are more likely to seek face-to-face communication or telephone conversations.[22] Another influence of technology is how we listen. In some cases, we are no longer listening but are reading instead. A significant number of Americans are online and spend less time listening to other forms of media. On the other hand, the use of iPods enable individuals to select their listening experience. According to Hayakawa, "The advent of new forms of technology has been accompanied by the onslaught of more forms of communication. The information overload that people have to deal with every day forces them to be selective about what and what not to believe."[23]

Summary

Communication is a learned skill. The more you attend to communication factors, the better you will communicate, build relationships, and make decisions. Communication is an area that must be improved through good practice of skills, training, and discussion about communication.

■ CHAPTER SUMMARY

The major domains of decision making include: (1) willful choice or rational models, (2) reality-based on the garbage can models, and (3) combination of willful choice and reality-based models. Willful choice models in decision making may be most effective when participants' goals are similar, time and information is available, and participants are trained well in the use of the model. Reality-based or the garbage can model in decision making may be most effective when time and information are limited, where structure/organization hierarchy is loosely coupled, and organized chaos is present.

The garbage can model is a decision-making process that attempts to find logic and order in the midst of decision-making chaos. There are three states of nature that contribute to the garbage can model, which immerse in ambiguity to include technology, preferences of participants, and attention of participants.

Decision possibilities in the garbage can model of "flight" (intentionally moving to another problem), "resolution" (using classical decision-making process to include the willful choice model), and "oversight" (activating a process before problem becomes apparent) are prominent categories in the model. Various methods of decision making include quantitative methods, qualitative methods, and triangulation (combination of both quantitative and qualitative methods).

Communication is a transfer of meaning by using symbols, gestures, body movements, and context to someone else. Media richness can reduce equivocality (ambiguity) within the organization's process of information. Confirmatory language and culturally competent communication are necessary communication skills of healthcare leaders in diversified workforces. Good listening skills build relationships with others because it shares empathy and trust.

Review/Discussion Questions

1. What organizational circumstances would a healthcare leader use— the willful choice rational decision-making model or the reality-based garbage can model?

2. Discuss what operational issues and changes in the external environment might cause healthcare leaders not to utilize the willful choice model.

3. Under what organizational conditions should the reality-based/ garbage can model be considered by healthcare leaders?

4. What is the difference between ambiguity and uncertainty in a decision-making model?

5. Discuss the four criteria for determining the coupling status in organizations.

6. What is meaning of "flight," "resolution," and "oversight" as decision-making possibilities?

7. Which of the tools for decision making (quantitative methods, qualitative methods, and triangulation methods) should be used in developing operating procedures?

8. What is the definition of communication?

9. How would you explain the difference in verbal, nonverbal, paralanguage, body language, and context when transferring meaning from one person to others?

10. Is it true that the shorter the time interval to exchange understanding, the less rich the information?

11. Would communicating a message of individual achievement with a person from Japan have a different meaning than with a person from the United States? Explain.

12. Why are goal listening skills so important to building relationships?

Case Study

The president of Community Medical Center was having a meeting with the chief of surgery concerning an operating room nurse who many thought had HIV/AIDS. The majority of surgeons in the surgical department had become quite concerned and requested the operating room nurse be removed from his duties in this department. The chief of surgery firmly stated that if the nurse was not removed from the operating room, then a significant number of surgeons (approximately 50) would admit all of their patients to the Community Medical Center's local rival hospital across the city. Such activities would not only affect the operating room, but also the emergency room, surgical inpatient floors, surgical ICU, and clinical departments such as radiology, clinical laboratory, respiratory, rehabilitation, pharmacy, etc. The possible effects could be millions of dollars in lost revenue and the immediate layoff of hundreds of employees.

When Community Medical Center approached the nurse involved about relocating to a non-patient area with the same pay, shift, and working hours, he refused to accept the offer. In addition, he had contacted a labor attorney specializing in the healthcare industry and mentioned that the attorney had advised that they would file federal litigation in accordance to violation of several federal laws.

Because of an internal leak, the president of Community Medical Center was contacted by the editor and publisher of the main local newspaper about this event. It was most unusual for the editor and publisher to discuss a story instead of sending a reporter but they indicated that this story was too important and could have national media exposure. They gave the president 24 hours to provide a news release. Such media attention would most likely not only have instant concern of patients and families who were presently scheduled for surgery but also long-term damage of the institution's strong reputation for quality of medical care.

You are the president of Community Medical Center so what decision-making models will be most effective in this situation and how are you going to communicate your decision to the surgeons, medical center employees, governing board, and to the public?

References

1. Ledlow G, Cwiek M. The Process of Leading: Assessment and Comparison of Leadership Team Style, Operating Climate and Expectation of the External Environment, *Global Business and Technology Association Proceedings*. Lisbon, Portugal; 2005.
2. Ledlow G, Cwiek M, Johnson J. Dynamic culture leadership: Effective leader as both scientist and artist. Global Business and Technology Association International Conference; In Delener, Nejdet, Chao, Chiang-nan (Eds.) *Beyond Boundaries: Challenges of Leadership, Innovation, Integration and Technology*, 694–740; 2002.
3. March JG, Weisinger-Baylon R. *Ambiguity and Command: Organizational Perspectives on Military Decision Making*. Marshfield, MA: Pitman Publishing; 1986.
4. Argenti PA, ed. *The Portable MBA Desk Reference: An Essential Business Companion*. New York: John Wiley & Sons, Inc.; 1994.
5. Jelinek M, Litterer JA. Toward entrepreneurial organizations: Meeting ambiguity with engagement. *Entrepreneurship: Theory and Practice*. 1995; 19 (3):137–169.
6. Swanson DL. Neoclassical economic theory, executive control, and organizational outcomes. *Hum Relat*. 1996;49(6):735–757.

7. Swanson DL. Addressing a theoretical problem by reorienting the corporate social performance model. *Acad Manage Rev.* 1995;20 (1):43–65.

8. Tsang EWK. Organizational learning and the learning organization: A dichotomy between descriptive and prescriptive research. *Hum Relat.* 1997;50(1):73–90.

9. Takahashi, N. A single garbage can model and the degree of anarchy in Japanese firms. *Hum Relat.* 1997;50(1):91–109.

10. Pablo AL, Sitkin SB. Acquisition decision-making processes: The central role of risk. *Journal of Management.* 1996;22(5):723–747.

11. Bennis W, Parikh J, Lessem R. *Beyond Leadership: Balancing Economics, Ethics, and Ecology,* revised edition. Cambridge, MA: Blackwell Publishers, Ltd.; 1996.

12. Van de Ven AH, Poole MS. (1995). Explaining development and change in organizations. *Acad Manage Rev.* 1995;20(3):510–541.

13. Locke EA, Latham GP. *Goal Setting, A Motivational Technique That Works!* Englewood Cliffs, NJ: Prentice-Hall, Inc.; 1984.

14. Kreps GL, O'Hair D, Clowers M. The influences of human communication on health outcomes. *Am Behav Sci.* 1994;38(2):248–257.

15. Lindeborg RA. Excellent communication. *Public Relations Quarterly.* 1994;39(1):5–12.

16. Daft RL, Lengel RH. Organizational information requirements, media richness, and structural design. *Manage Sci.* 1986;22(5):554–571.

17. Daft RL, Lengel RH, Trevino LK. Message equivocality, media selection, and manager performance: Implications for information systems. *MIS Quarterly.* 1987;September:355–366.

18. Frey LR, Botan CH, Friedman PG, Kreps GL. *Investigating Communication: An Introduction to Research Methods.* Englewood Cliffs, NJ: Prentice Hall, 118–138; 1991.

19. Beebe SA, Masterson JT. *Communicating in Small Groups: Principles and Practices* (5th ed.). New York: Addison-Wesley Educational Publishers Inc.; 1997.

20. Bentley SC. Listening in the 21st Century. *International Journal of Listening.* 2000;2(14):129–142.

21. Timm S, Schroeder B. Listening/Nonverbal Communication Training. *International Journal of Listening.* 2000;14(20):109–128.

22. Messaging Practices in the Knowledge Economy. *Pitney Bowes.* (Report obtained from Pitney Bowes, based on a 1999 study completed by the Institute for the Future and the Gallup Organization); 1999.

23. Hayakawa SI. The task of the listener. (Retrospect) Analysis of skepticism. *A Review of General Semantics.* 1999;56(2):110.

CHAPTER

13

Culture Values and Ethics

Rupert M. Evans, Sr.

Learning Objectives

- Identify the cultural structures in healthcare organizations.
- Explain functions of the four cultural structures in healthcare organizations.
- Differentiate culture and climate.
- Explain the differences between diversity and cultural competence.
- Define organizational values.
- Describe the different priorities and values of multiple constituencies.
- Describe the relevant principles of medical ethics.
- Describe the American College of Healthcare Executives Ethical Policy Statement.

■ INTRODUCTION

Organizational culture, values, and ethics as they relate to healthcare organizations are grounded in management theory and are essential competencies necessary for aspiring healthcare executives. Each of these topics deserves a thorough discussion separately, however, they all relate to each other in practice. A substantive examination of organizational behavior and dynamics requires an understanding of how culture, values, and ethics are an integral component of a high-performance healthcare organization.

This chapter will address each area separately, highlighting relevant theory, and discuss how these concepts can be put into practice.

■ WHAT IS CORPORATE CULTURE?

Organizational culture, or corporate culture, comprises the attitudes, experiences, beliefs, and values of an organization. Edgar H. Schein says it best: "Culture is the sum total of all the shared, taken-for-granted assumptions that a group has learned throughout its history." Culture has been defined as "the specific collection of values and norms that are shared by people and groups in an organization and that control the way they interact with each other and with stakeholders outside the organization. Organizational values are beliefs and ideas about what kinds of goals members of an organization should pursue and ideas about the appropriate kinds or standards of behavior organizational members should use to achieve these goals. From organizational values, the organization can develop norms, guidelines, or expectations that prescribe appropriate kinds of behavior by employees in particular situations and control the behavior of organizational members towards one another."[1] In healthcare organizations, management may try to determine a corporate culture. They may wish to impose corporate values and standards of behavior that specifically reflect the objectives of the organization. In addition, there will also be an extant internal culture within the workforce. Culture consists of basic assumptions and prescribed criterion for success that drives the organization and its practices, systems, structures, and other components that flow from them.

The culture of an organization is an amalgamation of the values and beliefs of the people in an organization. It can be felt in the implicit rules and expectations of behavior in an organization where, even though the rules are not formally written down, employees know what is expected of them. Management decisions on policy set up the culture of the organization. The organizational culture usually has values and beliefs that support the organizational goals.

The organization's culture is manifested in a variety of ways, and researchers have identified various types of culture.

■ THE HEALTHCARE SETTING

Work groups within the organization have their own behavioral quirks and interactions that, to an extent, affect the whole system. Task culture can be imported. For example, computer technicians will have expertise, language, and behaviors gained independently of the organization, but their presence can influence the culture of the organization as a whole.

Healthcare organizations, however, are similar to all organizations because they also have different types of cultures in force. Most healthcare organizations have at least four identifiable cultures: clan culture, entrepreneurial culture, bureaucratic culture, and market culture.

Clan culture defines the culture in an organization that is full of tradition and rituals, teamwork and spirit, self-management and social influence.[2] These characteristics are often found in your faith-based healthcare organizations such as Catholic Health Initiatives, headquartered in Denver, CO, and Ascension Health, which is the nation's largest Catholic and largest non-profit health system.

Bureaucratic culture is one that emphasizes rules, policies, procedures, chain of command, and centralized decision making. Organizational members and clients accept (conform to) its authority because the rules are defined and administered fairly. Rights and privileges protect individuals from organizational (officer) injustice—equity prevails regardless of "who you are." Rules include policies and standard procedures for implementing these. They are solutions to past problems demanding known responses (we avoid reinventing the wheel). Rules guide behavior, ensuring consistency at every level. Nine out of ten problems encountered are covered by regular procedures. This is a risk minimizing, consistent apparatus.[3] Healthcare organizations of the federal government, such as the Veteran Administration, the military, and state and local governmental facilities, all express the bureaucratic culture.

Entrepreneurial culture is expressed by healthcare organizations that value innovation, creativity, risk taking, and aggressively seeking opportunities. The organizational culture values change, individual initiatives, and autonomy. For-profit corporations, such as HCA, which is headquartered in Nashville, TN, and is the nation's largest investor-owned health system, and the new emergence of specialty hospitals, emulate entrepreneurial cultures.

Finally, market culture emphasizes sales growth, increased market share, financial stability, and profitability. All healthcare organizations, both not-for-profit and investor-owned, government and private, at some point embrace a market culture.

None of the cultural attributes identified can be put in discrete baskets, because as organizations grow and change, their respective cultures can also evolve and change with the organization's leadership.

■ HOW ARE CULTURE AND CLIMATE DIFFERENT?

There are hosts of scholars who study organizational cultures, and it would be naïve of this author to oversimplify the concepts, which warrant future study for a student who truly wishes to delve deeply into the concepts of organizational behavior. The theory behind organizational culture and climate is drawn from research in the social sciences by studying researchers like Gabrielle O'Donovan, Edgar Schein, Charles Handy, Geert Hofstede, and Daniel Denison, all of whom contributed to a body of knowledge that combined theory and practice. A good example is provided by Schein who defined culture as "a pattern of shared basic assumptions that the group learned as it solved its problems of external adaptation and internal integration that has worked well enough to be considered valid and, therefore, to be taught to new members as the correct way to perceive, think, and feel in relation to those problems."[4] Values and behavior, Schein argued, are more superficial representations of this underlying structure. Tagiuri and Litwin defined climate as "the relatively enduring quality of the total organizational environment that: (a) is experienced by the occupants, (b) influences their behavior, and (c) can be described in terms of the values of a particular set of characteristics (or attributes) of the environment."[5] To this definition, he added that climate is "phenomenological external" yet "in the actor's head." Tagiuri and Litwin's definition places more emphasis on the way in which the social environment is experienced by the actors, and Schein's definition places more emphasis on how the social environment is created by the actors; however, both authors focused on the collective cognitive representation of patterns of social learning over time. These two definitions also show similarities in other areas.

Both attempt to describe the holistic nature of social contexts in organizations, the durability of these organizational contexts over time, and the roots of these contexts in the organization's system of beliefs, values, and assumptions. Comparing these two definitions thus suggests that these two literatures may have a far more complex set of similarities and differences than those suggested by much of the organizational theory literature.

The further comparison of the definitions of culture and climate in these two bodies of knowledge support the idea that there are in fact both differences and similarities in the concepts of culture and climate in these two literatures. Fully understanding these concepts requires a more careful examination of the research that is actually done when authors use them.

■ WHAT IS THE THEORY BEHIND CULTURE AND CLIMATE?

Several examples help to illustrate how theorists in both areas have struggled with a highly similar set of generic issues. In theory, both perspectives try to address the problem of social contexts simultaneously being the product of individual interaction and a powerful influence on individual interaction. Organizations are made of individual interactions but are also a determining context for those interactions.[6]

These two theories are similar in other ways as well. For example, it becomes apparent when the "content" of traditional climate research is compared to the "content" of recent culture studies, the culture researchers would choose to describe culture in terms of comparative traits or dimensions. However, when they do, the content of the culture domain begins to take on a strong resemblance to the topics that climate researchers have been concerned with for decades. A good example is Hofstede's concept of power distance—the appropriate social and emotional distance that should be maintained between individuals of different status and power—is highly similar to the concept of "aloofness" introduced in one of the earliest studies of organizational climate.[7] They defined climate as a "belief and value structure members employ as they act in the organization."[8]

Ashforth (1985) also took a similar approach in his examination of the formation of organizational climates. The classical approach of Schneider and Reichers theorized the creation of organizational climates in such a way that fit well with the implicit assumptions about the situated nature of social contexts and the inherently problematic nature of comparison.[9]

Based on all of the state theories, what is the significant difference between the culture and climate? Denison states, "literature lies not in the nature of the phenomenon or the methods used to study it, but in the theoretical traditions that have been borrowed from other branches of the social sciences."[10] He goes on to illustrate that climate literature has its roots in the field theory of Kurt Lewin, whereas the culture literature is grounded in the symbolic interaction and social construction perspectives developed by George H. Mead in 1934 and Peter L. Berger and Thomas Luckmann in 1966.[11] Many of the differences between climate and culture can be understood by examining Lewin's basic concept of the relationship between individuals and their social environments and then considering the implications of this framework for the study of organizations.[10] Lewin expressed his basic formulation in terms of a simple equation:

$$B = f(P, E)$$ in which B = behavior, E = the environment, and P = the person.

Quite apart from the unending complexities of actually computing the predictions of such an equation, Lewin's framework makes a far more basic assumption that has had a strong influence on the study of organizational climates. According to Lewinian field theory, the social world can be neatly divided into B's, P's, and E's. Thus, in order to study a phenomenon such as organizational climate (or culture) from Lewin's perspective, the person must be, by definition, analytically separate from the social context.

■ VALUES AND BELIEFS THAT SUPPORT ORGANIZATIONAL GOALS

The culture of the organization, if it is positive and helpful, can help to motivate staff or at least prevent them from becoming dissatisfied. At International Business Machines Corporation (IBM), the attitude of management, to their employees, is an attraction to prospective staff and would probably help maintain the staff that they have. If the climate does not satisfy the needs of staff, then it will probably become a demotivator, that is, it would cause dissatisfaction and so people would become less inclined to want to work toward the organizational goals.

The culture of today's healthcare organizations consists of the systems of values and beliefs, which are characteristic of their society. These systems overlap significantly with the other components of culture, which were explored in proceeding paragraphs. For example, religious belief systems can affect the cultural significance of how patients are treated or how they receive treatment, or systems of morality can affect the cultural significance of whether or not the organization is a good citizen and adds to the overall benefit of their community.

Belief/value systems overlap so much with these other components of cultural systems largely because beliefs and values play such a pervasive role in culture. In Edgar H. Schein's definition of a growing, changing culture, belief and value systems pass on from generation to generation. Beliefs and values affect virtually every learned behavior; therefore, these systems are a central component of the larger cultural systems in which they exist and greatly influence how the organization executes its mission.[12]

Belief systems involve stories, or myths, whose interpretation can give people insight into how they should feel, think, and/or behave. The elaborate polytheistic mythologies of the ancient Greek and Roman civilizations are a good example of how belief systems can affect the daily lives of a society's members and the role they can play in giving significance to people's actions. The most prominent systems of beliefs tend to be those associated with formal religions; however, any system of belief in which the interpretation of stories affects people's behavior—a system of superstitions, for example—can be a living, contributing component of a given society's culture.

A value system differentiates right feelings, thoughts, and behavior from wrong feelings, thoughts, and behavior. Value systems can and very often do grow out of belief systems. For example, one could argue that the value system behind Good Samaritan Law (a law that protects off-duty medical personnel from being sued for malpractice when they assist someone in an emergency) is a direct descendant of the Christian belief system—a belief system whose story of the Good Samaritan gives the law its name. However, other value systems—those governing incest, for example—appear to exist independently of formal belief systems.

The purposes of healthcare organizations (HCOs) have not changed drastically over time. Benjamin Franklin, conducting the fund drives for the first community hospital in North America, the Pennsylvania Hospital founded in 1760, outlined five principles:

1. Samaritanism and support of the poor—a desire to aid the sick and needy because the aid itself has value or intrinsic merit. In advanced industrial nations, Samaritanism has two forms: tax-supported government programs and voluntary charity.
2. Personal health—a desire to improve the health of oneself and one's loved ones to deal more effectively with disease, disability, and death.
3. Public health—a desire for health as a collective or social benefit to prevent illness, ensure a healthy workforce and military force, and reduce the social burdens associated with disease, disability, and death.
4. Economic gain for the providers and the community—a desire to use the HCO as a source of income and employment and a desire to make the community, as a whole, economically successful and attractive as a place to live.
5. Control of costs and quality of healthcare—a desire to ensure certain levels of quality and costs for healthcare, recognizing that poor quality and inefficiency impair the achievement of the other four goals.

These five motivations are the permanent support for community HCOs. The debates that occur from community to community and from generation to generation are about the relative importance of each rather than the introduction of new ones.[13] Edgar Schein explains that culture can be thought of as existing in different levels. Level one, called an artifact, is the easiest to observe when you go into an organization. These are the things that you see, hear, and feel as you move throughout the organization. For instance, as you enter most faith-based organizations you immediately see religious artifacts, such as crosses and statues of the Virgin Mary or Christ. The individuals' observations and emotional reactions to the architecture, the décor, and the climate are based on how people behave toward each other.[14]

The second level is the espoused values of the organization. In most healthcare organizations, these are often written and posted with the mission and vision statements of the organization. These values express the beliefs of the organization and serve as a guide to behavior. They describe the organizations' values, principles, ethics, and visions and may even reflect the value system of the organization's founders.

The third and final level according to Schein (1999) is the "shared tacit assumptions." At this level, one has to think of the history of the organization. At this level, you find the value, beliefs, and assumptions of the founders and key leaders are taken into account, and how those factors made the organization successful (see Figure 13-1).

The culture of the organization plays a very significant role in how the healthcare organization executes its mission. In today's multicultural environment, the culture of an organization is the foundation for an organization's commitment and accountability for diversity and inclusion, both, which are important in ensuring that all patients are treated with dignity, respect, and in a culturally proficient and competent manner.

Diversity in Healthcare Management

Diversity in healthcare management is important to the U.S. healthcare system as a strategy to advance the effectiveness of healthcare organizations and help them achieve greater representation of underrepresented minorities in leadership, improve cultural competence, and decrease the racial and ethnic disparities that exist in the delivery of health services. There are many definitions of diversity such as the one stated by Dr. Roosevelt Thomas that diversity is the total collective mixture, made up of "main" ones and "others," it is not a function of race or gender or any other us-versus-them dyad, but a complex and ever-changing blend of attributes, behaviors, and talents.[15] Using this as a construct, in healthcare management we use the definition from the Institute for Diversity in

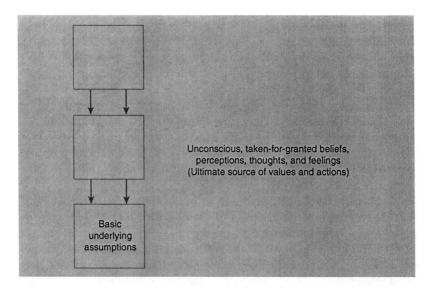

Figure 13-1 Observable Cultural Levels.

Health Management that states that healthcare organizations represent all aspects of society, including but not limited to race, ethnicity, national origin, gender, age, physical ability, sexual orientation, religion, and family status. Healthcare institutions should be totally inclusive organizations that value the differences in their staff and recognize that diversity adds value to the organization, its mission, and the quality of their programs and services.

The need for broad representation of minorities in healthcare management has been an ongoing concern for healthcare administrators and professional organizations, such as the National Association of Healthcare Executives (NAHSE), the American College of Healthcare Executives (ACHE), the American Hospital Association (AHA), and the Institute for Diversity in Healthcare Management (IFD).

A 1992 joint study by the American College of Healthcare Executives (ACHE), an international society of healthcare executives, and the National Association of Health Services Executives (NAHSE), an association of African American healthcare executives, compared the career attainments of their members. In 1993, ACHE and NAHSE published the results of the 1992 study in a report entitled, "Racial Comparison of Career Attainment in Healthcare Management: Findings of a National Survey of African American and Caucasian Healthcare Executives." The study documented that, although African Americans and Caucasians had similar educational backgrounds and years of experience in the field, African Americans held fewer top management positions, less often worked in hospitals, earned 13% less money, and were less satisfied in their jobs.[16]

In 1997, the Association of Hispanic Healthcare Executives (AHHE) and the Institute for Diversity in Health Management (IFD) joined ACHE and NAHSE in a repeat study to assess these indicators, by adding Hispanics and Asians to the study. These two studies have shown that, with minor exceptions, racial/ethnically diverse individual managers:

- Earned less than their majority counterparts
- Felt they received less respect than Caucasians from supervisors
- Felt they received less autonomy in doing their work than their majority counterparts
- Felt they experienced discriminatory acts in the workplace (such as not being hired or promoted)
- Felt that they had to be more qualified than their majority counterparts to get ahead in their organization

In 2003, the survey sponsors conducted a follow-up study and many of these findings revealed in the initial study remained present among racial/ethnically diverse individual managers. The follow-up study showed that more than 50% of the Caucasian healthcare leaders did not feel that diversity and inclusion were issues and that improvements were not necessary concerning the lack of qualified minority health-care leaders. Although some positive strides were observed nationally, researchers estimated that less than 2% of all senior executives were ethnic minorities.

This study is unique because a formal study of this magnitude had not been conducted before. Past research and data estimates are anecdotal at best. There are a few studies conducted on diversity-related measures (such as cultural competency) within healthcare organizations, but these studies aimed to assess the general climate of the environments and the support of diversity efforts. These studies focused on the organization and not on the individual. The ACHE study referenced above is one study geared toward the individual, but that study intended to assess the career attainment and overall satisfaction of minority healthcare executives only and was limited to members of select professional associations (i.e., ACHE, NAHSE, and AHHE). It did not provide a count of individuals in specific job categories by race/ethnicity, which is data that the profession highly needs. Further studies could provide the data needed by healthcare organizations to:

1. Determine whether or not their management staff truly represents a diverse racial mixture and, if not, identify where gaps exist.
2. Benchmark their diversity attainment against similar types of organizations (facility types).
3. Determine if their diversity attainment is appropriate for their geographical location.

This data will also be useful for healthcare associations and executive search firms eager to assess the universe of candidates available for memberships within their associations and for placing these candidates in healthcare delivery organizations. Understanding the number of mid- and senior-level executives in the field, for example, allows healthcare organizations, executive search firms, and IFD to determine where potential opportunities exist for succession planning so that organizations can develop strategies to advance minorities into executive ranks. Associations and executive search firms could become allies in the IFD's efforts to enhance the number of minorities in healthcare management by being co-advocates for encouraging more minorities to enter healthcare management and to highlight the need for more inclusive hiring and retention practices within healthcare delivery organizations.[17]

The richness of the diversity of one's community should be reflected in one's staff and in one's leadership. Therefore, there is a need to have people at the leadership table who understand the community and that can help the organization strategize about how to make the best business case for diversity. Businesses also need to decide who will get involved in training the frontline management staff and the rest of the staff on the need for diversity in their organization and how they can use that to build a more effective organization. By understanding, appreciating, and managing differences, leaders can actually build a better, richer, and higher performing organization.

The ranks of healthcare executives, physicians, pharmacists, laboratory technicians, and especially nurses are far less diverse than the general population, and based on statistics from the American College of Healthcare Executives, the American Hospital Association, and the American Organization of Nurse Executives, the mismatch is of staggering proportions.[18] This means, among other things, a lack of role models and mentors for members of minority groups, a probable concern that the chances of advancement in one's chosen healthcare profession are limited, and the strong possibility that some of the healthcare industry's "the best and the brightest" will seek careers in other economic sectors.

The top jobs in healthcare are still disproportionately held by Caucasian men and although this is a pattern common in almost all areas of American society, it has particularly negative implications for healthcare. For one thing, prospective healthcare leaders may be unwilling to commit to careers in a field that is unlikely to offer them the opportunity to fulfill their potential. For another, succession planning will suffer if current healthcare organization leaders are not willing or able to broaden the pool of aspiring executives. In 2002, the Institute for Diversity in Health Management warned that many healthcare organizations were struggling with the fact that although they are very diverse in some areas—housekeeping, food service, and plant management—their leadership structure does not reflect the diversity in their own workforce. Therefore, when potential employees look for role models, there are not any, and they will look outside their own organizations for advancement. It is extremely important for those who want to be the provider—and employer—of choice to have diversity in leadership.

Societal trends and a rapidly changing demographic picture are forcing many of our hospitals and healthcare organizations to realize that they will have to look for new insights, examples, and best practices to help them on their diversity journey. Frequently, organizations ask themselves questions of how an organization is to succeed in implementing a diversity program if they do not know how to build a business case for diversity.

Large healthcare systems are responding to the challenge. Take, for example, Trinity Health, a faith-based organization, which operates a network of hospitals at the community, regional, and national levels. Trinity Health is sponsored by Catholic Health Ministries, an entity established by the Catholic Church to oversee its healing ministry. Formed by the Sisters of Mercy Regional Community of Detroit and the Congregation of the Sisters of the Holy Cross, Catholic Health Ministries draws upon a rich history extending more than 140 years. Trinity Health is the fourth-largest Catholic health system in the United States. To support their culture, mission, and values, Trinity Health has developed a unified diversity and inclusion action plan. Table 13-1 is an outline of their plan.

Table 13-1 Unified Diversity and Inclusion Action Plan

Commitment and Accountability
- Ensure commitment from the Ministry Organizations, Trinity Health Board of Directors, and senior management that diversity and inclusion is a top priority for the future success of Trinity Health.
- Commit resources, both financial and human, that are necessary to ensure that diversity and inclusion remain high priorities for Trinity Health.
- Encourage and reward a courageous leadership team that is willing to take risks and create opportunities for our diverse associates and new hires.
- Hold managers accountable for creating an environment within their role of responsibility that supports diversity and inclusion by making it a part of their annual evaluations.

Training and Education
- Educate associates, physicians, and board members on the "why, what, and how" of diversity and inclusion.
- To the best of our ability, ensure that a patient's healthcare experience within a Trinity Health organization will be tailored to meet their cultural differences.

Recruitment
- Create recruitment strategies that support our ability to hire key talent throughout the organization.
- Provide clear metrics that measure and track the success of our diversity efforts.
- Ensure we have diverse associates (management and hourly) within our Ministry Organizations that represent the communities we serve.

Retention and Development
- Create retention strategies that support our ability to retain key talent throughout the organization. Create development/career plans for top talent across the organization.
- Identify leadership development opportunities for associates to learn and grow.

Communication
- Ensure incorporation of diversity and inclusion into internal and external communication materials that represent Trinity Health.

Community Partner
- Ensure that community organizations representative of diverse groups are partners regarding outreach and delivery of culturally competent care.

Source: Presentation by Joseph R. Swedish, President and Chief Executive Officer at the 50th Annual Congress on Healthcare Leadership, Institute for Diversity in Healthcare Management breakfast, March 21, 2007.

The business case for diversity is unique to each organization. The circumstances, environment, and community demographics of one organization cannot be generalized to another, and there is no "one size fits all" solution. However, there are some common elements that should be present in designing a business case for diversity. The key components should include the healthcare marketplace, available talent, and organizational effectiveness, which are all key drivers for the institutional investment in and commitment to diversity. To achieve growth, profitability, and sustainability the organization should:

- Expand market share while improving patient loyalty and satisfaction.
- Bridge the marketplace with the workplace by recruiting, developing, and retaining diverse talent.
- Create and implement workplace policies and management practices, which maximize talent and productivity, building a high-performance organization.

History illustrates that there is diversity in the healthcare marketplace, the talent pool, and the workplace. Our hospitals and healthcare institutions cannot afford to miss the opportunity to seek, retain, and cultivate the talent of their employees to compete in today's healthcare business environment. Failure to do so will mean the difference between being a provider and employer of choice and losing ground to a competitor.

Successful organizations have learned that in today's very dynamic healthcare environment, diversity is a competitive advantage for their organization. The *Fortune* Magazine Top 100 Companies have found that people of color bring strategic input to their organizations and generate productive dialogue. Different genders and races bring vital, diverse perspectives, which help their companies succeed.

■ THE ETHICS AND THE SOCIAL RESPONSIBILITY OF MANAGEMENT

Each of us has our own set of values and beliefs that we have evolved over the course of our lives through our education, experiences, and upbringing. We all have our own ideas of what is right and what is wrong and these ideas can vary between individuals and cultures.

As a manager, you bring your own concept of what is right and what is wrong. Every decision that you make, for better or for worse, is the application of these values to the question at hand. The pressures of organizational life make it more difficult. There are the pressures of productivity, competition, bosses, etc. Sometimes managers make decisions that conflict with their own or society's values because of what they see as the pressures of the business world. Dr. Thomas C. Dolan, president of the American College of Healthcare Executives, along with 44 physicians, nurses, healthcare executives, ethicists, academic policy analysts, and religious leaders, attended the Woodstock Seminar in Business Ethics to discuss some of the ethical dilemmas now facing healthcare providers.[19] The meeting was sponsored by the Woodstock Theological Center at Georgetown University; the seminar spanned 2 years and consisted of four conferences where we explored the question, "What are the most pressing ethical issues healthcare providers face?" The group identified the following common ethical dilemmas:

- Meeting patient needs with scarce resources.
- Providing the most appropriate care when providers profit from patient use of specific resources or when rules and regulations conflict with professional judgment.
- Acting in the best interest of the patient when reporting requirements may be in conflict with patient confidentiality.
- Making appropriate care decisions when patients' behaviors contribute significantly to their problems.
- Appropriately using new or unproven technologies

Through a series of often-heated debates, Dr. Dolan expressed that the group conceded, "while not everyone will act alike, all healthcare providers are obligated to make decisions within a basic ethical framework built on compassion and respect for human dignity, commitment to professional competence, spirit of service, honesty, confidentiality, good stewardship, and careful administration."[19]

But, what is the right thing to do when it comes to social responsibility, especially in the healthcare field, is one of the most crucial questions that leaders will face in this century. Is it a leader's job just to maximize profits? Or, should they be concerned with using their organization to carry out other social responsibilities such as controlling healthcare cost, improving quality, eliminating racial/ethnic disparities, employing disadvantaged groups, or managing diversity?

There are five factors that affect decisions made on ethical problems:

- The law
- Government regulations
- Industry and company ethical codes
- Social pressures
- Tension between personal standards and the goals of the organization

Who is responsible for acting ethically? You are! It is not the "company." It is not just the business owner. It is not only your manager. It is every person. Ultimately, each of us is responsible for our own actions, including being ethical.

John R. Griffith states, "Managers have two tools for promoting moral virtue in their organizations: by example and by using the pragmatic systems of the modern organization to promote moral ends. These mechanisms are not perfect. As to whether they are effective enough to be worth the effort, the answer is that we cannot afford to find out. To be a moral leader, you have to accept the challenge."[13] He goes on to say those leaders make moral decisions and show others that it can be done. "The more positive examples there are—and the fewer negative ones—the stronger the moral culture of the organization." Recognizing virtuous decisions multiplies the effect of example by the leader. Conversely, a lack of leadership examples and of reward for virtuous decisions destroys the moral culture of the organization.

There are three elements related to the business of ethics and the first is respect. Respect must be directed to people, organizational resources, and your environment. Respect includes behavior such as:

- Treating everyone (patients, staff, stakeholders, etc.) with dignity and courtesy
- Using the organization's supplies, equipment, time, and money appropriately, efficiently, and for enterprise use only
- Protecting and improving your work environment and abiding by the laws, rules, and regulations that exist to protect our world and our way of life

The second element of business ethics is the responsibility to your patients, your co-workers, your organization, and yourself. Included are behaviors such as:

- Providing timely, high-quality, safe, and cost-effective patient care
- Working collaboratively and carrying your share of the load
- Meeting all performance expectations and adding value

The final element is results. Essential in attaining results is an understanding that the way results are attained—the "means"—are every bit as important if not more important than the ultimate goals—the "ends." Using the phrase "the ends justify the means" is an excuse too often used to explain an emotional response, or action not well planned or carefully considered.[20]

All healthcare organizations are expected to perform at the highest level and provide the best quality care possible. However, you are also expected to accomplish it in a legal, moral, and ethical manner. If you lose sight of the distinction, you jeopardize your credibility, your organization, and your career.

By considering respect, responsibility, and results before taking action, you will avoid the following common rationalizations for not doing what is right:

- "Everyone else does it."
- "They'll never miss it."
- "Nobody will care."
- "The boss does it."
- "No one will know."
- "I don't have time to do it right."
- "That's close enough."
- "Some rules were meant to be broken."
- "It's not my job."

In the health services, business ethics involves much more than compliance with policies, laws, and financial regulations. These are major concerns with high visibility. It makes headlines when these are not obeyed. For those reasons, most organizations do not have problems with these issues. Instead, it is the "little things" that cause problems.

For the individual healthcare leader, it is the day-to-day, seemingly insignificant actions and behaviors by individuals that represent the largest area for ethics problems and the greatest opportunity for ethics improvement. This why most health professions establish guidelines for professionals to follow. The American College of Healthcare Executives has developed a detailed code of ethics and illustrated its preamble.

By following the code of ethics, you will be sure to set the ethical example in your organization. The leader's ultimate responsibility is modeling the behaviors you expect from others. To a large degree, you operate in a fishbowl. Employees are constantly watching you and learning from you. They rightfully assume that it is okay to do whatever you do. Regardless of what is written or said elsewhere in the organization, your behavior is the performance standard employees will follow. That is an awesome "comes with the territory" responsibility, but it is also an awesome opportunity to influence the ethics of your work unit and the entire organization. Giacalone and Thompson, stated ten reasons why leaders should model ethical behavior:[21]

- Reduces pressure on employees to compromise ethical standards
- Increases employee willingness to report misconduct
- Improves trust and respect at all levels
- Protects the positive reputation of the organization
- Encourages early detection of problem areas and ethics violations

- Fosters a positive work culture and improved customer service
- Provides an incentive and framework for ethical decision making
- Increases pride, professionalism, and productivity
- Enhances your ability to attract and retain high-quality and diverse employees
- Ensures the long-term viability of the enterprise

PREAMBLE

The purpose of the *Code of Ethics* of the American College of Healthcare Executives is to serve as a standard of conduct for affiliates. It contains standards of ethical behavior for healthcare executives in their professional relationships. These relationships include colleagues, patients, or others served; members of the healthcare executive's organization and other organizations, the community, and society as a whole.

The *Code of Ethics* also incorporates standards of ethical behavior governing personal behavior, particularly when that conduct directly relates to the role and identity of the healthcare executive.

The fundamental objectives of the healthcare management profession are to maintain or enhance the overall quality of life, dignity, and well-being of every individual needing healthcare service; and to create a more equitable, accessible, effective, and efficient healthcare system.

Healthcare executives have an obligation to act in ways that will merit the trust, confidence, and respect of healthcare professionals and the general public. Therefore, healthcare executives should lead lives that embody an exemplary system of values and ethics.

In fulfilling their commitments and obligations to patients or others served, healthcare executives function as moral advocates and models. Since every management decision affects the health and well-being of both individuals and communities, healthcare executives must carefully evaluate the possible outcomes of their decisions. In organizations that deliver healthcare services, they must work to safeguard and foster the rights, interests, and prerogatives of patients or others served.

The role of moral advocate requires that healthcare executives take actions necessary to promote such rights, interests, and prerogatives. Being a model means that decisions and actions will reflect personal integrity and ethical leadership that others will seek to emulate.

Source: American College of Healthcare Executives Code of Ethics: http://www.ache.org/ABT_ACHE/CodeofEthics.pdf.

■ CHAPTER SUMMARY

This chapter gives a detailed discussion of organizational culture, values, and ethics and how they relate to healthcare organizations. All of these concepts are grounded in management theory and are essential competencies necessary for aspiring or seasoned healthcare executives. The culture of an organization is an amalgamation of the values and beliefs of the people in an organization. It can be felt in the implicit rules and expectations of behavior in an organization where, even though the rules are not formally written down, employees know what is expected of them. Management's decisions on policy usually set up the culture of the organization.

The culture of today's healthcare organizations consists of the systems of values and beliefs that are characteristic of their society. These systems overlap significantly with the other components of culture, explored in proceeding paragraphs. For example, religious belief systems can affect the cultural significance of how patients are treated or how they receive treatment, or systems of morality can affect the cultural significance of whether or not the organization is a good citizen and adds to the overall benefit of their community.

The ethics of Diversity in Healthcare Management is important to the U.S. healthcare system as a strategy to advance the effectiveness of healthcare organizations and help them achieve greater representation of underrepresented minorities in leadership, improve cultural competence, and decrease the racial and ethnic disparities that exist in the delivery of health services.

Ethics teaches us that we each have our own set of values and beliefs that we have evolved over the course of our lives through our education, experiences, and upbringing. We all have our own ideas of what is right and what is wrong and these ideas can vary between individuals and cultures. By adherence to a code of ethics and considering respect, responsibility, and results before taking action, you will uphold high ethical standards in the performance of your duties.

Review/Discussion Questions

1. What are the four cultural structures in healthcare organizations?
2. What is the difference between culture and climate?
3. How can the culture and values of the organization impact diversity and cultural competence?
4. Why does the American College of Healthcare Executives have ethical policy statements?

Learning Activities

CASE: No African Americans Allowed—White Patient's Racism Rules at Pennsylvanian Hospital

African American workers at a major Pennsylvania Hospital were outraged when told they were not to enter the room of a white patient.

Supervisors at the nationally recognized hospital told its African American healthcare professionals, as well as food service and housekeeping staff, not to enter the patient's room or interact with the family.

Administrators said they broke hospital policy to avoid a potentially "volatile situation" by adhering to the request of the patient's husband, that only white employees enter his wife's room on the maternity ward.

"We were wrong," said a vice president at Abington Memorial Hospital. "We should have followed our policy. The whole incident has greatly upset many of our employees who perceived that we were acquiescing to the family's wishes."

Despite the hospital's policy that states "care will be provided on a nondiscriminatory basis," it seems as though patients are allowed to discriminate.

Catholic Health Care West's medical ethicist said the hospital failed in its responsibility to its employees and the community in order to accommodate a patient's racial preference.

"This was a fundamental disrespect of these professionals' skills and their fundamental dignities . . . a hospital needs to stand against this undercurrent of racism in our society."

The Philadelphia office of the Anti-Defamation League (ADL) said that prohibiting African American employees from carrying out the full scope of their duties is reprehensible.

"I don't see why and how a hospital could justify accommodating a request that the professionals attending to a patient be of a particular background," said Barry Morrison, director of the Philadelphia chapter of the ADL. "Certainly, it's demoralizing for the people who work there."

The American Hospital Association (AHA) acknowledged there have been several similar instances its staff knows about and that there are no fixed industry guidelines for hospitals to follow when such a request is made.

With nearly 5000 hospitals as members, the Chicago-based AHA is the largest hospital association in the United States. It would not offer hospitals a suggestion as to how to address that situation.

The supervisors at Abington Memorial were acting with good intentions and sought to deflect any confrontation between its African American staff and the white family. There was no incident reported during the woman's stay.

Since then, the hospital's president sent a letter to all its employees and volunteers apologizing for the situation, which he termed "morally reprehensible."

In addition to creating a diversity task force at the 508-bed hospital, which is located in Abington and services patients from Philadelphia and the surrounding primarily white suburbs in Bucks and Montgomery counties, it has hired consultants, and the hospital is revising its anti-discrimination policy.

Earlier in the year, the AHA bestowed upon the hospital the "Quest for Quality" award for raising awareness of the need for an organizational commitment to patient safety and quality.

AHA said hospitals are constantly evaluating how to provide the best treatment for their patients, while protecting and maintaining the dignity of its employees. They also said that a hospital's constant patient turnover sometimes subjected workers to society's underbelly.

Question to ponder: How do culture, values, and ethics come into play in this case? If you were the leader of this organization, how would you handle this situation?

References

1. Schein E. *Organizational Culture and Leadership*. San Francisco, CA: Jossey-Bass; 1985.
2. Hooijberg R, Petrock F. On cultural change: Using competing values framework to help leaders execute and transformational strategy. *Hum Resour Manage*. 1993;32(1):29–50.
3. Mintzberg H. *The Nature of Managerial Work* Englewood Cliffs, NJ: Prentice-Hall; 1980.
4. Schein E. *Organizational Culture and Leadership* (2nd ed.). San Francisco, CA: Jossey-Bass; 1992.
5. Tagiuri R., Litwin G. (eds.). *Organizational Climate: Explorations of a Concept*. Boston, MA: Harvard Business School; 1968.
6. Ashforth B. Climate formation: Issues and extensions. *Acad Manage Rev.* 1985;10:837–847.
7. Halpin A, Croft D. *The Organizational Climate of Schools* (Contract No. SAE 543-8639). August. Washington, DC: U.S. Office of Education; 1962.
8. Poole D. Future of public and private partnerships in the human services. In D Austin, Z Hasenfeld (eds.). Special Issue on the Future of Human Services. *J Appl Behav Sci.* 1985;21:393–406.
9. Reichers AE, Schneider B. Climate and culture: An evolution of constructs. In Schneider B. (ed.) *Organizational Climate and Culture*. San Fransico, CA: Jossey-Bass; 1990.
10. Denison DR. *Corporate Culture and Organizational Effectiveness*. New York: John Wiley & Sons; 1990.
11. Lewin K. *Field Theory in Social Science*. New York: Harper & Row; 1951.

12. Schein EH. *Organizational Culture and Leadership* (3rd ed.). San Francisco, CA: Jossey-Bass; 2004.
13. Griffith JR, Alexander JA, Foster DA. Is anybody managing the store? National trends in hospital performance. *J Healthc Manag.* 2006; 51(6):392–406.
14. Schein EH. *The Corporate Culture Survival Guide: Sense and Nonsense About Culture Change.* San Francisco, CA: Jossey-Bass; 1999.
15. Thomas RR. Beyond Race and Gender. *AMACOM.* New York, NY: American Management Association; 1991.
16. Evans RM. Sr., FACHE, President, Institute for Diversity in Health Management. Interview by K Grazier. *J Healthc Manag.* 2002;47(3):143–147.
17. Evans RM. Diversity: A common sense solution or a business imperative. *Forum Magazine,* March. Association Forum of Greater Chicagoland; 2003.
18. Dreachslin JL. *Diversity Leadership.* Chicago, IL: Health Administration Press; 1996.
19. Hofmann PB, Nelson WA. *Managing Ethically: An Executive's Guide.* Chicago, IL: Health Administration Press; 2001.
20. Perry F. *The Tracks We Leave: Ethics in Healthcare Management.* Chicago, IL: Health Administration Press; 2002.
21. Giacalone RA, Thompson KR. Business Ethics and Social Responsibility Education: Shifting the Worldview, the Academy of Management Learning and Education (AMLE). *Academy of Management.* 2006;5(3).

CHAPTER
14

Stakeholder Dynamics

M. Nicholas Coppola, Dawn Erckenbrack, and Gerald R. Ledlow

Learning Objectives

- Describe the parity of healthcare model.
- Describe vertical and horizontal organizations.
- What are the principal components of the managed care quaternion, and how to they relate to the logistical elements of the iron triangle?
- How does SARFIT help support and explain the value of the parity of healthcare model?
- How does an understanding of stakeholder dynamics support organizational survival?

■ INTRODUCTION

This chapter discusses stakeholder dynamics and the power stakeholders have on influencing policy and programs in healthcare organizations. Specifically, this chapter introduces the concept of the parity of healthcare.[1] A clear understanding of the parity of healthcare will assist organizations in aptly making policy decisions, forecasting issues with current operating procedures, and analyzing business case analysis from multiple perspectives. Additionally, the parity of healthcare model is useful to the leadership of the organization in creating mission guidelines, organizing resources, and delegating tasks. Furthermore, the model assists leaders in creating vision statements and metrics for the organization. Finally, failing to understand the parity of healthcare model and its utility in the healthcare analysis process may result in flawed or imperfect analysis of the environment for decision making and decision implementation. Students and experienced executives alike will find utility in the parity of healthcare model.

■ STAKEHOLDERS (ACTORS) IN HEALTHCARE

Philosophy about Stakeholders

Stakeholders are constituents with a vested interest in the affairs and actions of healthcare organizations. They are individuals, groups, or organizations, affected by the healthcare organization, who may seek to influence it. A well thought-out and implemented philosophy about stakeholders is prerequisite to a healthcare organization's strategic planning, resource allocation and utilization, customer service, and ability to cope with the external environment. Stakeholders can be classified into three groups. Internal stakeholders "operate entirely within the bounds of the organization and typically include management, professional, and nonprofessional staff."[2] Interface stakeholders "function both internally and externally to the organization" and include medical staff, the governing body, and stockholders in the case of for-profit healthcare organizations. External stakeholders such as suppliers, patients, and third-party payers, including government, provide resources. The healthcare organization needs them to survive. Other external stakeholders are competitors, special-interest groups, local communities, labor organizations, and regulatory and accrediting agencies.

Healthcare organizations must assess stakeholders to determine which are relevant, which are potential threats, and which have the potential to cooperate. Such assessment suggests appropriate healthcare organization behavior toward them, ranging from ignoring to negotiating to co-opting and cooperating, and suggests which of the conflicting priorities, needs, demands, and pressures they present should be addressed by the healthcare organization. Balancing the demands of multiple stakeholders with different interests is a major challenge. Levey and Hill suggest that the need for healthcare organization managers to balance demands can pose "moral dilemmas arising from responsibilities to patients, governing boards, [professional] staff, and community."[3] Balancing these demands maintains ethical values and social responsibility and prevents inappropriate demands made by single-interest stakeholders from predominating.

A stakeholder philosophy is consistent with continuous quality improvement. "For example, patients as consumers were passive stakeholders until this decade."[4] Now they are major stakeholders, as are third-party payers, who aggressively seek to influence healthcare organizations. External stakeholders are a fact, and responding to their legitimate interests while minimizing the effects of inappropriate demands is a necessity.

Healthcare Organizations

Healthcare organizations are dynamic, heterogeneous entities composed of numerous sub-organizations and processes, each of which is linked with other processes and departments in the environment. Various types of healthcare organizations are found in both the private (owned by private individuals or groups) and public (owned by government) sectors. Healthcare organizations may be institutions, the most prominent of which are hospitals and nursing facilities, or they may be programs and agencies such as public health departments and visiting nurse associations. All depend on their environments, the range of health services delivery, and various providers.

For healthcare organizations, policies are officially expressed or implied guidelines for behavior, decision making, and thinking within the organization. They help organizations attain objectives and thus must be consistent with the healthcare organization's mission. When determining policies, healthcare organizations must take into account the needs of the community, patients, providers, and insurers.

The primary objective of any healthcare organization is to provide quality patient care and a wide range of services to meet community needs. In order to provide these services, healthcare organizations must delicately balance cost, quality, and access. For example, a healthcare organization may be unable to hire the optimal labor force required to meet its mission if it does not have the operational funds needed to hire more staff. Alternatively, hiring more staff may not be the solution to an organization's efficiency requirements. Rather, performance of the organization may lie in its ability to hire the appropriate *mix* of staff within the available resources of the organization. In this regard, all elements of overall healthcare organizational performance are contingent on other elements in the environment.[5]

Patients

Traditionally, healthcare patients have been more interested in the indicators of satisfaction, access to care, facility accommodations, and service quality than how an organization is structured to provide that care. This was especially true if this healthcare actor had insurance resulting in little to no out-of-pocket cost. Now, however, a new era of healthcare consumerism exists. Patients, who have learned to expect more from the products and services they purchase, are beginning to benchmark their healthcare services against similar services they receive from the best organizations outside healthcare. Patients are using their experiences and observations to ask pointed questions. For example, if a package shipping company can answer calls in one ring, why cannot the insurance claim center? If an investment advisor can offer a convenient after-hours appointment within a week, why cannot a physician? If a company will accept, without question, the return of a product that does not fit properly, why would not the triage center trust a consumer who shares information about medical symptoms?

Healthcare has not kept pace with the expectations of increasingly demanding patients. Complaints about quality and access to care are common. Making convenient appointments with the "right" practitioner is still a challenge for the average patient. Administrative minutiae have become more time consuming than the actual delivery of healthcare services, and stories of medication errors and the lack of patient safety in different settings are increasingly prevalent. In the midst of this turbulence, organizations known for healthcare excellence—e.g., Harvard Pilgrim and many Blue Cross Blue Shield plans—are falling on hard financial times.[6] As a result, healthcare organizations that do not control costs, while managing patient's expectations of quality and access, will fail to receive the confidence of their patients and maintain financial viability.

As noted above, in today's modern world of healthcare insurance and managed care prospective payments, patients are worried less about the cost of care as opposed to access and quality issues. The concept of morale hazard is a critical economic confounder in this regard and can play heavily into the Damoclean (i.e., frail) relationship between actors within the managed care quaternion (to be discussed later).

For example, third-party payers may have case and risk management plans installed within organizational operating procedures that monitor and guide relationships between patients that are high or costly utilizers of healthcare. High utilizers are often the focus of morale hazard driven economically focused policy-making in frail organizations. It is in the best interests of the organization to deter overutilization of healthcare when appropriate. However, aggressively monitoring and restricting access to care—regardless if prudent or not—may result in the perception of a self-serving organization more interested in profit than quality and access to care.

Providers

One of the greatest fears that physicians have with managed care—and current organizational dynamics surrounding standards of care—is that they will lose control of their clinical practice autonomy. Physicians feel that any time spent away from direct patient care on additional bureaucratic requirements lowers quality. Additionally, providers view decreased patient contact as inhibiting access to patients. Organizations can alleviate some of this fear by continuing to solicit physician input in all policy analysis and decision making. For example, provider participation in policy-making and strategic planning is essential to program success. To discount physician involvement and influence in healthcare policy, such as the Clinton Administration did in 1992 when forwarding the Clinton Healthcare Plan, dooms policy implementation.

Marketing to providers is also an important step in encouraging participation and buy-in.[7] Too often, organizational leadership will concentrate marketing efforts on patients only without first getting stakeholder buy-in from internal physician executives. Physicians need to be enlisted as partners in the process of decision making in the organization. The incorporation of providers will improve organizational quality by helping to ensure the appropriateness of target activities. Providers' active participation will also improve the timeliness, safety, continuity, and efficiency of organizational strategy. Lastly, physicians that are involved in organizational dynamics and implementation are more likely to adhere to the guidelines designated.[8]

Providers are incentivized differently in regard to the delivery of services in today's modern managed care world than their counterparts of previous decades. Many providers find themselves working in capitated environments, with restrictions on referral decisions in complicated peer review clinical practices that may view additional testing for diagnosis as superfluous and redundant rather than thorough and careful. Contrary to the near autonomous environment that existed in the middle and later 20th century, physicians are bounded by practice guidelines, HEDIS standards, JCAHO accreditation benchmarks, and an increased practice of defensive medicine in the delivery of care. As a result, cost is still a major concern to the providers in the care continuum.

Working to achieve high-quality outcomes is generally the goal of practicing healthcare providers. Therefore, any discussion of policy-making or strategic planning with providers must involve a careful consideration of quality outcomes in order to active satisfactory buy-in.

Third-Party Payers

Large insurance companies may be more interested in healthcare costs as opposed to outcomes of healthcare. Furthermore, while interested in healthcare policy as a vehicle to lowering costs, the legislation that surrounds policy-making is only a means to an end of cost controls. However, purchasers of healthcare may see reasonable price controls as a quality indicator and demand to see comparative data from different organizations. Such has been the case lately with many car insurance companies who freely offer their prices for automobile insurance against competitors. This transparent and open system of pricing not only offers an imprimatur of honesty and candidness for the organization, but also can be perceived as an effort to promote a partnership in the insurance industry rather than a cost-driven industry.

Accordingly, comparative data in healthcare may include information to assist the purchaser to distinguish between healthcare organizations' quality outcomes to services delivered. The payer—if not an individual—

may also be concerned about the total cost per employer per year and acuity-adjusted disability periods if economies of scale are achieved to negotiate large-scale discount fees-for-services. As a result, healthcare organizations need a strategy to know ahead of time how to implement a strategy-based partnership with outside purchasers, seen as a cooperative relationship rather than a utilitarian profit-driven one.

Payers want to provide the lowest cost possible for healthcare and are usually willing to sacrifice the time costs of patients in order to achieve that goal. Accordingly, access is a secondary issue to the cost of care and the quality trade-off is only marginally discussed after the cost of care. While risk-managed issues certainly come into play with large-scale healthcare based plans, unfortunately the payer of care will often go with the lowest physician bidder who can validate equally effective healthcare outcomes in an environment of acceptable access. Such is the paradox and dilemma of being a large-scale healthcare payer.

Employers

The employer may also be the purchaser or payer of healthcare in today's complex world of managed care. However, the employer is more often the conduit to a healthcare plan that ultimately reimburses for the cost of care. In this regard, because healthcare is a prospective commodity that is paid for in advance, employers' concerns revolve around productivity in the workforce and the quality and timeliness of care over purchase issues since care is prepaid. Employers are generally concerned with the time away from work to receive care, as well as the payer's willingness to resolve disputes for care reimbursement at the lowest level possible.

Employer contracts are frequently highly specific in regard to the allotted time away from work an employee is able to take for healthcare. Generally, sick leave is allotted in both paid and unpaid amounts. For example, employees are offered a specific number of days per year that paid sick leave will be allowed. Generally, organizations will allow one-half day per month, or six days per year of paid sick leave. Unpaid sick leave will vary from organization to organization. Regardless, employers are concerned with productive hours away from the employment location and will normally be drawn to healthcare plans with a variety of services offering lower access at a decreased cost.

■ UTILITY OF PARITY OF HEALTHCARE IN STAKEHOLDER DYNAMICS

Horizontal Organizations

One of the most difficult leadership skills for healthcare executives to master is viewing healthcare organizations as horizontal organizations. Horizontal organizations are organizations that have cooperative relationships with multiple outside agents and actors. A healthcare actor is any individual, group, or organization that exerts influence on an entity. An agent is a principal lobbyist or representative of a healthcare actor that is trusted with making decisions or statements on behalf of the actor. When poor relationships are in place, actors and agents working in concert can exert so much pressure on organizations that the organization is placed in a position to adopt the will of outside parties rather than acting in its own interest. As a result, it is the goal of every healthcare executive to ensure that harmonious and affable relationships are maintained within the horizontal structure.

From a reductionist point of view, horizontal organizations seek to maintain a level of homeostasis with all elements internal and external to the establishment. In horizontal organizations, it is not possible to operate and survive without forming cooperative relationships with multiple outside actors and agents. As a result, horizontal organizations must maintain a careful balance between mutually exclusive organizational needs and the simultaneous needs of external stakeholders. Failing to balance these simultaneous priorities may lead to organizational failure or loss of competitiveness (also called market share or market penetration).[9]

For example, a healthcare organization that only views healthcare from a business-driven perspective (defined as concentrating on rates of return as the primary goal), may find over time that it has lost competitive advantage with organizations as well as the trust and confidence of customers. Such was the perception of the healthcare industry by the U.S. population in the 1980s and early 1990s. The introduction of managed care principles, such as gatekeeper access, specialty care referral, and preauthorization, resulted in customer perceptions of large, uncaring healthcare organizations more concerned with keeping people away from healthcare rather than fostering care for the ill.

A recent organizational example is found in traditional big-oil companies in 2005 and 2006, where 100% increases in less than 1 year (and higher in some areas) for fuel created distrust for these organizations among consumers. Compounding this perception were record-breaking, billion dollar profits for the fuel companies as well as exorbitant personal salaries and bonuses for executives. These outcomes resulted in a perception of greed and self-fulfillment by consumers for big-oil companies that resulted in the Democratic Congress of 2007 revoking certain tax incentives for these organizations.

Despite these examples, healthcare organizations cannot afford to become too altruistic and empathetic. For example, engaging in an abundance of uncompensated and charity care may fail to promote organizational survival, prosperity, and growth. Clearly, balance is necessary in a healthcare organization participating in a horizontal environment.

Vertical Organizations

The horizontal organization is in stark contrast to the vertical organization. The vertical organization builds a monument unto itself and seeks to minimize reliance on any and all outside stakeholders and actors. In the true sense of organizational dynamics, there are actually few true vertical organizations. As a result, when we speak of vertical organizations, we refer to organizations that attempt to control the environment first rather than living in the environment and becoming a participatory member within the community.[10]

One of the last great vertical organizations was the Ford Motor Company of the early 20th century. Henry Ford not only built cars, he also owned dealerships, transportation companies, steel mills, oil refineries, rubber plantations, tire manufacturing warehouses, fuel companies, and leather and tanning industries. Henry Ford attempted to control all aspects of automobile manufacturing. This philosophy eventually failed; however, many organizations still try to minimize reliance on outside environmental actors and agents.

Some early healthcare organizations, such as the initial Kaiser Health Maintenance Organization (HMO) closed panel model of the early 1940s, also attempted to replicate the vertical organization structure. However, in today's dynamic healthcare environment, few organizations can be mutually exclusive while simultaneously relying on no outside influence. For this reason, we offer healthcare executives a model to guide decision-making and problem-solving development. We call this model the parity of healthcare.

Parity of Healthcare

The parity of healthcare is a unique model that juxtaposes two mutually exclusive models together in an interrelated medium that allows leaders to forecast the effect of new policy decisions on various factors that affect the organization in horizontal environments. The two models within the parity of healthcare are the managed care quaternion and the iron triangle (Figure 14-1). To understand the utility of the parity of healthcare, it is first necessary to present an overview of both the managed care quaternion and the iron triangle of healthcare.

Kissick's Iron Triangle

Kissick developed the concept of the iron triangle in the early 1990s during the managed care revolution in America.[11] Kissick coined the term iron triangle to demonstrate the difficulty in selecting priorities for healthcare as they relate to healthcare costs, healthcare quality, and access to healthcare. Kissick suggested that an understanding of these resource elements would assist managed care organizations in setting logistical priorities.

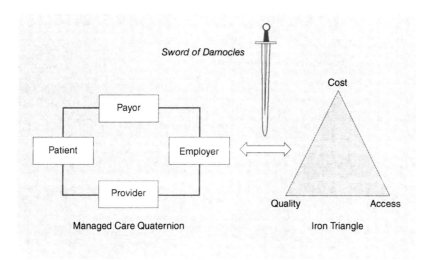

Figure 14-1 The Parity of Healthcare.

For example, Kissick recognized that cost is only one important resource to the healthcare industry. In the iron triangle, costs form one angle of the three points, with quality and access comprising the other two resource priorities. These three factors together are kept in balance by the expectations, cultural goals, and economics of the society that supports the industry. Any angle (or factor) in the triangle can be increased, but only at the expense of the other two. For instance, quality in the American healthcare industry can be improved through great expenditures in additional technology or in training allied healthcare providers; however, the increased expenditures may result in restricted access to only those who can pay for the higher quality of care. As a result, the normal increase in one factor may adversely affect some combination of equifinality of the other two.

Healthcare leaders have used the concept of the iron triangle for over a decade to guide strategic plans, organizational vision, and mission statements. Furthermore, the iron triangle has become a staple and core competency in most accredited health and business graduate school programs in America. Every young graduate student in American should be familiar with the iron triangle and be able to relate it accordingly to resource priorities in organizational analysis.

Optimally, it is every healthcare leader's goal to deliver high-quality care, while simultaneously increasing access to services and lowering costs. However, as health leaders try to make improvements in one area, there is often a trade-off consideration in another area. For instance, increasing access to pharmacy benefits by opening an after-hours pharmacy window may improve access for patrons and can be seen as a quality initiative; however, it may not generate enough new revenue to pay for itself. If the pharmacy window continues to draw scarce resources from other areas in the healthcare facility, its growing drain on the overall fitness of the organization may result in negative influence on other areas—perhaps in professional development and training opportunities. In this case, the decrease in continuing health and medical education opportunities may result in lower quality outcomes for customers. The decrease in quality outcomes may be the result of the organization failing to take advantage of industry best practices that peer organizations have implemented due to their emphasis on professional development and training.

This complicated relationship forces healthcare leaders to think conceptually and in nonlinear manners. As a result, healthcare leaders must make careful executions with new policy ideas or agendas in order to maintain an effective balance between healthcare costs, quality, and access. The cost, quality, and access trade-offs of interrelationships among actors must be considered.

Kissick's model is a vital tool to healthcare leaders; however, the model itself fails to take into account outside actors and agents. In this regard, it is incomplete by itself for dynamic organizational analysis. For this reason, we offer a companion model, the managed care quaternion, and tie both together in a new model we call the parity of healthcare.

Managed Care Quaternion

The principal actors or stakeholders within the managed care quaternion (MCQ) are payers, providers, patients, and employers. Coppola developed the MCQ model in the early part of 2003.[1,12] The MCQ has gained popular support within governmental organizations and some state Medicaid agencies as an aid to healthcare planning and policy-making, as well as forecasting future healthcare needs. Furthermore, the MCQ concept is slowly working its way into the mainstream of healthcare education. It will be an important model for healthcare executives to become familiar with as a tool for decision making in the next decade.

Organizations and organizational leaders cannot be successful if they do not understand the wide-ranging impact of stakeholder influence. Too often in healthcare policy-making and strategy analysis, organizations become overly concerned with isolating themselves (i.e., the organization) as the principal actor around which all other factors revolve. Such was the case with Enron and WorldCom who viewed customers, allies, employees, and investors as tertiary catalysts and insignificant stakeholders in the quest for growth and wealth. Healthcare organizations are no different—regardless of for-profit or not-for-profit status. Stakeholder dynamics are critically important in organizational survival and success.

In order to be successful in the competitive economy of the 21st century, healthcare leaders must be cognizant of stakeholder dynamics and how the principal actors and components of each interrelate and affect one another.

The Relationships between the MCQ and Iron Triangle in the Parity of Healthcare

Perhaps the most significant struggle the U.S. healthcare system has grappled with since the inception of managed care as an accepted healthcare paradigm to the present is the ineffable balance between the business priorities of care and the stakeholder needs of outside actors. These relationships can be conceptually viewed in the parity of healthcare model. For example, as previously mentioned, the MCQ has been used since 2003 to help explain the complex interactions among employers, patients, providers, and payers in regard to partisan and competing views about healthcare. Moreover, these healthcare actors also have dissimilar views in reference to Kissick's iron triangle. The triangle is comprised of logistical factors of cost, quality, and access.

As presented, since each MCQ actor may have different views associated with Kissick's cost, quality, and access options, the potential number of outcomes can be difficult to negotiate. Table 14-1 demonstrates the complexity of this, and assists in explaining why sustained consensus is difficult in developing health policy.

As we can see from Table 14-1, even a slight variation in the prioritization of iron triangle options results in a myriad of inter- and intra-competing priorities from actors that can be hard for even the actors to

Table 14-1 Parity of Healthcare Competing Priorities	
Payer	**Patient**
Cost-Quality-Access	Access-Cost-Quality
Access-Cost-Quality	Quality-Access-Cost
Quality-Access-Cost	Quality-Cost-Access
Quality-Cost-Access	Access-Quality-Cost
Access-Quality-Cost	Cost-Access-Quality
Cost-Access-Quality	Cost-Quality-Access
Employer	**Provider**
Access-Quality-Cost	Quality-Cost-Access
Cost-Access-Quality	Access-Quality-Cost
Cost-Quality-Access	Cost-Access-Quality
Access-Cost-Quality	Cost-Quality-Access
Quality-Access-Cost	Access-Cost-Quality
Quality-Cost-Access	Quality-Access-Cost

resolve within themselves, let alone in tandem with another actor along the continuum of care.

The challenge facing healthcare professionals in regard to employers, patients, providers, and payers is in maintaining high satisfaction with each actor along the continuum of care as they relate to aspects of cost, quality, and access. For example, in regard to quality, a primary care clinic without extended and weekend office hours may be regarded as low quality by the patient and employer, but high quality by the payer and the providers that work in the clinic. However, if employers and patients continue to perceive lack of extended and weekend office hours as low quality, dissatisfaction with the overall health plan may result. A worst-case scenario might result in the termination of the health contract. As a result, health professionals are in a constant struggle to maintain high satisfaction with all elements of the MCQ.

Another example of the complexity of relationships can be seen by revisiting the example of construct development in the "Anatomy and Physiology of Theory" chapter earlier in this book. For example, we learned earlier about propositions and offered the propositional phrase of the "Right to Bear Arms" as an example of the complex nature surrounding the difficulty with understanding the meaning of multi-construct propositional phrases. We suggested that for over 200 years the greatest scholars and minds in our country have debated on the true meaning of our founding fathers' objective in granting the "Right to Bear Arms" to the people.

However, in the aforementioned example, the propositional phrase, the "Right to Bear Arms," has three constructs applied to one unit of analysis—"people." On the other hand, understanding and applying the parity of healthcare is (perhaps) four times as complex due to the addition of four distinct units of analysis competing over three different logistical priorities. The factorial nature of competing priorities within the parity of healthcare results in over 500 potential combinations of echelon rankings among all actors. With the complexity associated with forecasting only one actor's priorities over a sustained period of time, it becomes clear why it is so challenging for healthcare administrators and leaders to accurately predict all future needs.

Sword of Damocles

Compounding the complicated relationship between actors and priorities in the parity of healthcare is the *sword of Damocles*. In Greek mythology, the sword of Damocles represents "ever-present peril." It is also used as a metaphor to suggest a (sic) "frailty in existing relationships." For example, in the parity of healthcare, the sword of Damocles represents an inability of any one actor to reach sustained consensus in reference to priorities of cost, quality, and access. With healthcare priorities constantly changing due to environmental demands, it is no wonder why agreements on healthcare policy are difficult to reach. However, an understanding of the parity of healthcare can be helpful to healthcare leaders for strategically forecasting threats to relationships amid actors and balancing priorities among actors.

As a result, healthcare planners must be cognizant that solutions developed to solve healthcare problems in the current environment may not be solutions to tomorrow's new issues. As environmental demands continue to place pressures on the relationships within the parity of healthcare, healthcare leaders must renegotiate priorities. Healthcare planners and leaders should be aware of this fact and view change as a new opportunity for success and not problems to dynamic environments.

■ THE SARFIT MODEL

Structural contingency theory provides additional tools for supporting and validating the utility of the parity of healthcare model. For example, the underlying assumptions of contingency theory are that organizational structures are open and are not organizationally egalitarian, there is no one best way to organize an organization, and any one way of organizing is not equally effective in another organization. Furthermore, the postulate acknowledges, for example, that one set of organizational relationships in the parity of healthcare might work in one organization with one set of environmental conditions and constraints; however, the same set might not work in a similar organization with its own set of conditions and constraints, regardless of the similarity of the organizations.[13]

A derivative of contingency theory is the structural adaptation to regain fit (SARFIT) theory.[14] The SARFIT theory suggests that the goal of all organizations is to organize themselves as efficiently as possible, to achieve high performance. When high performance is not achieved, the SARFIT theory suggests that the organization undergoes a re-evaluation of its internal processes for producing services and products. As a result, the theory suggests that if elements in the parity of healthcare are not organized efficiently, the organization must re-evaluate priorities and relationships to achieve higher efficiency and performance in future times.[15]

For example, in healthcare organizations, efficiency is usually viewed as the effective use of inputs to generate outputs. In other words, the more that effective inputs are used to generate outputs, the more efficient the organization will be.

Because the fit of organizational characteristics to contingencies leads to high performance, organizations seek to maintain fit and regain fit when they are out of synch; consequently, they are shaped by their contingencies as they struggle to maintain performance. Such adaptation occurs over time. As a result, performance can be measured by examining the various contingent factors associated with the organization, in a systems-oriented approach.[16]

According to SARFIT, organizational performance can be investigated by examining selected constructs and their contingent relationships. The SARFIT model recognizes that not all contingencies place similar demands on organizations. The more varied the types of environments confronted by the organization, the more differentiated its structure needs to be. However, the more differentiated the organization is, the more difficult it becomes to manage its sub-units. Eventually, productivity is diminished if the organization cannot find the right fit to meet those demands.

Contingency theory and the SARFIT theory posit that different organizational forms can adapt to the same environment. Those organizations that adapt most readily have the advantage. Adaptation includes achieving an effective balance between the organization's external environment and internal strategies—similar to our analysis of the managed care quaternion and the iron triangle.

In healthcare organizations, internal strategies include possessing the appropriate technology at the appropriate time, maintaining and hiring appropriate skill levels of individuals, and ensuring that those individuals perform the right tasks at the right time. Contingency theory suggests that the organizations most likely to survive are those that are the most effective at making such adaptations. As a result, understanding the ineffable balance between the managed care quaternion actors and logistical elements of the iron triangle within the parity of healthcare model are critically important.[16,17]

■ PARITY IN POLICY AND STRATEGY

Health policy refers to actions taken by an organization to achieve specific goals and objectives. Health policy decisions often affect the entire scope and practice of the delivery of medical care within society and result in practices and procedures that affect the overall conditions and effectiveness of services provided.[18] Failing to take charge and make accurate and timely decisions in reference to policy-making may result in mission and organization failure.[19] Understanding principal component actors in policy-making is critical to organizational survival and is impossible if not correctly applied.[20]

Often underrepresented in policy-making is the necessary precursor of effective strategic planning. Strategic planning provides a structured process for reaching consensus among different actors and for documenting the thinking that resulted in the original process of consensus making. This is particularly important in understanding the parity of healthcare. For example, strategic planning must be a consensus-driven group process. Strategic planning absolutely requires that key strategic thinkers periodically come together to share ideas and develop a map for the organization.[21]

Understanding the parity of healthcare in stakeholder dynamics assists healthcare leaders in prioritizing scarce healthcare resources and programming those resources against the practical reality of rationing and delivering care to individuals and organizations.

■ CHAPTER SUMMARY

This chapter introduced various stakeholders and the influences they have on healthcare organizations and the parity of healthcare model. The parity of healthcare is a composite model composed of two derivative models called the managed care quaternion and the iron triangle. The managed care quaternion is composed of four stakeholders (actors). These actors are patients, providers, payers, and employers. The iron triangle is composed of three logistical elements of costs, quality, and access. The manner in which the actors and logistical priorities relate to one another is complicated and dynamic. This relationship is constantly in jeopardy of changing due to the frailty of the relationships. These relationships are affected by the sword of Damocles, a Greek metaphor for suggesting frailty in stability of relationships.

Organizations are constantly trying to maximize inputs to create outputs. The structural adaptation to regain fit (SARFIT) model supports the parity of healthcare model insofar that the SARFIT theory is based on the drive of all organizations to be productive and organize relationships as efficiently and effectively as possible.

Healthcare leaders can use the parity of healthcare to forecast priorities and maintain balanced relationships in the dynamic world of healthcare delivery.

Review/Discussion Questions

1. How would you apply the parity of healthcare model in healthcare organizations?
2. Would you describe modern healthcare organizations as vertically or horizontally organized? Why?
3. Compare and contrast the managed care quaternion and the iron triangle.

Learning Activities

Case Study: The Dilemma of the Uninsured in the United States

In the years 2001 through 2007, an estimated 14.6–16% of the American population, or 41.2 to 49.1 million people, were uninsured. In 2004, this number had grown to 48.1 million uninsured. "For the first half of 2004, the most recent Medical Expenditure Panel Survey–Household Component (MEPS-HC) estimates available, 19% (48.1 million people) of the non-elderly population was uninsured."[22] In comparison, approximately 240.9 million Americans had health insurance coverage in that same year.[23,24] Young adults (18–24 years old), American Indians, Alaska Natives, and residents of New Mexico and Texas were most likely not to have health insurance as compared to other groups.[23] The dire situation of the uninsured can be better understood by this panoply of facts from 2001:[24]

- The number and percentage of people covered by Medicaid rose from 10.6% to 11.2% in 2001, but 30.7% of the poor or 10.1 million people lacked insurance (including lack of Medicaid coverage), and women were more likely to take part in Medicaid than men.
- 8.5 million (11.7%) children are uninsured.
- Employed persons were more likely to have insurance than those unemployed, but among the poor, employed persons were less likely to be covered.
- Firms employing fewer than 25 people were less likely in 2001 to offer health insurance as compared to 2000.
- For people *without health insurance* for the entire year in 2001:
  - 23.3% earned less than $25,000, 17.7% earned between $25,000 and $49,999, 11.3% earned between $50,000 and $74,999, and 7.7% earned $75,000 or more;
  - For those between 18 and 64 years of age, 17% worked sometime during the year, 16% worked full time, 22% worked part-time, and 24.7% did not work, while a total of 118,776,000 million Americans worked full time and 23,698,000 worked part-time;
  - 27.6% did not have a high school diploma, 17.4% had a high school diploma, 14.4% had some college without a degree, 10.8% had an Associate degree, and 7.3% had a Bachelor's degree or higher.

In 2004, the situation has worsened, especially for certain populations:

- Minorities were substantially more likely than whites to lack health insurance. Among people under age 65, 36.2% of Hispanics/Latinos, 21.9% of black non-Hispanics or Latinos single race, and 19.1% of other single race/multiple race non-Hispanics or Latinos were uninsured during the first half of 2004 compared with 14.5% of white non-Hispanics or Latinos single race.[25]
- Persons who never married accounted for 24.1% of the non-elderly population but 37.5% of the uninsured population. People who were

married were the least likely to be uninsured: 15.4% of all persons under 65 who were married were uninsured.[25]

- Hispanic or Latino children were more likely than children of other racial/ethnic groups to be uninsured in each year from 1996 through 2004. In 2004, 21.8% of Hispanic or Latino children were uninsured compared to 14.5% other single race/multiple race non-Hispanic or Latino, 10.5% black non-Hispanic or Latino single race, and 8.4% white non-Hispanic or Latino single race.[26]

It is important to emphasize that many *working* Americans lack health insurance coverage.[27] "Among people aged 18 to 64 who were employed full time, about 15% lacked health insurance. However, the rate was 21% for people in the same age group who worked part time. Poor workers were even less likely to have insurance. Almost half (48%) of poor, full-time workers were uninsured in 2000."[28] People without health insurance for the longest periods of time share these characteristics: (1) lack higher levels of education; (2) are 18- to 24-year-olds, followed by 25- to 34-year-olds, and then 35- to 44-year-olds; (3) are non-employed followed by intermittently employed people.[29] In Chicago, the working poor are the most likely to be uninsured; approximately 33% of the uninsured in Chicago have annual incomes between one and two times the federal poverty line (between $16,600 and $33,200 for a family of four).[30] The majority of the uninsured in Massachusetts are employed, earn between $15,000 and $25,000 per year, and are most likely to be under the age of 35.[31]

To compound the problem, a study by the Center for Health System Change reported that at least 7.4 million adults with chronic conditions lacked health insurance in 1999.[32] The combination of uninsured Americans with chronic conditions, and the uninsured with acute episodic conditions, puts a Herculean burden on the healthcare system. People without insurance (chronically and acutely ill) tend to wait to seek healthcare; subsequently, their episodic and non-continuous care increases the acuity of their primary complaint and often is complicated by co-morbidities. The lack of continuity of primary care for the uninsured is a serious problem and as time moves forward, this problem becomes larger and more complex. At the front lines of care for the uninsured is the local hospital emergency department.

Case Study: Overburdened Emergency Departments Threatened by the Problem of Uninsured

Emergency departments across the nation are in crisis because of the "perfect storm" caused by the gargantuan uncompensated care burden of the uninsured, lower reimbursements, and government regulation (such as EMTALA).[33] The Emergency Medical Treatment and Labor Act (EMTALA), an unfunded mandate passed into law in April, 1986, requires emergency departments of participating Medicare hospitals to screen and treat anyone with an emergency medical condition. The viability of hospitals is severely compromised by an emergency department function that reels as the rank of the uninsured grows.[33] Unless something is done (to include dealing with the nation's uninsured), average Americans will find it increasingly difficult to access emergency care in their communities.[34,35]

Americans with chronic disease and without health insurance significantly add to the overuse and abuse of hospital emergency rooms.[35] Sixty-three percent of uninsured Americans with chronic diseases have incomes less than 200% of the poverty level as compared to 18% of the insured.[35] Emergency departments are overburdened by inappropriate use by the nation's uninsured chronically ill.[35] The uninsured utilize the emergency departments of local hospitals at twice the rate of insured persons.[35] The care provided in the emergency department is not the most effective, efficient, or efficacious for primary or acute care needs.[33] The results of years of emergency department misuse include over 1100 closed emergency departments in the past decade, exhausted staff, physicians refusing to work in the ER, and inefficient primary care.[33] Emergency departments are in serious trouble given the state of healthcare, regulation, and the uninsured (uncompensated care). It is not unusual for many hospitals around the country to simply, and often unexpectedly, close their ERs for a short time to reduce growing financial losses.[36] A significant number of emergency department patient visits are from the nation's 42 million Americans without health insurance.[33]

The financial burden of uncompensated care is severe for hospitals and physicians across the nation. "Nationally, an estimated 150,000 people owe $50,000 or more in unpaid medical bills and an estimated 20% of the 1.4 million bankruptcies each year are due at least in part to high medical expenses."[30] In Michigan, "hospitals reported charges of over $1.1 billion for uninsured and uncompensated care in 2000 with associated costs of $456.2 million after accounting for recoveries, offsets, and private payment receipts."[36]

Georgia hospitals report spending over $1.28 billion in indigent or uncompensated care each year.[37] Missouri hospitals incurred $364.6 million in uncompensated care costs in 1995.[38] "Wisconsin hospitals recently reported a 60% increase in uncompensated care since 1996 and nearly a quarter of them (the hospitals) lost money on patient care in 2001."[39] Over 82% of California emergency departments reported financial losses totaling $325 million in 2000, over $8 million more than in 1999, and this financial burden has created an environment that fosters closing emergency rooms; in fact, 10 emergency departments closed in 1999 and more than 60 have closed since 1990.[40]

Physicians are also burdened by the uninsured. According to the California Medical Association, physicians in that state lost an estimated $130 million in 2001 due to the uninsured, uncompensated care burden.[41]

Case Study: Business Feels the Consequences of the Uninsured Problem

Not only do healthcare costs reduce our nation's ability to compete in the global marketplace, but also the loss of productivity due to illness or injury is of concern to any business. For the uninsured, time away from work further complicates family financial issues but also decreases overall productivity of the nation. Median time away from work in 2000 due to illness and injury was 6 days (median for males = 6 days; females = 5 days).[42] A total of 1,664,000 days away from work were reported (those that were reported) in 2000.[43] In 1996, temporary illness or injury resulted in 1,234,000 people between the ages of 20 to 64 years to miss work.[44] Using the median days missing work per person (6 days) and the number of people missing work due to temporary illness or injury (1,234,000) by the percentage of Americans without health insurance (14.6% and removing the 24.7% of the uninsured that did not work), a crude estimate of workdays lost is calculated to be nearly 814,000 days attributed to uninsured working Americans. If those Americans had health insurance, how many days of missed work and productivity could have been avoided? If only 20% of those lost workdays of the uninsured could have been avoided, over 160,000 workdays could have been added to the nation's productivity.

How do you evaluate the problem of the uninsured from a stakeholder perspective? Use the template or model below to summarize your thoughts and discuss this problem with others.

Describe the issue based on the topic/content area/change in your own words (2–3 sentences) (the uninsured Issue is the case study in the chapter):

How does this topic/content area/change impact the following major stakeholder groups? Fill in Table 14-2 below (you can copy and paste the symbols if using a computer).(3 points)

Table 14-2 Thought Worksheet

Stakeholder Group	Overall Perspective ☺ ☺ ☹	Impact on Cost from Specific Stakeholder Perspective ↑ ↓	Impact on Quality from Specific Stakeholder Perspective ↑ ↓	Impact on Access from Specific Stakeholder Perspective ↑ ↓
Example	☺ or ☺ or ☹	↑	↑	↓
Providers: Hospitals				
Providers: Physicians				
Consumer: Employers				
Consumer: Patient				
Third-Party Payers (Insurers)				
Government				

From the table above, explain what is the healthcare industry perspective on this issue over the next 3 years? Look at the topic, individually, from a cost, quality, and access point of view and then summarize the overall industry perspective in four to five sentences below.

Cost: _____

_____

Quality: _____

_____

Access: _____

_____

Overall industry perspective (integrate cost, quality, and access perspectives):

_____

_____

_____

_____

References

1. Coppola MN, Harrison J, Kerr B, Erckenbrack. D. The Military Managed Care Health System. In Kongstvedt PR, Gaitherburg MD (eds.). *Essentials of Managed Care* (5th ed.). Sudbury, MA: Jones and Bartlett Publishers; 2007.

2. Fottler MD, Blair JD, Whitehead CJ, Laus MD, Savage GT. Assessing key stakeholders: Who matters to hospitals and why? *Hosp Health Serv Adm.* 1989;34(Winter):527.

3. Levey S, Hill J. Between survival and social responsibility: In search of an ethical balance. *J Health Adm Educ.* 1986;4(Spring):227.

4. Blair JD, Whitehead CJ. Too many on the seesaw: Stakeholder diagnosis and management for hospitals. *Hosp Health Serv Adm.* 1988;33(Summer):154.

5. Harrison JP, Coppola MN. The Impact of Quality and Efficiency on Federal Healthcare. *International Journal of Public Policy.* 2007;2(3/4):356–371.

6. Ramsaroop P, Ball MJ, Beaulieu D, Douglas JV. *Advancing Federal Sector Health Care.* New York: Springer-Verlag; 2001.

7. Coppola MN. Ensuring physician input can ease HIPAA preparation and implementation. *Healthc Exec.* 2003;Jan/Feb:54–55.

8. Coppola MN, Burke D, Dianna M, Rangappa S. Physician Practice Awareness and Preparedness for HIPAA: A National Survey. *Group Pract J.* 2002; 51(5):13–19.

9. Daft RL. *Organization Theory and Design* (8th ed.). Cincinnati, OH: South Western College Publishing; 2003.

10. Scott WR. *Organizations: Rational, Natural, and Open Systems* (5th ed.). Englewood Cliffs, NJ: Prentice-Hall; 2003.

11. Kissick WL. *The Past is Prologue, in Medicine's Dilemmas: Infinite Needs Versus Finite Resources.* New Haven, CT: Yale University Press; 1994.

12. Coppola MN. *The Managed Care Quaternion.* San Antonio, TX: Army-Baylor Graduate Program in Health & Business Administration, Fort Sam Houston; 2004.

13. Lawrence PR, Lorsch JW. *Organization and Environment: Managing Differentiation and Integration.* Boston, MA: Harvard Business School Press, 250–264; 1967.

14. Donaldson L. *The Contingency Theory of Organizations.* Thousand Oaks, CA: Sage Publications; 2001.

15. Donaldson L. The normal science of structural contingency theory. In Clegg SR, Hardy C, Nord WR (eds.), *Handbook for Organization Studies.* Thousand Oaks, CA: Sage Publications; 1996.

16. Coppola MN. *Correlates of Military Medical Treatment Facility (MTF) Performance: Measuring Technical Efficiency with the Structural Adaptation to Regain Fit (SARFIT) Model and Data Envelopment Analysis (DEA).* (August) Richmond, VA: Dissertation for the award of the PhD in Health Services Research, Medical College of Virginia Campus, Virginia Commonwealth University; 2003.

17. Donaldson L. Strategy and structural adjustment to regain fit and performance: In defense of contingency theory. *Journal of Management Studies.* 1987;24(1):273–296.

18. Longest BB Jr. *Health Policymaking in the United States* (3rd ed.). Chicago, IL: Health Administration Press; 2002.

19. Coppola MN. The four horsemen of the problem solving apocalypse. *Army Medical Department Journal.* 1997;July/August, PB 8-97-7/8:20–27.

20. Coppola MN, Hudak R, Gidwani P. A Theoretical Perspective Utilizing Resource Dependency to Predict Issues with the Repatriation of Medicare Eligible Military Beneficiaries back into TRICARE. *Military Medicine.* 2002;167(9):726–731.

21. Swayne L, Duncan W, Ginter P. *Strategic Management of Health Care Organizations* (5th ed.). Malden, MA: Blackwell Publishing; 2006.

22. Rhoades JA. The Uninsured in America, 1996–2004: Estimates for the U.S. Civilian Noninstitutionalized Population under Age 65, Agency for Healthcare Research and Quality. *Medical Expenditure Panel Survey, Statistical Brief # 84,* June, 2; 2005.

23. United States Department of Commerce. Health insurance in America: Numbers of Americans with and without Health Insurance Rises, *Census Bureau Reports.* Washington, DC: Economics and Statistics Administration, Bureau of the Census; 2002, http://www.census.gov/Press-Release/www/2002/cb02-127.html. Retrieved on December 5, 2002.

24. Mills R. *United States Department of Commerce Health Insurance Coverage: 2001.* United States Census Bureau, September; 2002.

25. Rhoades JA. The Uninsured in America, 2004: Estimates for the U.S. Civilian Population under Age 65. *Agency for Healthcare Research and Quality, Medical Expenditure Panel Survey, Statistical Brief # 83,* June, 2; 2005.

26. Rhoades JA. Health Insurance Status of Children in America, 1996–2004: Estimates for the U.S. Civilian Noninstitutionalized Population under Age 18. *Agency for Healthcare Research and Quality, Medical Expenditure Panel Survey, Statistical Brief # 85,* June, 1–2; 2005.

27. Coppola MN, Croft T, Leo E. Understanding the uninsured dilemma: A necessity for managed care survival. *Med Group Manage J.* 1997;44:72–82, 100.

28. United States Census Bureau. Population Profile of the United States: 2000. *People at Risk: Health Insurance Coverage.* Ch. 15; 15-1–15-2; 2000.

29. United States Census Bureau. *The Official Statistics.* June 22; 1998:5.

30. Seifert RW, Sokol K. The Uninsured in Illinois and Chicago: Close to 2 Million Face Barriers to Health Care. *The Access Project,* October; 1999.

31. O'Sullivan MJ. Caring for the uninsured in Massachusetts. *Hospital Topics.* 1998;76(1):20–24.

32. Parker C. Study: Chronic conditions, coverage gaps = health risks and ER overuse. *American Hospital Association (AHA) News.* 2002;38(7):3.

33. Carpenter D. Our overburdened ERs. *Hosp Health Netw.* 2001;75(3):44.

34. Menninger B. State of emergency. *HealthLeaders.* 2002;5(11):34–38.

35. Parker C. Study claims increasing ER diversions threaten nation's health care quality. *American Hospital Association News.* 2001;37(19):1.

36. CRC Memorandum. Health Insurance Coverage and Uninsured/Uncompensated Care in Michigan Hospitals. *Citizens Research Council of Michigan.* 2002;No. 1061, June:1.

37. Rust G. *Georgia's Health Safety Net: Access to Primary Care for Georgia's Uninsured and Underserved.* Atlanta, GA: National Center for Primary Care at Morehouse School of Medicine: 2000.

38. Burda D. Uncompensated Care Costs Rose in '95 for Missouri Hospitals. *Mod Healthc.* 1996;26(49):14.

39. The Receivables Report. *Uncompensated Care on the Rise.* Vol. 17, No. 10. 10; 2002.

40. Health Forum. Regulatory update. *Health Facilities Management.* 2001; 14(12):36.

41. Fujimoto DR. A shot in the arm for emergency rooms. *Business Journal Serving Fresno & the Central San Joaquin Valley.* 2002;September 13, Issue 322981:1–2.

42. United States Department of Labor. *Percent distribution of nonfatal occupational injuries and illnesses involving days away from work by selected worker characteristics and number of days away from work 2000;* 2001. Retrieved on December 3, 2002. http://www.bls.gov/news.release/osh2.t07.htm.

43. United States Department of Labor. *Bureau of Labor Statistics, Injuries, Illnesses, and Fatalities;* 2001. Retrieved on December 3, 2002. http://www.bls.gov/iif/home.htm.

44. Weismantle M. *United States Department of Commerce. Reasons People Do Not Work: Household Economic Studies 1996.* Economics & Statistics Administration, U.S. Census Bureau. 2001;70–76:2.

CHAPTER

15

Organizational Dysfunction and Pathology

David R. Graber

Learning Objectives

- Understand the numerous factors that can contribute to dysfunction in a healthcare organization.
- Identify key cultural and psychological aspects of healthcare professional groups that contribute to separation and a lack of cohesiveness within the organization.
- Understand leadership and management deficiencies that are common in healthcare organizations.
- Identify conflicting cultures within the organization and the tendency of healthcare organizations to have values and cultures that are not in synchrony with their environments.

■ INTRODUCTION

Many lenses can be used to view dysfunction or pathology in organizations. One lens focuses on the leaders and managers within the organization. While dysfunctions certainly exist and persist at lower levels of organizations, it is the domain and the responsibility of managers to take the needed actions to create a positive environment that minimizes their negative impact. Consequently, the primary foci of attention of writers and academics have been on the CEO or the leader of the organization and, to a somewhat lesser extent, on the mid- and lower-level managers within the organization.

The CEO or organizational leader is responsible for not only establishing the policies and programs of the organization, but also for creating, or at least upholding, the vision and the culture of an organization. Dysfunction can be a reflection of the hubris, egotism, and subsequent groupthink[1] of the CEO and upper management team who, by acts of commission, undermine the organization. Writers on leadership have consistently noted the causal link or connection between deficiencies of leaders and subsequent organizational dysfunction. Kets de Vries and Miller stated, "Our experience with top executives and their organizations revealed that parallels could be drawn between individual pathology—excessive use of one neurotic style—and organizational pathology, the latter resulting in poorly functioning organizations."[2]

On the other hand, the leaders of an organization may not have a clear neurotic style, be well intentioned, and hope for positive organizational attributes, such as engagement, empowerment, trust, and creativity, yet not know how to infuse or instill these in the organization.[3] In such cases, their omissions and the lack of needed action results in the failure to restore the organization to healthiness. Expressed differently, organizations may become dysfunctional due to pathological leaders or due to incompetent or partially competent leaders.

Partially competent leaders may lack clarity or be ambiguous about the organization's goals, vision, and culture. Such leaders may value engagement, trust, and empowerment, but also value control and predictability. They may use participative management on minor issues and switch to an authoritarian style on major issues. Employees then become uncertain or distrustful of the leaders' intentions in the face of varying and changing organizational goals and directives, and conflicting or inharmonious programs and policies.

Healthcare organizational leaders may be deficient in several primary domains including values, vision, culture, awareness of how to motivate humans, developing relevant reward systems, and competence and capacity to effect needed changes. When many of these domains are problematic or undeveloped, then a pathological or dysfunctional organization exists. This article will discuss the relevance of these domains to effective organizational functioning and offer suggestions as to how these contributors to organizational pathology can be remedied.

Healthcare organizations possess unique structural, cultural, and motivational features that pose a unique challenge to creating a unified culture with all organizational members feeling included and motivated. One of these features is the diversity and heterogeneity of employee or professional groups in many healthcare organizations. These professional groups, with their own values and reward systems, pose a challenge for managers who wish to create a unified culture.

■ HEALTHCARE ORGANIZATIONAL GROUPS

A major challenge to creating and maintaining a healthy organization is management's limited authority over professional, licensed personnel such as physicians, nurses, and therapists. Physicians are often not employees of healthcare organizations, yet have considerable power and influence. In hospitals, although physicians may have little or no formal organizational authority, they often give directives or orders to individuals not under their jurisdiction.[4] In a recent presentation at a class of the author's, the manager of special imaging in an academic medical center stated that he reported to two supervisors, the director of radiology (his line supervisor) and the physician's chairman of the radiology department, both of whom asserted authority over him. He noted that other high-level managers, such as vice presidents of information and finance, also expected compliance and assistance. Such fractionalization of supervision generally demands considerable accommodation by a mid-level manager to the varying goals, values, and concerns of unique and dissimilar supervisors and is common in large healthcare organizations.

In many healthcare organizations, physicians are a powerful subculture existing outside of the institutional culture; they expect deference and take action individually or jointly when their interests are threatened. When physician interests are not closely aligned with the healthcare organization, organizational dysfunction will occur on a daily and even continual basis.

Alexander and Morlock described several key cultural differences between physicians and healthcare executives.[5] Physicians tend to have a stronger professional identity or ego than healthcare managers. Healthcare executives are expected to position the organization for the future, with middle to long-term frame of action. Physicians are primarily focused on meeting the immediate needs of patients and tend to have more of a short-term frame of action. There are exceptions, but physicians' principal sense of professional duty is toward serving individual patients. Alexander and Morlock noted that executives also consider service to patients within the organization as important, but they also must be concerned about providing services and programs to the greater community.[5] Executives were described as viewing resources as limited and being highly aware of the need to allocate scarce resources effectively. Conversely, physicians were noted to generally consider resources as critical for quality of care and for serving their own patients.

Although physicians are undoubtedly key actors in healthcare organizations, they are not the only element in the considerable heterogeneity of these organizations. Subcultures exist in very disparate settings in healthcare, such as in the distinct motivational and working conditions of a hospital laundry department[6] and the unique culture observed in the humor, teamwork, and "bonding" of operating room staff.[7]

Nurses have less influence than physicians do in most healthcare organizations and, in contrast to physicians, are generally organizational employees. Hence, the capacity of healthcare managers to motivate and engage nurses would appear to be greater than is possible with physicians. However, primarily due to professional education and socialization, the worldview of both physicians and nurses differs from that of managers. Nurses have been noted to possess stronger values of altruism and compassion than healthcare administrators.[8] As mentioned above, physicians often view patient care issues, organizational resources, and community service in a different light than healthcare managers.

These distinctions and differences in professional subcultures, which possess unique values and desired behaviors, are greater in healthcare than most modern organizations. Healthcare managers must confront this challenge that is intrinsic to and embedded in healthcare organizations. In this sense, an innate pathology exists in healthcare that can only be remedied by insightful management, which understands the motivations and values of a number of different professional groups and creates reward systems that are valued by these groups. Failure to do so inevitably will result in conflict, demotivation, and lack of engagement within the organization.

■ COMPLEXITY AND WORK INTENSITY

In 1982, Smith and Kaluzny's influential book *The White Labyrinth* noted the enormous complexity of the U.S. healthcare system and the considerable skills, competencies, and acumen needed to be successful as a manager or clinician in the system.[6] The complexity of healthcare has only increased since this publication. Complexity, intensity of work, and a multitude of diverse responsibilities is true of many jobs in healthcare.

As described in the first section of this chapter, healthcare workers, clinicians, and managers must be aware of and satisfy multiple influential authority figures and may have several supervisors. The rapid pace of change in healthcare has been a major challenge for healthcare managers and employees. Throughout the 20th and early 21st century, mergers and acquisitions were common in healthcare. Clinical practice guidelines and benchmarks were introduced, as well as new management models or operational models (e.g., quality management, Studer Group interventions). Job redesign and major downsizing initiatives, as well as major changes in reimbursement and information technology, have and continue to be more the norm than the exception in healthcare. Many of these major change initiatives have not come without detriment to employee motivation and performance.

Over 10 years ago, Filipczak noted that front line workers are "dog-tired of all the changes foisted on them by managers. . . ."[9] In the words of management, ". . . we switched from change to change almost as fast as we could read about them in business magazines."[9] There seems to be little evidence that managers typically consider the capacity of employees to undergo and embrace consistent, consecutive, and major change initiatives. Healthcare workers must continue to carry out demanding jobs in the face of major changes that require compliance, cooperation, and often, substantial job modifications on their part.

Continual change in healthcare has exacerbated another major factor, one not unique to healthcare, but one that is endemic in healthcare—job overload and understaffing, and the significant morale and motivational costs that accompany this malady. Job overload and work intensity has contributed to a high prevalence of burnout in the health professions. Burnout is considered rife in the health professions and is evidenced by literally hundreds of academic articles on the topic since the 1970s.

Maslach and Freudenberger coined the term *burnout* to denote a type of stress response in the helping or service professions, among professional groups such as nurses, educators, and social workers.[10,11] The three major negative features of burnout are exhaustion, cynicism, and feelings of ineffectiveness. Maslach and Leiter noted that burnout is not so much due to personal weaknesses or the inadequacies of an employee, but is built or embedded into an organization.[12] In short, organizational features, presumably under the influence of managers, create the burnout environment.

In contrast to organizational dysfunctions that are sourced in the leaders of an organization, in burnout environments the leaders may create the conditions that foster burnout, yet personally remain unaffected by the burnout that is rife in the organization.

Thus, an established feature of many healthcare organizations is a burnout environment that may affect a high proportion of staff and clinicians in the organization. In the experience of the author, burnout is a widespread pathology in healthcare, often fueled by an organizational insensitivity to staff. Consequently, it is not surprising that many healthcare organizations have been unable to eradicate burnout or even effectively control burnout.

■ AMBIGUOUS AND CONFLICTING CULTURES

Healthcare organizations typically include employees or participants who belong to distinct professional groups, with their own identities and areas of concern that may or may not align with those of the organization. Similarly, healthcare organizational values may not reflect the values of the general public and key stakeholder groups. An organizational focus on efficiency and profitability is usually necessary for survival. However, if this focus becomes the raison d'etre of the organization, then the organization will not be compatible with or embraced by the community.

Americans have always valued individuals with an ethic of selfless service and organizations that truly provide compassionate healthcare.

The majority of Americans raised in Christian traditions were exposed from an early age to such stories as those of Christ healing lepers, the crippled, and the blind man, and the story of the Good Samaritan. In the past century, Albert Schweitzer and Mother Theresa's Sisters of Charity received world-wide acclaim. In early American history, many hospitals had religious affiliations. The widespread almshouses founded by benevolent societies or religious groups also may have contributed to values held by many Americans that there should be access to care for all, and the provision of healthcare should be something greater than a purely financial or economic enterprise. Thus, the proprietary or corporate model of healthcare that is devoid of a social or humanistic ethos conflicts with American values. Similarly, healthcare professional groups that have embraced technology and rationality at the expense of humanism and compassion may find themselves ill-equipped to work with patients.

Within the healthcare organization, conflicts between professional groups are embedded and built in to the system. This article has described value and cultural differences between different professional groups in hospitals, such as nurses, physicians, and administrators. Even within professional groups, cultural differences exist. Hojat et al. studied two groups of medical students and identified their specialty 25 years after graduation.[13] Physicians were noted to belong to one of two groups: (1) people-oriented specialties, such as family medicine and general pediatric physicians; and (2) technology-oriented specialties, such as surgical specialties, oncology, and cardiology physicians. Analyzing scales administered in medical school, physicians in the technology-oriented specialties had shown a greater focus on economic rewards and a lesser focus toward interpersonal relationships and the community than physicians in the people-oriented specialties had. The authors noted that personal values at the inception of medical education were associated with the nature of later physician practice. Such distinctions in values among physicians and within or between professional groups are a key ingredient in the diverse subcultures that exist in healthcare organizations.

When a healthcare organization does not succeed in establishing a strong, overarching culture with members feeling a sense of belonging and loyalty to the overall good of the organization, then small and great dysfunctions will exist throughout the organization. See an example of this in a communication to the author from a hospital CEO. (S.H. Fine, personal communication, February 22, 2007):

> In the "non-system," that of most formalized hospital medical groups, there is constant infighting and maneuvering among constituencies (e.g., cardiologists, vascular surgeons and radiologists fighting over who will "own" peripheral endovascular procedures). The cardiologists care not how their push for expanding the definition of "cardiology" to include interventional work in areas of the body distal

to the heart may impact upon the ability of the hospital to maintain a viable vascular surgery or interventional radiology service, and the GI physicians care not how stripping away the better paying, lower risk endoscopy procedures may impact upon the hospital's ability to maintain proficiency and capability to deal with the more complicated and emergent cases. In short, many parties don't particularly care about how changing one element may impact upon the rest of the organization. However, there are certainly other groups and individuals who commit to the mission and values of the organization, and set aside or modify opportunities to maximize personal gain in favor of supporting the broader community.

Consequently, physician groups may be competing with each other, and also acting against administration and the good of the hospital with little concern for the greater good or the need to maintain a financially viable workplace. Another casualty in the professional arrogation of influence or turf may be the quality of care received by the patient.

■ HEALTHCARE MANAGEMENT AND ORGANIZATIONAL DYSFUNCTION

Kets de Vries and Miller described various types of neurotic organizations.[2] One is the *dramatic* organization that may have a bold, charismatic leader, yet still be fundamentally unsound. The *paranoid* organization typically insists on control mechanisms and both external and internal organizational intelligence for protection and sustainability. The *compulsive* organization is characterized by dogmatism, inflexibility, and submission to orders and initiatives. The *depressive* organization is pessimistic, with members feeling helpless, at the mercy of external events, and often inhibited or indecisive in action. In the *schizoid* organization, many members are cold, unemotional, and withdrawn. They may be indifferent to praise or criticism and largely uninvolved with their organization.

The reader with healthcare experience may recognize one or more of these types of neurotic organizations. Each of these types of organizations may manifest due to a leader possessing a particular neurotic quality. Much has been written about the "dark side" of charisma and how a charismatic personality can severely harm or even destroy an organization.[14,15] Certainly, many charismatic personalities have greatly influenced healthcare delivery. Florence Nightingale's charm, insight, organizational skills, and self-abnegation during the Crimean War essentially created the modern model of nursing.[16] On the other hand, leaders like Richard Scott of Columbia/HCA have been enormously destructive to their organizations. Due to external forces, negative publicity and lawsuits, and the need to comply with regulatory and accreditation standards, some organizations may gravitate toward a paranoid model. Healthcare organizations that fail to motivate or engage employees and who fail to develop a sense of membership among diverse professional groups may also incline toward dysfunctionality.

In healthcare, there are powerful forces that may propel organizational leaders toward a neurotic style. In fact, these forces are so substantial that failure to respond to them may automatically begin to engender a negative environment. Healthcare organizations are replete with dualistic or segregated areas of influence and responsibility. These have been discussed in this article and include management authority versus clinical authority; organizational allegiance versus professional allegiance; substantial external forces dictating change versus organizational-based change initiatives; and community values versus efficiency and financial values and imperatives.

■ CONCLUSION

To avoid neurosis and dysfunction, healthcare organizations must begin to develop a comprehensive approach to management that addresses the entrenched, structural challenges to optimal functioning that have been described in this chapter. Healthcare organizations should seek to hire and promote employees that care for patients and other employees and have the capacity to provide patient-centered care. Many organizations extol this attribute, but few have an intense focus on achieving a humanistic, caring environment. Such a patient orientation is a foundation for the quality care that the community expects. A patient-oriented culture will be aligned with American values and is likely to ultimately contribute to the prosperity of the healthcare organization. Until healthcare organizations achieve a caring culture, they will not be fully recognized and valued by the community and will continue to suffer from the pathology manifested in an uncaring, sterile environment.

Healthcare organizations should find mechanisms for integrating the diverse professional groups within a functional and recognizable organizational culture. One step toward achieving this is to formulate common overarching values that have meaning and relevance to all organizational members. It is also important to create distinct reward systems for healthcare professionals, such as physicians, nurses, and therapists. Due to the high preponderance of clinical or unit managers within healthcare organizations without management training, many healthcare organizations are deficient in managers who know how to run a meeting, deal with conflict, give performance appraisals, and competently carry out the essential functions of management. This can be remedied by instituting in-house training in management. Programs to develop physician leaders may also be adopted. Another approach used successfully in some hospitals is to use leadership assessment tools that give as much weight to personal characteristics like honesty, humility, and caring as to technical skills and knowledge (G. Mikitarian, personal communication, February 18, 2007). Such programs may help an organization to develop servant leaders or the Level five leaders identified by Collins.[17] Level five leaders are said to possess humility and to be unassuming, yet have an intense professional will and focus to transform the organization from a good one to a great one.

These are some of the steps that will reduce the chances that an inherently unbalanced, neurotic, or self-absorbed personality will take over all or part of the healthcare organization. A strong culture that values solid, caring management and that has institutionalized some of the programs described here will be unlikely to tolerate individuals who seek to sidetrack the organization and promote themselves. This chapter has argued that neuroses are common and often entrenched in healthcare organizations.

Countering these negative influences and patterns is not simple and does require an intense focus by management. However, creative and consistent management programs and clear organizational values can be effective as *treatments*. To put it simply, this is the right thing to do and is what organizations should do to better serve sick and disabled individuals who need quality care and a caring environment.

■ CHAPTER SUMMARY

Dysfunction in healthcare organizations may stem from neurotic, harmful leaders or may arise from well-meaning, but ineffective leaders. Healthcare professional groups may contribute to organizational dysfunction due to management's failure to address the dissimilarities in their work and their varying values and cultures. The demanding nature and stresses of work in healthcare experienced by a large proportion of an organizational workforce may contribute to a pathological healthcare environment. Healthcare organizations with cultures that do not match community values will not be adapted by the community and will fail to achieve their potential. External forces such as governmental and political influences, as well as legal threats, may contribute to neuroses in healthcare organizations. Healthcare organizations may develop optimal functioning through employee and management training and engagement and working to develop a unified culture.

Review/Discussion Questions

1. What are the internal cultural forces that can contribute to organizational pathology?
2. How do job overload and job intensity affect employees and the healthcare organization?
3. How can leaders or managers who will exemplify and contribute to a healthy organization be developed?
4. What values should a healthcare organization embrace and enact to be accepted by the community and by the individuals it serves?

References

1. Janis I. *Groupthink* (2nd ed.). Boston, MA: Houghton Mifflin; 1982.
2. Kets de Vries M, Miller D. *The Neurotic Organization: Diagnosing and Changing Counterproductive Styles of Management.* San Francisco, CA: Jossey-Bass; 1984.
3. Kerr S. On the folly of rewarding A, while hoping for B. *Academy of Management Executive.* 1995;9(1):7–14.
4. Scott R. Managing professional work: Models of control for health organizations. *Health Service Research.* 1982;17(3):213–239.
5. Alexander J, Morlock LL. Multi-institutional arrangements: Relationships between governing boards and hospital chief executive officers. *Health Service Research.* 1985;19(6Pt1):675–699.
6. Smith DB, Kaluzny AD. *The White Labyrinth.* Ann Arbor, MI: Health Administration Press; 1986.
7. Cushman (Producer). *Hospital Corporate Cultures* (Film). Los Angeles, CA: Hospital Satellite Network; 1984.
8. Thorpe K, Loo R. The values profile of nursing undergraduate students: Implications for education and professional development. *Journal of Nursing Education.* 2003;42(2):83–90.
9. Filipczak B. Weathering change; Enough already. *Training.* 1994;September, 23–29.
10. Maslach C. Burned-out. *Human Behaviour.* 1976;5:16–22.
11. Freudenberger HJ. Staff burnout. *Journal of Social Issues.* 1974;30(1):159–165.
12. Maslach C, Leiter MP. *The Truth about Burnout : How Organizations Cause Personal Stress and What to Do About It.* New York, NY: Jossey-Bass; 1997.
13. Hojat M, Brigham T, Gottheil E, Xu G, Glaser K, Veloski J. Medical students' personal values and their career choices a quarter-century later. *Psychological Reports.* 1998;83:243–248.
14. Hogan R, Raskin R, Fazzini D. The dark side of charisma. In Clark KE, Clark MB (eds.), *Measures of leadership.* West Orange, NJ: Leadership Library of America; 1990.
15. House RJ, Howell JM. Personality and charismatic leadership. *Leadership Quarterly.* 1992;3(2):81–108.
16. Gillian G. *Nightingales: The Story of Florence Nightingale and her Remarkable Victorian family.* New York: Ballantine Books; 2004.
17. Collins J. *From Good to Great: Why Some Companies Make the Leap and Others Don't.* New York: Harper Business; 2001.

Organization Development and Change

"He who loves practice without theory is like the sailor who boards ship without a rudder and compass and never knows where he may cast."

Leonardo da Vinci

16

Transformational Change and Development

Jim Whitlock

LEARNING OBJECTIVES

- Understand the relationship of organization development and change.
- Differentiate between transitional change and transformational change.
- Apply analytical approaches to assessing organizational change.
- Understand the significance of organizational culture to the effective implementation of change initiatives.
- Apply concepts of *systems thinking* and team building to the implementation of change initiatives.

■ INTRODUCTION

Healthcare emerged from the shadows of social responsibility in the mid-1960s to address a new and challenging environment. Events occurring in the mid-1990s signified the end of "one kind of history."[1] Although healthcare was not considered an industry until mid-century, the focus has always been on clinical knowledge as opposed to economic productivity. However, the challenges of the 21st century reinforce the need for solidarity and balance between radical reform and incremental changes to the healthcare system.

Healthcare, unlike other industries, is highly fragmented and subject to constant and unpredictable change.[2] The industry response to change has been complicated by the unique relationships with its stakeholders and the control they exert on strategic initiatives. These relationships can and do create barriers to change.

The events of the 1960s and 70s, specifically technological advances, the Medicare/Medicaid program, and the entrance of investor-owned companies into healthcare, have transformed the healthcare environment from a local social responsibility to a national economic industry. Consequently, differing viewpoints relative to the scope and speed of the necessary changes have created frustration and produced limited benefits. Steven Shortell's model in Figure 16-1 demonstrates the relationship between the scope and speed of change as the healthcare industry struggles to transform a highly fragmented delivery system. [3]

Incremental changes associated with state healthcare reform efforts have been narrowly gauged and rapidly implemented, compared to the broad and radical initiatives proposed by the Clinton Administration in 1994. Health policy analysts in the 1990s predicted an evolutionary and incremental rate of change, focusing on benefit packages that would cover more Americans and include accountability mechanisms for all stakeholders.[3]

As healthcare began the transition to an industry, organization development (OD) practitioners, such as Tannembaum, Argyris, McGregor, Shepard, Burkhard, and others, were advocating for a "total organizational culture change program. . . ."[4] The emphasis of this new approach was the worker/supervisor relationship. Peter Drucker's prediction of an "employee society" and a resulting "knowledge worker" in 1950 is evidenced by the results of OD research in the 1960s and correlates with the current transformation trends of the healthcare industry. Research in

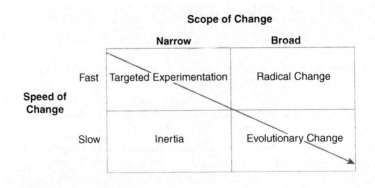

Figure 16-1 Assessing Approaches to Change.

OD provides a basis and a variety of models from which effective change in healthcare organizations can occur. Rothwell and Sullivan report findings from the research field that suggest:

- Expertise is not just held by experts, but exists throughout the organization—especially by those who are closest to the problem.
- "Resistance to change" does not have to be a given. When people are involved in the change process, not only does cooperation increase, but the quality of the outcome dramatically improves.
- It is possible to solve not only the problem at hand; even contentious issues can significantly increase individual, team, and organizational ability to function more effectively. This is the "development" in organization development.[5]

Change models reflect a simplified process in the initiation and implementation of change strategies. Most models are rational models, emphasizing planning and problem solving or sociological models that focus on changing unique situations, rather than change per se.[5] We will consider both types in this review.

■ ORGANIZATIONAL DEVELOPMENT: FRAMEWORK FOR CHANGE

Healthcare's Changing Environment

Change within the healthcare industry is occurring at an exponential rate. Although change is not new to healthcare, the underlying reasons for change are diverse compared to other industries. Consumer perception that healthcare is a right has inspired regulatory changes that affect both access and quality of care, adding to the already escalating costs. The entry of investor-owned companies into the acute-care markets in the late 1960s has created a challenging and changing healthcare environment, which threatens the survival of those unable to adjust to the trends of the industry.

Other factors contributing to unpredictable changes in the healthcare industry include the exclusive expertise of the providers, the physician/hospital relationship and related referral patterns, the absence of a traditional competitive market, and the fragmentation of the industry.[6]

Consistent with the *whitewater* changes occurring in the industry, healthcare is in a state of transformation and restructuring, integrating a vast network of diverse enterprises. The consolidation of healthcare networks appears to have peaked around 1996; however, in 2003, 100 hospitals were involved in 68 mergers and acquisitions.[7] These and other changes have forced healthcare leaders to reconsider traditional systems for delivering care and the subsequent need to transform the industry.

Organization Development and Change Management

Organization development (OD) is a relatively new concept of organizational improvement strategies. Its evolution in the 1950s and 60s was inspired by researchers such as Kurt Lewin in 1946 (the grandfather of applied behavioral science), Wilfred Bion and his work with the Tavistock laboratories in 1948, and Douglas McGregor's Theory X and Theory Y in 1954. Building on their research, practitioners Dick Beckhard and Herb Shepard are credited with coining the term "OD" in 1957.[5] Although the concept is new, the healthcare industry has adopted it as a framework for developing strategies of sustained change initiatives.[8]

Rothwell, Prescott, and Taylor report six key trends of change that have the greatest impact on the workplace: (1) changing technology, (2) increasing globalization, (3) continuing cost containment, (4) increasing speed in market change, (5) growing importance of knowledge capital, and (6) increasing rate and magnitude of change.[9] The changing technology of the healthcare industry requires rapid advances in human know-how and the growing importance of *knowledge capital*. The continuing decline of profit margins and escalating cost demand flexible cost containment strategies that can be implemented quickly and effectively. In an effort to respond to these demands, the healthcare industry is focusing its strategic management efforts around an emerging second-generation concept of OD. These strategies include organizational transformation, organizational culture, the learning organization, high-performance work teams, and total quality management (TQM).[10]

Defining Change

The concept of *change* is far too broad to justify any one definition. Extenuating circumstances and unpredictable shifts within the healthcare industry require a strategic management model that addresses both *change* and *changing*. Visionary leaders must be alert to external change and have the organization prepared to respond by changing internally. Consequently, everyone in the organization plays a role in change management.

Among the many definitions of change reported in the literature, transitional and transformational changes provide the most practical distinction relative to the scope and depth of change. Transitional change, sometimes referred to as developmental change, is associated with the incremental adjustment or "tweaking" of processes. These changes may or may not influence the variables and methods of measurement within the system but are designed to improve the system outcomes. Transitional change initiatives are planned and typically occur at divisional levels of the organization, representing a bottom-up process of change. Effective transitional changes integrate with other organizational changes to achieve the overall goals and objectives.

Transformational change is associated with organizational restructuring and represents a broad and complex radical shift, as the organization "reinvents itself." Although strategies associated with transformational change are controllable, the forces that drive the change are not. Consequently, healthcare providers unprepared to make the shift in a timely manner generally do not survive.

Change Models

An effective change process, whether incremental (transactional) or organization wide (transformational), generally follows a definable sequence of events. Depending on the scope and depth of the change initiatives, the process can be very complex and difficult to organize. A simplified representation of the phenomenon is best depicted by modeling the various change interventions; creating a picture of the phases through which the changes travel. Two approaches typically applied to the development of a change model include the *rational* approach, which focuses on planning, problem solving, and execution and a more subjective sociological orientation applicable to an organization-wide transformation.

Many different models have been designed to inspire effective change and assist leaders in the implementation. Kurt Lewin, an early behavioral science practitioner, designed a model for industry in the early 1940s that focused on the forces driving and resisting change initiatives. His *force field analysis model* is still used by many organizations to demonstrate the unfreezing, moving, and refreezing of behavior consistent with early change philosophy.

The *action research model* represents a philosophy of change, which incorporates employee participation, engagement, and empowerment into the change process. A more contemporary model, the *appreciative inquiry model*, focuses the attention of the organization on the positives (things that are going right) as opposed to the traditional negatives (things that are going wrong).[5]

Although there is no best model to ensure sustained organizational change, there is consensus that change is best represented as a cyclical process with no beginning, middle, or end; the objective being to create a *learning organization* that continually reinvents itself, based on external and internal environmental forces. Figure 16-2 reflects the common phases associated with organizational change.

A simplified linear model in Figure 16-3, developed by W. W. Burke, suggests three phases of a change initiative: pre-launch, launch, and post-launch. Each phase incorporates essential activities that lead to the next phase and terminates as the organization incorporates the change into the system. In the pre-launch phase, the external and internal environments are assessed and the need for change is established. The launch phase incorporates data collection and collation to justify the change initiative. This

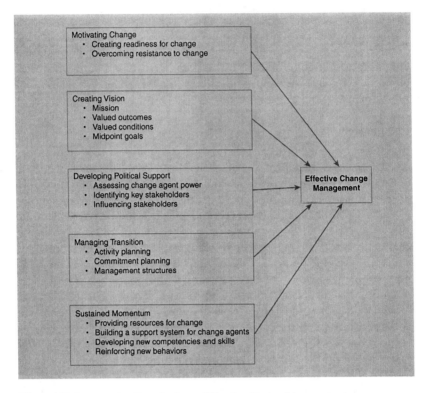

Figure 16-2 Activities Contributing to Effective Change Management.

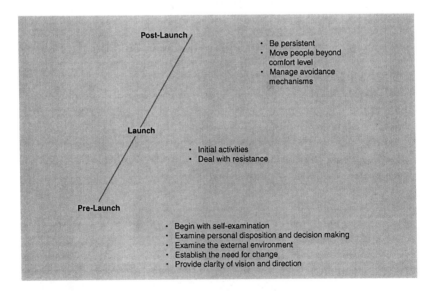

Figure 16-3 A New View of the Action Research Model.

phase focuses attention on communicating the vision to all stakeholders, both internally and externally. Ultimately, the change is incorporated into the organization (institutionalized) and becomes an element of the organization culture.

Ironically, the early change models were not designed for the rapid, chaotic, *whitewater* change that the healthcare industry is experiencing. Consequently, Roland Sullivan and William Rothwell expanded the Burke model to reflect the more appropriate cyclical nature of the contemporary *learning organization* by adding phases of *scanning, acting,* and *reacting,* in a cyclical format (Figure 16-4).[5] Although the expanded model addresses the phases and steps through which effective change must proceed, it assumes leadership skills and establishes an organizational culture prior to the launch phase of the initiative. However, incorporating the many different variables into a simple model would result in a complex and busy representation that could be confusing and frustrating to management, especially since most change models are top-down directed and give little consideration to middle management.

In reviewing the numerous alternatives to change models, commonalities emerge. Most agree that an awareness of the need for change is an initial step in the process, resulting from internal and external analysis of the relative environments. Data collected from the environmental assessments lends credibility to the need for change and is used to communicate

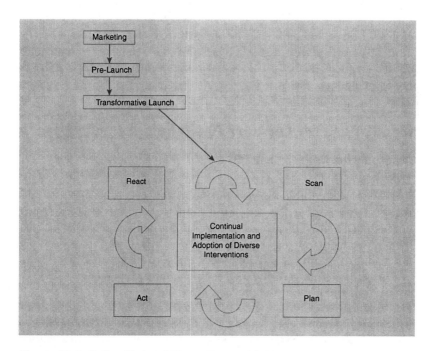

Figure 16-4 Sullivan/Rothwell Change Process Model.

the vision to the stakeholders of the organization. Representing organizational divisions, change teams are empowered to act on behalf of the organization in the development of innovative alternatives that complement the change initiatives. Ultimately, the selected alternatives are implemented and institutionalized. Monitoring and benchmarking ensure the effective outcome of the initiative and provide a base from which the process recycles.

As significant as they are to the process, change models cannot ensure that behavioral change will occur or be sustained over time. There is agreement in the industry that fundamentally changing the values and belief systems of the employees is essential to survive in a competitive, yet compassionate market.[11] Consequently, the effectiveness of organizational change lies with the leadership and senior management. The culture of the organization is a reflection of the leadership and an expression of the values that drive the mission and vision.

Although involving people throughout the organization in the change process is advocated by Rothwell's research, preparing those to be empowered to act on behalf of the organization is both critical and difficult. Empowering those who do not wish to be empowered is an assurance of failure. Consequently, establishing a clearly defined representation of the process, a unique model, customized for the organization, will not only support the initiative but also help to keep the process on track throughout the various phases. Figure 16-5 represents one alternative that incorporates the transformational philosophy of organization-wide change with the transactional philosophy of integrated operational change. The model also correlates the leadership and management competencies needed to efficiently move the organization through the respective phases of the change process.

■ CREATING THE CAPACITY TO CHANGE

Assessing the Need to Change

Whitewater change inspires strategies that produce a "quick-fix" mentality for solving problems. Recognizing that there are unique situations that do require immediate attention, transforming the organization is not included among them. Stakeholders in the healthcare system are demanding valued-added services at all levels of the organization and are not willing to wait while providers decide how to effectively deliver them.

Operational frameworks, such as total quality management (TQM), continuous quality improvement (CQI), and reengineering, have not proven effective in reducing costs or significantly improving the quality of care. The micromanagement of these initiatives by top management represents a barrier to sustained and discontinuous change programs, leaving a perception of the "flavor of the month" change

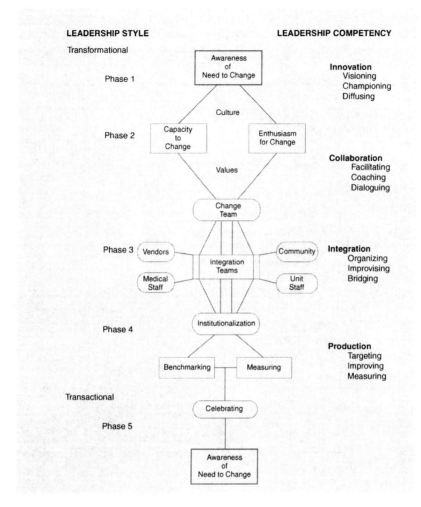

Figure 16-5 Leadership Style and Competency.

process. The justification for failed change initiatives is typically applied to the radical and somewhat unpredictable *whitewater* changes previously described, suggesting "it's hard to remember that the objective is to drain the swamp, when there are alligators nipping at our heels." However, healthcare leaders must not lose sight of the mission of social responsibility to those they serve, the patients and potential patients of the service area.

As the transformation of the healthcare delivery systems continues to evolve, the acute care hospital has shifted from a central focus in the delivery system to that of a primary stakeholder, alongside the physician community, the insurance and managed care companies, and the community at large. Healthcare providers have also experienced a corresponding loss of influence associated with decision making and environmental change.

The awareness of the need to make radical changes in the organization becomes most obvious in the evolution of new and diversified healthcare markets. Although the local hospital continues to be the perceived focal point for healthcare needs, the breadth and depth of network providers has inspired significant changes in the external environment. A good example is the decision by the American Hospital Association to change the name of the organization to "Hospitals and Health Networks."[12]

Identifying Change Initiatives

The decision to change goes beyond the boardroom and the senior manager's office suite. Change initiatives threaten the balance of power held by primary stakeholders in the organization. The perceived threat of losing power creates a barrier to change, while those who stand to gain power will likely embrace the desired changes. Consequently, the awareness of the need to change must address the diverse interests of all stakeholders if consensus is to be achieved. Complete agreement among stakeholders is seldom achieved.

One alternative approach to reaching consensus is the application of the previously described appreciative inquiry philosophy. By focusing on creative outcomes and individual stakeholder benefits, organizational values can be clearly articulated.[13] Successful healthcare organizations are continually monitoring the external environment in an effort to anticipate and predict forces of uncontrollable change. When the responsibility for identifying these forces is expanded to the primary stakeholders, the potential for effective and timely implementation of organizational change is enhanced.

Change Leaders

This chapter is not about defining leadership or identifying effective attributes of good leaders; it is about leading change. The term "leadership" is ambiguous, at best, and suggests positions of power, authority, and control. The phenomenon of leading change incorporates a diverse set of leadership skills that must be applied through each phase of the change initiative if the process is to succeed. The change agents must exert appropriate influence on the system to ensure that anticipated behavioral changes are endorsed and supportive of the intended transformational effort.

Researchers debate the question as to whether change leadership is the property of an individual or the property of the associated social system.[14] A suggested response to this debate is, "it depends." Figure 16-5 demonstrates the discontinuous process of transformational change and the incremental phases through which the process proceeds, beginning with an awareness of the need to change and terminating with the institutionalization of the change initiative. Each phase represents sociological interventions that require the application of different skill sets by the change leaders, whether individuals or groups. Few, if any, individuals in leadership positions possess all of the competencies required to influence behavior necessary to sustain transformational change. Consequently, the responsibility is distributed throughout the organization, in the form of "change agents." The application of desired leadership competencies depends on the respective phase of the change initiative. Leadership styles relative to Phase 1 are more transformational, while Phase 4 requires a more transactional approach. The ideal relationship provides for the integration of both styles, depending on the situation.

Transformational Leadership

Effective organizational change begins with a common vision, inspired by a transformational leader, capable of championing and communicating their vision to all of the organization stakeholders. Attributes typically associated with successful transformational leaders include:

- A self-perceived change agent
- A prudent risk taker
- One who is sensitive to the needs of others
- One able to articulate core values
- One who is flexible and open to learning
- One with cognitive skills consistent with analytical problem solving
- Intuitive thinkers with vision[14]

Phase 1 of Figure 16-5 identifies the leadership style and desirable competencies needed to influence system stakeholders in recognizing the need to change. The transformational leader serves as a mentor through which the values of the change initiative are communicated and support groups are identified. From these groups arise the "champions of the cause" who, by expanding the capacity for learning to those around them, create the beginning of a learning organization. The learning organization represents discontinuous (cyclical) and sustained transformational change. In effect, all members of the organization become change leaders in some respect.

Changing Organization Culture

In their book, *Diagnosing and Changing Organizational Culture*, Kim Cameron and Robert Quinn recognize the high failure rates of planned organizational change in the 1980s and 1990s. They attribute these failures to neglected organizational culture and conclude that the three major change initiatives, TQM, reengineering, and downsizing, fell short or failed completely due to slow, laggard, wrong-headed change efforts that did not assess or attempt to alter the organizational culture.[15]

The response of healthcare systems to these conclusions is mixed. A study of nine healthcare systems attempting major transformational change initiatives under a grant from the Woods Johnson Foundation and Pew Charitable Trust (Strengthening Hospital Nursing [SHN]: A Program to Improve Patient Care), reported that only a few change leaders considered culture an important part of the initiative.[11] A continued review of vertically integrated initiatives by Stephen Shortell in 1996 recognized that these efforts have given way to a vertical disintegration and supports the need for healthcare systems to assess and diagnose the current culture of the organization before attempting to implement radical changes.[3]

In the unique healthcare environment, cultural values may vary significantly within the organization. Clinical staff (nursing, technical, and physician) may feel that upper management does not understand the value of quality of care, while upper management feel that clinical staff do not appreciate the value of functional operations that produce needed revenue and sustain profitability. Cultural elements, regardless of the industry, have common relationships; some are tangible and easily defined, while others are not as easily defined or intangible. Figure 16-6 categorizes the elements and provides a means of integrating the relationship between the two. The inputs directly affect the outcomes. The intangibles (culture related) influence the outcomes both directly and indirectly. Consequently, it is imperative that these elements work together if radical change is to be sustained.[2] While it is not within the constraints of this chapter to define the various assessment tools for addressing specific cultural characteristics, the reader is directed to the reference list for further attention to the subject.

The Learning Organization

The goal of organizational transformation is to create a culture that embraces the capacity to change, not incrementally but continuously. Consequently, individuals within the organization must integrate their cultural values with those of the organization and vice versa; the ultimate objective being the "learning organization" that prescribes to "lifelong" learning for both the individual members and the organization.

Organizational change initiatives that are sustained over time are representative of "learning organizations." Peter Senge describes five disciplines that compose the core of the learning organization:

- Personal Mastery—learning to expand our personal capacity to create the results we most desire, and creating an organizational environment, which encourages all its members to develop themselves toward the goals and purposes they choose.

- Mental Models—reflecting upon, continually clarifying, and improving our internal pictures of the world, and seeing how they shape our actions and decisions.

- Shared Vision—building a sense of commitment in a group by developing shared images of the future we seek to create and the principles and guiding practices by which we hope to get there.

- Team Learning—transforming conversational and collective thinking skills, so that groups of people can reliably develop intelligence and ability greater than the sum of individual members' talents.

- Systems Thinking—a way of thinking about, and a language for describing and understanding, the forces and interrelationships that shape the behavior of systems. This discipline helps us see how to change systems more effectively, and to act more in tune with the larger processes of the natural and economic world.[16]

Systems Thinking

To appreciate the value of "systems thinking" one must first understand the interrelatedness of elements that define a "system." Obviously, the elements will differ depending on the system. However, the behavior of all systems follows specific common principles that guide the process. Systems thinking is not top-down or bottom-up but a participative relationship between management and operations.[16] The more effective organizations are in defining and articulating their systems, the more likely they are to sustain organizational change.

Inputs		
Tangible		**Intangible**
Cash		Mission
People		Values
Policy/Procedures		Vision
Strategy		Inspiration
Plant		Leadership Style
Information Systems		Motivation
Outputs		
Tangible		**Intangible**
Profit		Culture
Market Share		Commitment
Products		Morale
Customer Satisfaction		Job Satisfaction
Growth		Team Spirit
Productivity		Pride/Joy/Trust
Quality		Quality

Figure 16-6 Relationships between Tangibles and Intangibles.

The healthcare industry is part of a complex adaptive system composed of many different agencies and related subsystems.[2] Each of these agencies and related stakeholders respond independently to the external forces that drive change in their respective organizations. Subcultures within an organization follow a similar philosophy when external forces interfere with operations, causing distraction, confusion, and frustration and negatively influencing the organization's capacity to change. The concept of a "tragedy of commons" described in Peter Senge's 1990 book *The Fifth Discipline* emphasizes the disastrous results produced when individual gain takes priority over the common good or well-being of the whole. Global warming, created by the desire of individuals to drive bigger cars or manufacturing plants that increase production by expelling unfiltered poisonous gases into the atmosphere, is an analogy more relevant to the healthcare organization that is unable to effectively integrate the elements of the system to produce the best outcome for the patient. Subcultures within the organization battle for precious resources at the expense of other subcultures, without concern for the ultimate benefit to all. Creating the capacity to make radical change within the organization begins with a vision that benefits all stakeholders and, when effectively communicated and actively demonstrated, results in the "learning organization." The "collaborative" competencies highlighted in Phases 2 and 3 of Figure 16-5 are prerequisite to building a strong and receptive culture that responds to external forces and inspires internal innovation.

Communicating Change

Effective leadership communication that reaches all employees is a challenging responsibility that must be addressed prior to, during, and after the proposed change. John Kotter in his article *Leading Change: Why Transformation Efforts Fail* declares, "Transformation is impossible unless hundreds or thousands of people are willing to help, often to the point of making short-term sacrifices. Employees will not make sacrifices, even if they are unhappy with the status quo, unless they believe that useful change is possible. Without credible communication, and a lot of it, the hearts and minds of the troops are never captured."[17] Regardless of the scope and depth of anticipated change, leadership must assess the current internal communication practices of the organization and ensure that they are sufficiently strong to support the effort. For the purpose of this discussion, communication strategy is directed to transformational change initiatives as opposed to incremental or business unit change. However, the basic steps of getting started, doing the work, and producing results represents a relatively simple overview of the communication plan. This plan is most effective when implemented by a communication change team (CCT). Communication challenges that leadership must confront in the selection and establishment of teams is presented in Figure 16-7.[18] Members of the CCT should be representative of all primary stakeholders and not restricted to middle or senior managers. Front-line employees provide a definite benefit to ensure an organization-wide "buy-in" of the change. However, care in the selection of the CCT is necessary to represent the culture of the organization. Members should, at a minimum, reflect open-mindedness, honesty, and interpersonal relations and facilitation skills. Although the CEO and other senior managers may not serve on the CCT, their responsibility to supporting the initiative must be recognized by everyone in the organization. The CEO must openly endorse and champion the process and ensure that senior management facilitates the implementation of the CCT recommendations. This typically occurs in Phase 2 of the change-communication action plan.

Knowing both what you want to communicate and how effective you are in the communication process is determined by monitoring the front-line staff and listening to their feedback. Focus groups and surveys are effective tools to ensure that what was communicated and what was interpreted are the same. Independent communication teams within the organization also provide an opportunity for front-line staff to express misunderstood communication or seek clarification.[18]

Although the formal action plan is a critical part of the effective change communication process, the informal communication links cannot and

Work Phases

Getting Started
- Selecting team members and communicating to them individually and collectively the reasons for their selection
- Establishing the team charter and confirming the understanding/acceptance of it by all team members
- Making sure that roles and expectations of team members are clear and accepted
- Setting ground rules for the way the team will work
- Creating a team communication protocol

Doing the Work
- Guiding or facilitating team meetings
- Giving feedback (positive and negative) as work is done
- Coordinating the work done by team members: making sure everyone is department informed
- Dealing with and resolving conflict
- Keeping people outside the team informed of what the team is doing when appropriate

Delivering the Results
- Preparing the presentation or report of the team's work
- Delivering the presentation or report
- Debriefing the experience of the team (what went well and what did not)
- Closing out the team, if appropriate

Figure 16-7 Teamwork Phases and Challenges: Leadership Communication Challenges.

should not be ignored. Information from the top-down is slow and typically communicated in writing through newsletters, bulletin boards, or policy releases, which are seldom read with any confidence of understanding the implications of the proposed changes for the individual employee. However, the "grapevine" flourishes when information is slow or organizational change is evident. Unfortunately, the information processed through the "grapevine" is seldom the message that management wants to convey. Consequently, it is important to monitor the informal channels and respond quickly when information is incorrect or misinterpreted.[19]

Simply communicating the facts is not sufficient to influence behavioral change. Transformational leaders communicate in a way that shifts the thinking and understanding of others. Bennis and Nanus refer to this as "meaning through communication." An open dialogue between and among various elements of the organization is essential to ensure commitment to the change. Communication should not just share facts and data but challenge the way the members of the organization view things, incorporating the lives of individuals into the change initiatives.[20]

Building Change Teams

One of the more effective strategies for communicating and initiating radical change is the development of change teams. Team development is designed to produce an outcome, not provide input to the process. Effective teams incorporate the purpose of the change initiative with the fit to the overall organization, and the dynamic tensions associated with the change.[2]

Figure 16-5 addresses the leadership style and competencies associated with effective team building. Issues associated with building change teams require both individual and organizational consideration. Initiatives that overlook or do not include members of the hierarchy, specifically middle management, face the potential for subconscious resistance by these individuals. James Champy declares middle management as the "Death Zone" of radical change if not incorporated into the change process.[21] Consequently, the quality of the leadership becomes a factor in the potential effectiveness of the change team.

Poorly designed teams with no clear objective and a limited knowledge of the team's role in the change process become a liability rather than an asset. Before engaging teams in the change process, the organization should conclude that:

- The team approach is the most appropriate strategy.
- The team members have been adequately trained in the dynamics of problem solving and process management.
- Employees are accustomed to working in teams and understand the ground rules and methodology of conflict resolution.
- The organization possesses essential technology to support the team communication needs.[18]

Criteria for selecting individual team members should be relative to the assigned tasks. While the overall change team is responsible for receiving and integrating the recommendations of the subordinate teams, the membership should also be diverse and represent the primary stakeholders. Teams should be functional in size and represent diverse skill sets. Large teams become more difficult to manage and are typically less effective than smaller ones. However, if the team is too small to represent the needed diversity of the group, effectiveness is compromised.

Effective teams function best when the project goals are clearly defined and to some extent measurable within the time frames allotted. When team members understand their respective roles and responsibilities, and how they integrate with the overall change plan, they tend to be more productive, more innovative and are more likely to champion the change initiatives. Although the subordinate change teams, representing the various departments of the health system, are not in a position to change the entire organization, their successful contribution to the process spurs others to accept and contribute to the overall process. Competencies from Phases 3 and 4 define the most effective skills leaders must employ in this process. Note that the application of these competencies begins to integrate the transformational style of leadership with the transactional style.

Institutionalizing Change

In Phases 4 and 5 of the transformation process (Figure 16-5), the organization begins to incorporate the recommended changes resulting from the assessment and diagnosis of external and internal forces driving the process. The objective is to move the change from "innovation" to "an accepted way" of doing things on a day-to-day basis. When consistency in *decision making* by all elements of the organization is realized, the change is said to be *institutionalized*.

Medical centers, in particular, can be thought of as multiple organizations within an organization; each with its own set of rules, policies, and decision-making processes, ruled by an informal authority (medical staff). Unlike other industries, the hierarchy of authority does not necessarily reflect the level of influence, depending on the nature of the decision. Consequently, effective transformational change within a healthcare system becomes difficult to implement and more difficult to measure. The constraints of this chapter do not provide for a detailed review of the many different tools available to monitor and adjust the change initiatives. However, Phase 5 of the process is critical if the change is to be sustained as a "way of life" in the informal organization. Hospitals function 24 hours a day, 7 days a week. Each shift within the schedule represents a separate and unique informal group, which requires individual consideration when institutionalizing change. Consequently, feedback groups and surveys will be essential to test the effectiveness of the change process. Monitoring should not be restricted to internal quantitative measures but include both external stakeholders and industry competitors. Externally, the transformation should link the organization to the community and not just to the patients they serve. Internally, the board and senior management of the organization must learn to practice "CEO curiosity."[16] That is, asking, "Are we doing what we should be doing, or are we doing what we want to be doing?" This and other questions establish a basis for the question, "Do we need to change?" If the answer to that question is "yes," the next question must be, "Does our organization have the capacity to change?" If the process described by Figure 16-5 has been effectively applied, a natural process of consistent decision making will occur. In either event, the organization must never assume an accurate understanding of the external forces that influence radical changes.

■ CHAPTER SUMMARY

The *whitewater* change occurring in healthcare, inspired by external environmental forces, challenges leaders in the industry to implement radical changes in their organizations. These changes are transforming medical centers from local service industries to global networks of providers. Because of the exponential rate of change, organizations are revisiting the mission vision and values that form their organizational culture and preparing to respond in the short-term to competitive and regulatory forces.

Unlike transitional or developmental change, which tends to reposition or adjust systems of operation, transformational change is organization wide and designed to redefine the organizational behavior of individuals and create a "learning organization." Organization development practitioners have developed several general models that provide guidance to organizations initiating radical change, each of which utilize common phases of process development. Although these models do not ensure the success of the initiative, they incorporate competencies unique to each of the phases outlined in the process and provide change leaders a means of monitoring progress toward the objectives. Figure 16-5 represents one alternative to these models.

Critical to the success of transformational change is the leadership style of the CEO and senior mangers responsible for change initiatives. Service industries, including healthcare, have begun to shift from a traditional *transactional* leadership style to a more *transformational* style, which encourages participation of everyone in the organization. Attributes of both styles have relevance to radical change and effective leaders balance the application of these competencies throughout the process.

Equally important to effective change is the development of a *communication strategy* to ensure clear and articulate demonstration of the vision, mission, and goals of the organization. Communication change teams provide an integrated relationship of idea exchange that when selectively defined enhances the potential for organization-wide buy-in of the cultural shift. These teams form the basis for the application of *systems thinking* and the evolution of a *learning organization*. The learning organization represents the foundation upon which the organization can build a defense to external environmental forces and create innovative responses to *whitewater* change.

Review Questions

1. Organization development practitioners have identified six key trends related to change. Using these trends, compare and contrast the healthcare and non-healthcare service industries.

2. Define "change." Distinguish between *transitional* (incremental) change and *transformational* change. Give examples of each.

3. Describe a "change model." Why are change models important to the transformational change initiatives?

4. What role does leadership play in creating a "capacity for change" throughout the organization?

5. What is meant by "institutionalizing" change? How do organizations assess the effectiveness of this process?

6. What is a "learning organization"? Why is this concept important to the transformational change process?

7. What challenges face the leader of a CCT?

8. Describe the phases of a discontinuous (cyclical) change model. Why is the discontinuous nature of these models relevant to transformational change?

9. What considerations are relevant prerequisites to engaging work teams in the change process?

10. Compare and contrast the attributes of a transformational leader with those of a transactional leader. Which attributes are considered more desirable for leading and sustaining radical changes?

References

1. Drucker P. *Post Capitalist Society*. New York: Harper/Collins; 1993.
2. Atchison T, Bujak J. *Leading Transformational Change:The Physician-Executive Partnership*. Chicago, IL: Health Administration Press; 2001.
3. Giles RR, Anderson DA, Erickson KM, Mitchell JB. *Remaking Health Care in America: Building Organized Delivery Systems*. San Francisco, CA: Jossey-Bass, Inc.; 1996.
4. French W, Bell C. *Organization Development: Behavioral Science Interventions for Organization Improvement* (6th ed.). Upper Saddle River, NJ: Prentice Hall; 1999.

5. Rothwell W, Sullivan R. *Practicing Organization Development: A Guide for Consultants* (2nd ed.). San Francisco, CA: Pfeiffer; 2005.
6. Zirkle T, Peters G. *Healthcare Commentaries: Almanac of Essential Facts.* Boulder, CO: Healthcare Commentaries; 1993.
7. Swayne LM, Duncan WJ, Ginter PM. *Strategic Management of Healthcare Organizations.* Malden, MA: Blackwell; 2006.
8. Borkowski N. *Organizational Behavior in Health Care.* Sudbury, MA: Jones & Bartlett; 2005.
9. Rothwell W, Prescott R, Taylor M. *Strategic Human Resource Leader: How to Prepare Your Organization for the Six Key Trends Shaping the Future.* Alexandria, VA: The American Society for Training and Development; 1998.
10. French W, Bell C. *Organization Development: Behavioral Science Interventions for Organization Improvement* (5th ed.). Saddle River, NJ: Prentice-Hall; 1993.
11. Rundall T, Starkweather D, Norrish B. *After Restructuring: Empowerment Strategies at Work in America's Hospitals.* San Francisco, CA: Jossey-Bass; 1998.
12. Aaronson W, Balotsky ER. *Community Hospitals and Networks* New York: Marcel Dekker, Inc.; 1999.
13. Draveky E, Preston J. *Managing Change.* New York: Marcell & Dekker; 1999.
14. Yukl G. *Leadership in Organizations.* Englewood Cliffs, NJ: Prentice Hall; 1994.
15. Cameron K, Quinn R. *Diagnosing and Changing Organizational Culture.* Reading, MA: Addison-Wesley; 1999.
16. Senge P. *The Fifth Discipline Fieldbook.* New York: Doubleday Dell; 1994.
17. Kotter J. *Leading Change: Why Transformation efforts Fail.* Boston, MA: Harvard Business Review; 1996.
18. Barrett D. *Leadership Communication.* Boston, MA: McGraw-Hill/Irwin; 2006.
19. McConnell C, Liebler J. *The Effective Healthcare Supervisor* (4th ed.). Sudbury, MA: Jones & Bartlett; 2004.
20. Kent T. Leadership. In Kilpatric A, Johnson J (eds.) *Health Administration and Policy.* New York: Marcell and Dekker, Inc.; 1999.
21. Champy J. *Reengineering Management.* NY: Harper-Collins; 1995.

Team Building and Development

Jo-Ann Costa

Learning Objectives

- Introduce the popularity of teams in organizations. Discuss teams in general, and why teams are more effective than individuals.
- Introduce interdisciplinary/multifunctional teams, their composition and purpose, and why they have value.
- Identify and discuss optimal behaviors for team success; benefits of teams to organizations and to individuals for their participation.
- Review the evolution of a rudimentary team and stages of development as a backdrop for team building.
- Address the importance of team building, ongoing training, and atmosphere critical for peak performance. Support with activities and exercises that foster team building.
- Discuss the team's obligations to the organization to develop an action plan, management presentation, and metrics using learned team-building skills.
- Discuss organizational obligations (internal team-building mechanisms) that reinforce the team's value, including rewards and recognition.
- Discuss team-building trends in leading-edge companies to demonstrate the ongoing improvements in team building that inspire other business models.

■ INTRODUCTION

Teams are cropping up in organizations at a faster rate than ever before. Among the reasons for this are the higher value that today's workers place on learning new knowledge and skills that lead to personal and professional growth than a decade ago. Being a team member contributes to the creation of knowledge and skills by exposing participants to a wide perspective of views, often from multiple disciplines and across business units.

One need only read the employment ads from the *Wall Street Journal* or study recruitment efforts across the nation, wherein businesses are seeking creative thinkers, consensus builders, and team players, to see that teams are valued.

It is apparent that the corporate world recognizes the values and expectations of today's workers as we witness teams fast replacing yesterday's hierarchical decision-making processes and corporate structures flatten. An example of this can be seen in the way organizations recruit new employees as shown in an increasing emphasis on team interviews of job candidates. Candidate evaluations almost always consider the candidate's experience and ability to be team players and a good fit with the organization's culture. By its very nature, the team interview reflects a culture that promotes teams and collaborative actions.

The business world is creating more and more opportunities to learn new skills by fostering teams that recognize employees for team behaviors and initiative. The healthcare field is not an exception to this phenomenon.

■ TYPES OF TEAMS

Many images come to mind when thinking of the word "team." One might picture a team of adventurers climbing Mt. Everest or a sporting event where two groups are in competition to win a game. There are many different types of teams with different compositions and purposes.

In business as well as in the healthcare field, a team may be flexible—either temporary or permanent—and generally speaking, it can turn out more work in less time than individuals working independently can. A team can keep the forward momentum of its work going when a team member is absent. Within the context of a team, information is shared and coordinated, synthesized, communicated, and re-communicated without dependence on any single individual. It can also be said that when a team is empowered, and when it is comprised of the right people and skills, it can be self-managing.

To narrow the possibilities, and for illustrative purposes, the type of team that will be the focus of this chapter is the type of team that includes members from more than one discipline and/or department that meets on a regularly scheduled basis for as long as it takes to achieve any given goal and measure it for success. The life cycle of this type of team need not be finite as it may continue its existence for follow-on projects as required.

The purpose of an interdisciplinary and/or multi-departmental team can be to:

- Examine a specific problem or issue.
- Study and/or act upon some matter.
- Investigate and analyze the efficacy of a process.
- Address a work initiative.

Whatever the composition and purpose of a team, it is the bonding, training, and growth of the team that will be emphasized here, for without proper tools, the mere formation of a team is only the beginning of what can be a long, enriching process for its members.

■ THE TEAM ADVANTAGE

As you read this chapter, think about success, how hard-won it can be, and about the times you focused on a single idea to achieve a goal.

If you have relied solely upon your own resources, talents, and intelligence in a work or learning environment, can you imagine for a moment how much more successful you could be by multiplying the chances of achieving your goals by involving others? Consider how the ideas and energies of others can shape your conclusions and perhaps even shorten deadlines associated with finalizing a project.

Asking for help may be the last thing you want to do, but imagine that expert help is available. Suppose that the expert's intention is to partner, encourage, motivate, and assist you in moving a project forward. Now take it a step further and say that there is an implicit requirement for the expert to jump in and share the workload with no hesitation to tackle the tougher issues. These experts even hold themselves equally accountable for the work product! What if there are even more of these experts in your corner, all working toward the same end, with the same passion for excellence as you?

Sounds nice you say, so what is the catch?

The only catch is that a potential team member must examine some fundamental questions about his/her work behaviors and be willing to learn.

- How do you feel about sharing credit for success?
- Are you the type of person who needs to be noticed and in the limelight?
- Are you the type of individual who prefers the comfort of numbers?
- Are you open to different approaches to problem solving?
- Do you enjoy discourse and the building of ideas?

The reason I want you to think about these questions is that you will automatically bring your preferences and individuality into a team setting. Many new team members find the strangeness of teams and the unfamiliarity of its members intimidating, preferring to remain alone rather than having to form new relationships or change behaviors in order to integrate successfully.

Team members must be deeply committed to one another's personal growth and the team's success. Team members need to collaborate in all aspects of their tasks and goals, sharing in planning, organization, goal setting, assessment of performance, resource allocation, and establishing measurement metrics. In organizations where teamwork is encouraged, it is also a powerful endorsement of the organization's belief that teams are valued and successful.

But wait! Do not automatically assume that becoming a member of a team is an identity-losing proposition. In the context of a fully functional team, members contribute personal resources without losing their individuality. If anything, team members grow personally and professionally, become more valuable, and learn important aspects necessary for career advancement. In cross-functional teams, members learn about the operations and issues of other departments. In interdisciplinary teams, members come to know and respect the jobs of others and appreciate where everyone fits in the larger organization.

Successful teams are comprised of dedicated individuals who create something larger than themselves. That is the beauty of teams. It is the richness of complementary individual talents that makes a variety of approaches valuable. As ideas build upon one another, the real synergies of a team emerge. And, as people stop vying for attention and differences are sorted through, the team begins to take on a life of its own in its journey to meet its objectives. It is when seemingly monumental tasks are reduced to less formidable status that the team relaxes into a comfortable rhythm and teamwork can happen. Thus, in a healthy team, the best qualities of human interaction unfold in a shared quest to accomplish common goals.

Another way to think about teams is that they are much like an extended family. It only takes one dysfunctional member to spoil it for the others. Cooperation is necessary within families, as well as respect and civility. This is not to say that disagreement is a bad thing, quite the contrary, but the key to good relationships in any setting is in the manner of discourse and conduct. The same is true for teams in healthcare organizations.

■ BENEFITS OF TEAMS

High-performing teams can be attractive to management and individual team members alike. When teams learn to produce at higher levels through mutual cooperation, everyone takes notice.

One of the reasons teams have grown in popularity in care giving is that there are very concrete, measurable benefits that result from good teamwork including new solutions to old problems and the ability to identify sound approaches that address regulatory requirements. Whether the business issue is service, process improvement, or cost reduction, teamwork is critical to both workable relationships and the bottom line.

Teams maximize the organization's human resources, for in teams, each member learns to be more effective through the coaching, help, and leadership of all the other members. All members, not just the individual, feel success and failures alike. Because failures are *not* blamed on individual members, they have the courage to take more risks in a team setting and more ideas are forthcoming.

The greatest lesson learned by team members is: Teams consistently outperform individuals. And, the second greatest is: Individuals may be considered for career advancement as a result of broadening their knowledge of the organization and acquiring teamwork skills.

When members are properly selected, trained, empowered, and given the nod to participate fully from their management, individuals grow professionally, learn to behave in ways that get results, appreciate the power of synergistic efforts, and take their knowledge and training with them back to the everyday work group where it has the potential to spread.

■ TEAM COMPOSITION

Let us say you have been asked to participate on an interdisciplinary/ cross-functional healthcare team outside your normal work group. Likely, you have been selected because:

- You are a self-starter.
- You possess a required skill or expertise.
- You and your unit have a stake in the outcome of the team's performance and eventual recommendations.

Ideally, team membership will consist of a group of professionals such as you, no greater than 10 to 12 members, with a designated leader. The team may be smaller in number, but larger numbers can slow the process.

Often interdisciplinary/multi-departmental teams are formed to bring about the best ideas from all stakeholders representing those departments having a vested interest in the outcome of the team's work as well as individuals who possess a special expertise required for understanding a matter.

Your team may have a facilitator as well as a leader. The facilitator coaches the team leader and team members, teaches team-building skills, and helps with logistics (meeting times, locations and dates), the problem-solving process, and team dynamics such as conflict resolution and decision making. In addition to these tasks, the facilitator will work toward helping the team to become self-reliant so that it no longer requires outside facilitation.

■ TEAM EVOLUTION

Envision if you will a three-layer cake (TLC) (see Figure 17-1). The top layer represents the designated leader/leaders, who may also serve as facilitators, providing structure and process. These individuals can be appointed by the boss, elected by the group, or they may be volunteers. How these individuals are designated really does not matter; what matters is that they possess critical teamwork training and leadership skills to guide the team.

The second layer represents the vocals; those that like to talk, possess high energy, produce tons of ideas, and have difficulty not interrupting others. From this layer usually emerges one or two other, as-yet unofficial, leaders.

The third, or bottom layer, represents the observers; those who are waiting for the vocals to cease competing for attention. Most likely, the observers are watching the deeds and listening to the words of others while forming opinions about those representing the first two layers.

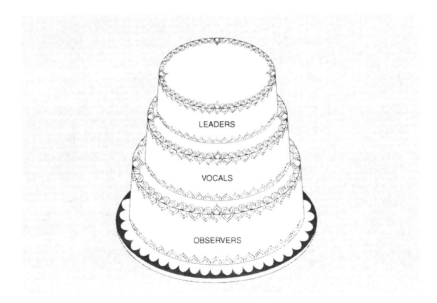

Figure 17-1 TLC Initial Team.

There is more going on with the observers than would appear as they consider all that is said and sit quietly by waiting for the vocals to tire or for the leader to acknowledge one of them. Eventually, someone in this group will speak up and that encourages others in the group to make their opinions known as well.

In short, the TLC initial team model represents a team formation in its most basic form. It is the most likely team formation you will encounter in the first few meetings of your new team.

As the team matures, an inversion of the TLC initial team model occurs.

In a mature team, the leaders often end up representing the bottom layer of the cake, perhaps taking on an occasional role of facilitator, minute-taker, or the tasks of housekeeping and announcements, while new leaders may have emerged from either the vocals or observers, or both. These last two groups will likely merge and may even swap roles as the dynamics change and the team grows.

The differences in the TLC initial team model and the TLC mature team model (see Figure 17-2) are three-fold:

1. New leaders have emerged from the ranks of vocals and/or observers.
2. The distinction between the vocals and observers is blurred.
3. The initial leaders have become inactive, letting others assume responsibility, thus acknowledging the new, self-directed team.

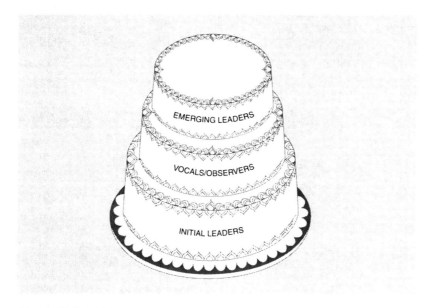

Figure 17-2 TLC Mature Team.

■ STAGES OF TEAM DEVELOPMENT

The evolution of team development can best be described by a model developed by Bruce Tuckman in 1965, wherein he identified four stages of group development and later added a fifth in the 1970s. Let us look at the progression of Tuckman's model, for it clearly captures the fundamentals of team progression.

Tuckman's Team Development Model

1. FORMING: In this stage, the group is assembled, members get acquainted and understand the task at hand.
2. STORMING: This represents a period where members become more comfortable with one another and vie for leadership and status in the group, often engaging in arguments.
3. NORMING: Here they reach agreement on rules to achieve the goal and how the group will operate.
4. PERFORMING: This stage is where the group becomes effective at reaching conclusions and implementing recommendations.
5. ADJOURNING: As the project concludes, the group begins the process of disbanding.

Tuckman's first four stages build upon one another. Just as with all stages of human development, one must crawl before they can walk, and walk before they can run.

Tuckman also explains that as the team develops maturity and ability, relationships develop and the leader changes leadership style. The leader may start with a directing style, but as he/she moves through coaching, participating, and delegating, the leader will become almost detached. At this point, the team may produce a successor leader.

A similar model can also be found in the Tannenbaum and Schmidt continuum model where the authority and freedom extended by the leader to the team increases while the control of the leader is reduced.

■ BUILDING TEAM FUNCTIONALITY

At first, any newly formed group of people will experience excitement and anticipation as well as anxiety about the task that lies ahead. In addition, finding one's place within the team can be a concern for some.

Without the proper training, the first couple of team meetings can be defining moments as the dynamics of personality, interaction with others, process, and the unknown can act as inhibitors to the performance of the team. Some team members may show up with an agenda that is all for change as long as their department is not affected. Others may feel that change is not desirable for the opposite reason.

There is really no magic to successful teamwork. It is a matter of on-going training, preparation, communication and dialogue, hard work, and a commitment to checking egos at the door so that the work of the team comes first.

People will become energized and perform around a cause that matters to them, so it is important that organizations have meaningful work for the team and the team believes that it has value to the organization.

One of the best methods for beginning to build a cohesive team is for the organization to set aside time for individuals to meet informally with no objective except to get to know one another. A quiet, relaxed environment is a must, with no dress code. This important time can be seen as a mini-retreat lasting from 2 to 4 hours, including a casual lunch or dinner. The purpose of the retreat is to get to know one another and exchange information, understand what views are held about the organization, and how each person thinks he/she might fit in.

At the retreat, a facilitator leads the initial introductions and makes the members comfortable. He/she may also lead the group through "icebreakers" to get the ball rolling. Icebreakers serve to:

- Create a positive atmosphere.
- Help people relax and get to know one another.
- Break down social barriers.
- Energize and motivate.
- Nudge people to think beyond the ordinary and conventional.

A retreat is an opportune time to team-build through planned activities. Many team-building tasks are like kids' games, others are novel, complex tasks designed to achieve specific goals. Among the more popular activities today are outdoor adventure games such as rock climbing, obstacle courses, and treasure hunts, which require cooperation, discussion, problem solving, and dependence on one's teammates.

Whatever activity is chosen, in the hands of an excellent facilitator even the simplest game can become a significant learning experience. And after the team-building exercises are completed, sharing what has been learned and experienced is an important part of team building. At this time, participants' discussion and reflection about how they approached a situation, their likes and dislikes, as well as how they felt while participating can be voiced.

1. Here are a few examples of team-building activities: Activity: *Goal Setting*

    The team members can establish the goal setting for the socialization retreat and later be asked if they think they met the goals. (People tend to be more committed to goals they set themselves.)

2. Activity: *Getting to Know You*

A good way to for members to get a sense of other team members' interests, credentials, experience, and desires is for the facilitator to ask each person a set of questions that can be read back to the group.

- Why are you interested in becoming a member of the team?
- What strengths do you believe you bring to the team?
- What do you want to learn from the team experience?
- Describe any experience you may have on other teams.
- What are your special interests/hobbies/fields of expertise?
- Other than the objective, what else would you like your team to accomplish?

3. Activity: *Building Relationships*

The retreat is a perfect setting to begin to build relationships using personalized interviews. Ask members to pair off and interview one another for 10 to 15 minutes after which partners introduce one another to the rest of the group, repeating as much information as they can remember about their partner.

4. Activity: *Cooperation*

The game of Matching Squares is an example of what can be done to demonstrate cooperation among team members. Cut squares of colored paper into odd shapes and a piece is given to each member. Members work with others with pieces of like color to form a perfect square. Do this in silence with no talking permitted.

5. Activity: *Brainstorming*

The facilitator proposes a hypothetical problem and the team is required to brainstorm. Record key words and phrases without judgment. Do not discuss or criticize ideas. There is no hand raising, just a calling out of ideas. The group then chooses from the list those ideas that will work best to address the problem.

6. Activity: *Create Your Own Group Activity*

Ask team members to design and present a new team activity. This is a challenging exercise requiring many of the elements of teamwork—communication, goal setting, planning, cooperation, and creativity.

7. Activity: *Naming the Team*

The importance of naming the team cannot be underestimated. A "we" identity is powerful tool for bonding and building team spirit. A strong team identity is a critical factor that can make a difference in the team's success. I recommend that this idea be advanced early in the team's training as it has the effect of focusing individuals on belonging to a larger body having a common goal. The team should *always* name itself and *all* of the members should have a say-so in this activity. It is reinforcing for the team to see its name and purpose prominently posted somewhere at the front of the meeting room, at every meeting.

Later in the team's development, the team's identity and goals will become preeminent. Team members will gain an intrinsic understanding that their effectiveness and survival are built upon each other's cooperation and collaboration rather than upon competition; that building consensus and finding areas of agreement rather than focusing on areas of conflict results in solutions everyone can support.

■ ONGOING TRAINING = SUSTAINABLE KNOWLEDGE

It is imperative to practice team building until the skills are second nature to the team. This may require warm-up exercises at the beginning of the first few meetings for reinforcement or separate team-building sessions if the team continues to remain in the storming stage of Tuckman's team development model.

Team building is an ongoing process, a long-term strategy, an activity that is never finished. Team-building techniques can be used at any time and can be helpful when:

- Members appear to be drifting away from the group.
- Conflict or infighting occurs.
- The team has been inactive for a while.
- The team needs a break from its work.

As members begin to embrace and embed desired team behaviors, they will begin to head, with some degree of confidence, in the direction of the goal.

■ PROBLEM SOLVING

The development of a high-performing team requires a grab bag of tools, not the least of which is problem solving. During the process of reaching any given goal, there will be obstacles to achieving success, questions will arise, and more than one path may force choices to be made.

There are many problem-solving models and they may have any number of steps, but a typical model includes the following:

1. Definition of the problem
2. Information and data gathering about the problem

3. Analysis of the problem, including process flow, cost benefit, regulatory and legal implications, etc.

4. Solution development, testing, and implementation

5. Results monitoring and measurement

6. Modifications as required

■ CONTINUOUS REINFORCEMENT: THE VALUE OF THE TEAM'S WORK

From the outset, team members need to believe their work has value. Not enough can be said about this. No one wants to think that the time and energy they are spending to solve a problem or revamp a process would not result in an action or change for the better, and it will be up to the leader to convey and reinforce how important the work of the team is to the organization. If this is not done, lackluster performance can almost be guaranteed. So it follows that during all meetings of the team, the "value claim" must be underscored and supported with frequent feedback from the leader, who is a surrogate speaker for the larger organization.

■ GETTING DOWN TO BUSINESS

Unlike previous social and team-building meetings that may have been scheduled, the launch meeting is one in which the team can begin its mission.

If it has not already been addressed in the training phase, develop a standard of behavior, such as a Code of Conduct. At this juncture, a statement of the goal and its importance to the organization should be stated and an action plan begun to be developed.

A. *Code of Conduct:* The team can be facilitated by either a member of the team or a professional facilitator to establish its own rules, which may include:

- Attendance and promptness issues
- Discouragement of interruptions and cell phone use in the meeting room
- Issues of confidentiality about team members
- Non-disclosure of preliminary ideas to anyone outside the team
- No blaming
- Factual analysis over emotions
- Open discussion and equal participation
- Everyone works, no slackers permitted
- Ownership of the team's work and decisions

Discussing these other rules may be useful:

- *Loyalty* to the group, requiring encouragement and support from all members of the team
- *Competition* is welcomed, but not when an individual pursues his/her own concerns at another's expense.
- *Compromise* is permitted if the objective of the compromise is to find a mutually acceptable solution that partially satisfies both parties.
- *Conceding* is discouraged when an individual does so to sidestep an issue or gives in to another, more forceful individual. When this happens, the person conceding may no longer "own" the solution.

A "trust discussion" may also be helpful where the team leader asks for trust attributes from the members (i.e., "do what you say you'll do," "give your team members the benefit of a doubt," "trust yourself as well as others," "we're all in this together," "listen and don't interrupt").

An upfront discussion of these issues will go far in removing inhibitors and helping the group achieve its goals. The team will perform, often beyond expectations when:

- A foundation is laid for common understanding and commitment to the goals
- Effective training is undertaken to help break down the barriers to communications
- Team-building exercises are learned and practiced
- Accommodation, cooperation, and good manners among individuals prevail and a Code of Conduct is developed as a guide
- Trust issues are openly discussed.

B. *The Action Plan:* Team development of an action plan not only utilizes and reinforces team-building skills, it is essential to have one in place in order for the team to take appropriate sequential steps that will move them in the direction of their goal. Together, members of the team outline (see Table 17-1):

- Goals (what is to be done?)
- Objectives (specific outcomes)
- Process (how it will be done?)
- Resources (who will do it?)
- Deadlines (when—timelines and accountabilities)
- Results (data, measurements, and conclusions)
- Recommendations (presentations and buy-ins—both stakeholders and management)
- Follow-up (continuous measurable improvement)

Table 17-1 Goals vs. Objectives

Goal = Reduce time and cost to admit a patient.

Objective = 1. Reduce intake time for each patient by 20%.
2. Reduce cost of intake by 25%.

The action plan is fleshed-out as the team moves along in its work, updated, changed, and constantly brainstormed, serving as a roadmap for the team as they go along. Action plans should always be visible and addressed at each meeting of the team to establish timelines, monitor progress, and provide ongoing guidance.

■ DEFINING SUCCESS

How do teams know they have succeeded? The obvious answer is "Mission accomplished!" But beyond meeting the goal or objectives, the team must determine how to measure its success. This means a quantitative look at the results. For example, sales are easy enough to measure as are increases and decreases in consumer complaints and lawsuits. There are project cost metrics, productivity metrics, quality metrics, and customer satisfaction metrics that can be used. However, all too often results are not immediately available, appearing sometime in the future as new processes and ways of operating prove out. Over time, however, measurements will emerge as the team continues to monitor and assess whether or not it has successfully addressed a quantifiable goal.

When the team is tasked to achieve a less clearly measurable goal, the team must continue to ask if they have succeeded. A good example of this might be a team goal to increase employee morale. In this case, coming up with measurements may require additional brainstorming sessions. One of the measurement tools might be tracking voluntary terminations, as a reduced turnover rate would support the team's success. Regardless, the team must establish "how" they will know they are successful, checking their assumptions along the way for clarity and continued fit. The application of previously learned team-building skills and activities will help the group achieve these metrics.

■ BEYOND METRICS

A team should examine four additional questions.

1. What are the lessons learned?
2. How can the lessons be applied to the next problem or issue?

3. What new skills were acquired?
4. What skills and information am I, as an individual, going to take away with me and apply in my work every day?

> **Achieving the goal is the business of the team. Learning from the process and applying that learning is the business of the individual.**

■ SELLING THE SOLUTION: MANAGEMENT BUY-IN

At some point, the team will have concluded its business and determined that it has done everything it can to satisfy the goal and objectives of the team. This is the time for a final report to management and it should take the form of a professional presentation. It is also at this time that management will recognize the team and show appreciation for its work whether or not it chooses to follow the recommendations of the team.

It is important to touch upon an appropriate recognition and reward system for good teamwork within the organization. Recognition and rewards are critical motivators and team members, as well as other future team candidates, will notice whether this is done. This is an essential ingredient in the organization's team-building repertoire and part of the organization's responsibility to the team. Every organization should determine for itself a system appropriate to the needs of its employees and unique culture. But whatever the system may be, it should be immediate, sincere, and meaningful.

Now, let us continue our discussion of the management presentation. Expect the team to present a well-thought-out, comprehensive report of their activities, conclusions, and recommendations.

As you may have noticed, team-building skills are used over and over again as the team moves toward its purpose. The management presentation is no exception. Members of the team will include the following components when developing their presentation:

- Purpose of the project
- Team members and their roles
- Introduction, history, and background of the issue
- Data and metrics
- Methods, components, and analyses employed to reach conclusions
- Issues, concerns, and buy-in of affected departments and other stakeholders
- Conclusions

- Recommendations
- Use ongoing assessment measurements and assign who will be responsible for reporting

■ BACK ON THE EVERYDAY JOB

Many team members thrive in a team environment, sparked by the energy of the team and the close relationships that are built working together over the life of the project. Some miss the team environment when the project has ended, perhaps not expecting to experience the same energy once they return to their normal duties.

While we have discussed the formation and training of teams as it relates to multi-functional and/or interdisciplinary teams, we have not addressed the everyday work or departmental team that awaits the member's return.

There are important aspects of the team experience that can be taken back and applied on the job, for rarely does a person work alone, without need of cooperation and input from others. This is where the *skill and knowledge capital* learned while serving on the team can earn dividends. Achieving these dividends requires both the transfer of training and the follow-on support of the organization.

We know that a department is a collection of individual performers the manager must guide and motivate in a common direction for a common purpose—another type of team effort. But unless the department is able to tap into the potential for true teamwork, output will rarely be greater than the performance of the individuals.

Anyone who utilizes team-building training learned from a broader team experience will be better prepared to cooperate and collaborate with his/her co-workers, undertake problem solving with others, and be a valuable role model and teacher in any work environment. Thus, the investment the organization has made in team building pays off for both parties.

■ TRENDS

Peter Drucker coined the term "knowledge worker" in his 1959 book, *Landmarks of Tomorrow*. The term is used to describe individuals who add value by processing existing information to develop additional information to clarify and solve problems benefiting the organization. Although there is a range of definitions for the term, it can be generally agreed that knowledge workers use their intellect to convert their ideas into products, services, or processes.

As Drucker states in his 1998 Forbes article, *Management's New Paradigms*, "What motivates workers—especially knowledge workers—is . . . they need, above all, a challenge. They need to know the organization's mission and to believe in it. They need continuous training. They need to see results. . . ."

From a practical perspective, two types of knowledge workers exist.

1. Core knowledge workers, and
2. Everyone else

The core knowledge workers are often categorized as those in the management of information such as information officers, librarians, systems analysts, and so on.

Everyone else includes doctors, nurses, dentists, pharmacists, administrators, technicians, managers, etc.

There may not be a fine line to divide the two, but it is helpful to know that everyone is a knowledge worker to some degree, and knowledge is the responsibility of everyone.

To take a closer look at the idea of knowledge workers and how some operate in today's business world, it is useful to understand the team building taking place inside a leading-edge company—Google. Although many of the employees at Google are engineers, many of their methods apply to all sorts of knowledge workers.

Google uses seven key principles:

- *Hire by committee.* Every applicant who interviews at Google talks to at least half a dozen interviewers from both management and potential colleagues. All opinions count, making for a fair hiring process and pushing the standards higher. Google believes that if they hire great people and involve them intensely in the process, they get great people.
- *Cater to their every need.* As Drucker says, the goal is "to strip away everything that gets in their way." Google provides a standard package of benefits, but adds first-class dining facilities, gyms, laundry rooms, massage rooms, haircuts, carwashes, dry cleaning, commuting buses, etc.
- *Pack them in.* Almost every project at Google is a team project, and teams have to communicate. At Google, they make it easy to communicate by placing team members within a few feet of each other. Thus, virtually everyone shares an office for immediate access—no telephone tag, no email delay, no waiting for a reply. They also provide many conference rooms for detailed discussions so office mates are not disturbed. Even the CEO shared an office at Google for several months after he arrived. Sitting next to a knowledgeable employee was an incredibly effective educational experience.
- *Make coordination easy.* Close physical proximity makes it easy to coordinate projects. In addition, each "Googler" emails a snippet once a week to his/her work group describing what he/she has done

in the past week, facilitating an easy way to track, monitor progress, and synchronize work flow.

- *Eat your own dog food.* Google workers use the company's tools. The most obvious is the Web with an internal web page for every project and task, all indexed and available to project participants as needed. They also use their own tools, some of which are later rolled out as products after being beta-tested within the company.

- *Encourage creativity.* Google engineers can spend up to 20% of their time on a project of their choice, pending approval and some oversight, but basically, Google wants to allow creative people to be creative. They provide an ideas mailing list, something like the old suggestion box, where people can post ideas. The software allows for everyone to comment on and rate ideas, permitting the best ones to percolate to the top.

- *Strive to reach consensus.* At Google, the role of the manager is that of an aggregator of viewpoints, not the dictator of decisions. Building a consensus can take longer, but always produces a more committed team and better decisions.

- *"Don't be evil."* Much has been written about Google's slogan, but they really try to live by it, particularly in the ranks of management. As in every organization, people are passionate about their views. At Google, they work at creating an atmosphere of tolerance and respect.

- *Data driven decisions.* At Google, almost every decision is based on quantitative analysis and their internal systems are built to manage this information. They have dozens of analysts who collect and measure performance metrics and plot trends.

- *Communicate effectively.* Every Friday, "all-hands" meetings are held with announcements, introductions, questions and answers, and refreshments. This allows management to stay in touch with what their knowledge workers are thinking and vice versa. Google has a remarkably broad dissemination of information within the organization with very few serious leaks. Contrary to what some may think, Google believes it is the first fact that causes the second: a trusted workforce is a loyal workforce.

While Google has focused on managing creativity and innovation, this is not at the expense of managing their day-to-day operations. Those who plan, implement, and maintain their growing systems must also have a strong set of incentives. At Google, operations are not just an afterthought: They are critical to the company's success and they want to have just as much effort and creativity in this domain as in new product development.

Google recognizes they must stay in touch with the needs of their workers, as their rapid growth stage will give way to a maturation of the company. As such, communications procedures must keep pace with their increasing scale as a global organization. Benefits and a work environment will also need to be structured to be attractive to all ages.

■ CHAPTER SUMMARY

As we have seen in the Google example, continuous creativity and improvement in team building has taken place since Tuckman's Team Development model was published. And while Tuckman's stages of team development and human behavior may still hold true, every business is unique. This factor must compel organizations to examine and improve upon what has gone before. One thing is for certain, given the right set of people and organizational support, teams are effective and to maximize the human potential embedded within teams, healthcare organizations must continue to provide an atmosphere in which they can flourish.

Review/Discussion Questions

1. What is the purpose of teamwork, and why are teams able to produce more than a single individual?
2. Name the five stages of team development as identified in Tuckman's model.
3. Discuss the composition of interdisciplinary/multifunctional teams. Explain why the mix is valuable in healthcare organizations.
4. What is the value of a team-building retreat?
5. What relationship skills are learned in team-building activities? Why is "naming the team" an important aspect of team building?
6. Why is it important for the team to develop its own Code of Conduct?
7. Discuss the benefits and value of teams to healthcare organizations and to the individual members.

Learning Activity

Case Study: Not Built Here

A business director of a California mental health facility was weary of handling volumes of paper to comply with the organization's obligations to satisfy state and local reporting requirements and ensure future funding. He decided to create a consolidated form for every department, to be input at a central location, intended to decrease the amount of time he/she and the staff spent preparing reports. Through the grapevine, word soon spread that the director intended to change various forms and processes, eliminate others, and possibly create new ones.

The Financial Information Manager, responsible for intake to determine a patient's ability to pay, resented the rumored changes as his/her under-staffed function could barely keep up with a burgeoning patient load. The Billing and Collections Office Manager agreed with the colleague as there was a ripple effect of whatever happened in the financial intake area.

Busy and uncomfortable with calling their superior with their concerns, the two managers sent a joint email to the director telling him/her that they needed more staff to deal with this proposal. The disarmed director responded that he/she did not know what they meant by "his/her proposal." Meanwhile, both managers gave their combined 21 employees a "head's up" about the impending additional work.

Before long, mental health social workers, doctors, and nurses also heard about the director's "new proposal" as it affected everyone in some manner. Calls and letters of protest begin to surface in both the offices of the director and his boss.

Case Study Questions

1. What went wrong? How could the two managers have handled their concerns differently?

2. How should the director have handled his/her idea, and who should have been involved? Would an interdisciplinary/multifunctional team have been valuable at the outset? Might a better idea have surfaced?

3. What team-building methods could be used to correct this course and bring about solutions that most of the staff could support?

4. How would you have gone about answering the email of the two managers?

References

Tuckman B. *Tuckman Forming Storming Norming Performing Model.* 1965. Accessed December 30, 2006 from A. Chapman (webmaster) Businessballs.com. http://www.businessballs.com/tuckmanformingstormingnormingperforming.htm.

The Wilderdom Store. *Team Building Activities, Initiative Games, & Problem Solving Exercises.* 2006. Accessed January 25, 2007. http://wilderdom.com/games/InitiativeGames.html,.

TeamTechnology.co.uk. *How to Improve Teamwork.* 1995. Accessed January 25, 2007. www.teamtechnology.co.uk/tt/h-articl/team-building-part2.htm.

Teambuilding Inc. *The Team Facilitator.* 2007. Accessed January 29, 2007. http://www.teambuildinginc.com/tps/020f.htm.

Schmidt E, Varian H. *Google: Ten Golden Rules.* In MSNBC Newsweek Issues 2006. Assessed February 10, 2007. http://www.msnbc.msn.com/id/10296177/site/newsweek/.

NHS National Electronic Library for Health. *What Is a Knowledge Worker? Knowledge Management.* Accessed February 11, 2007. http://www.nelh.nhs.uk/knowledge_management/ km3/knowledge_worker.asp.

McConnell CR. *The Effective Healthcare Supervisor* (6th ed.). Sudbury, MA: Jones and Bartlett Publishers; 2007.

CHAPTER

18

Physician Leadership and Development

Sudha Xirasagar

Learning Objectives

- Understand the importance of a clinical leadership process in healthcare organizations for meeting quality and cost benchmarks.
- Gain a better understanding of physician motivations and behavior, physician leader-follower dynamics, and the challenges of clinical leadership.
- Know the training needs of physician leaders and potential leadership development paradigms that can address physician leader-follower dynamics.

■ CLINICAL PERFORMANCE: THE KEY TO HEALTHCARE REFORM

Quality and Cost: Key Concerns in the U.S. Health Reform Agenda

The rising cost of healthcare in the United States is rapidly jeopardizing healthcare for many Americans whose income lags behind healthcare cost inflation. It is also seriously undermining the U.S. government's fiscal balance, and jeopardizing its Medicare and Medicaid commitments toward the baby boomers who will rapidly swell the ranks of the elderly over the next decade. Spiraling cost is also undermining the competitiveness of U.S. goods and services in today's global economy, jeopardizing the Gross

Domestic Product (GDP) base that is essential to finance all healthcare, including Medicare and Medicaid. In addition, there are quality concerns, with some experts estimating that 90% of all healthcare, 50% of cesarean sections, 30% of antibiotics used in common infections, and 30% of hysterectomies are either unnecessary, redundant, or reworked.[1] Patient safety is another issue: Even teaching hospitals show a 7% medication error rate, an estimated 98,000 Americans die, and more than one million patients suffer injuries each year due to care process failures, and only about half of U.S. doctors use known "best practices" for their patients.[2–6] These issues force physicians' role and performance to the center stage, because almost all healthcare decisions, directly or indirectly, are driven by physicians, about 75% according to some estimates.[7–9]

Incentives Alone Cannot Impact Clinical Performance

The fiscal and market pressures to contain costs, as well as quality and safety concerns, have caused health insurers and the Center for Medicare and Medicaid Services (CMS) to pursue quality-based purchasing policies. These policies put the onus on the provider to prove their quality credentials. The CMS's demonstration project on pay-for-performance requires hospitals in the selected demonstration areas to report their performance on 21 measures of clinical care quality. Based on these reports, CMS reimburses an additional 2% increment over the standard Medicare rate to hospitals performing in the top 10%, a 1% increment for those in the next 10% rung of performance, and a penalty of 1–2% reduction for those that grossly underperformed on these indicators. Apart from CMS, more than 80% of HMO enrollees in the United States are served by HMOs that use such quality-based purchasing.[10] Thus, providers, particularly hospitals with their capital intensive facilities, have their survival at stake if they fail on the quality measures. Most healthcare decision making, and perhaps, the clinical team culture that impacts these outcomes substantially, rest with physician decisions and behaviors. Yet, universally, rarely have healthcare organizations initiated measures to allocate responsibility and accountability for clinical outcomes to their physician community, and rarely do they provide the needed inputs for a meaningful leadership process among physicians. As for payers, their assumption, thus far, has been that behavior will follow the money: Put the incentives in place, and you will start seeing results.

Contrary to this assumption, the experience of Medicare's pay for performance has shown that the monetary incentive, (and penalty for failure) has made very modest, if any, impact on hospitals' quality performance.[11] This brings us to the question, what is it about physicians and their relationships within healthcare organizations that causes hospital managements, almost without exception, to shy away from initiating clinical leadership development?

■ WHY PHYSICIAN LEADERSHIP IS NEEDED

Let us first examine a central premise of this chapter, that effective physician leadership development is critical to address the fundamental issues of healthcare cost, access, quality, and patient safety. Many "excesses of managed care" documented in the mid-to-late nineties (the heyday of managed care) suggest that in the absence of effective physician engagement in the cost management process, corporate profit motives may rule over the practice of medicine to the detriment of true professional as well as social interests.[8,12,13]

Since the late nineties, the HMO-style dominance over healthcare has receded significantly, but the cost pressures continue to mount, and concerns over quality have become more audible. Fearing the stigma and backlash against managed care of the nineties, payers have turned to indirect means of extracting provider accountability for outcomes. Medicare and other HMOs' pay-for-performance (PFP) initiatives demand accountability in the form of aggregate outcomes for a hospital's total patient panel. However, the hospital, in turn is unable to transfer accountability for the same numeric outcomes to individual physicians. This is because each physician's patient panel outcomes are driven by individual patient's clinical severity (both measured and unmeasured), tailored treatment to individual's needs, and biological variation in response. Yet collectively, outcomes of a group of physicians' patient panels should conform to the quality standards (which are aggregate outcomes demonstrated by clinical trials/outcome studies) provided there is a professional culture of practicing evidence-based medicine and little inclination to practice according to individual physician's preferences. The call for aggregate clinical outcomes thus calls for physicians in leadership positions to assume responsibility for ensuring a collective accountability among their physicians for clinical outcomes and for delivering aggregate results. Why has this not happened so far?

■ UNDERSTANDING PHYSICIAN BEHAVIOR

Many have termed "physician manager or leader" an oxymoron.[14] Physicians in leadership or "managerial" positions, such as department heads or medical directors of group practices or hospitals, face many formidable challenges. Yet, they have generally assumed that providing the evidence for best practices should be adequate for their "rational" colleagues to change their practice patterns. Evidence shows that this leap from information to practice does not happen without "leadership-like" inputs to facilitate the change.[15–17] It requires a leader to engage physicians as peers, based on understanding physician values and interests, and identifying with the total clinical practice setting.[18]

Physician Values and Accountabilities

Physician practice behavior is driven by a mix of values, interests, and accountabilities that often place conflicting demands on their clinical decision processes, which in turn impact patient outcomes.[19] Understanding these complex accountabilities enables one to understand why financial incentives and disincentives alone cannot produce high-quality care, and why it takes a critical mass of physician leaders to take our health system where we want it to be.

As professionals, physicians have fiduciary accountability (i.e., they are expert agents for the patient). Given that the layperson is unable to choose between diagnostic and treatment options on their own, the physician is duty bound by their professional oath to act in the best interest of the patient. Second, in a managed care environment, when payers are stressing cost controls, the physician becomes accountable to the managed care payer, to produce the most cost-efficient results for the total patient panel, rather than for the individual patient. These two accountabilities could place conflicting demands on clinical decisions.[20] Third, the physician practices in a scientific discipline, and therefore has scientific accountability to advance the science of medicine. This motivation may also conflict with the earlier mentioned accountabilities, for example, note the consistently high cost of care in academic institutions relative to non-teaching settings. Fourth, physicians have legal accountability; not only must they act in the best interest of the patient, but also demonstrate thus, beyond all doubt (which may be needed in the future in a court of law if sued by the patient). This concern predisposes to defensive medicine, leading to unnecessary testing and referrals. Fifth, physicians have personal accountability; self-interest to maximize their income as a rational economic being.[18] Overarching all these motivations is an implicit awareness that professionalism should at all times supersede individual self-interest. All of these accountabilities and values are perfectly valid within themselves. What we measure and judge are patient outcomes, the end-result of physicians' clinical decisions, which, in turn, reflect each physician's preferred combination of these accountabilities and values.

The responsibility of each healthcare organization (hospital, group practice, independent practice association, etc.) is to improve its physicians' care quality to ensure the aggregate benchmark levels desired by payers. This means herding their physicians to keep up with and practice evidence-based medicine while internally balancing their individual perceptions and preferences regarding these multiple accountabilities. Since all these accountabilities are perfectly valid in themselves, the most appropriate route to influencing physician practice patterns for outcomes would be to involve clinical leadership by one of their kind, who understands where they are coming from and can guide the process toward a collective accountability.

Challenges in Leading Physicians Toward a Common Vision

Combine the above mix of accountabilities with the universal physician mindset that demands (and receives) non-negotiable, professional autonomy. This explosive mix of values and autonomy seems to doom physician leadership processes from the start. The medical profession's autonomy is rooted in its highly specialized work, combining expertise with complex, rational-intuitive judgmental processes.[21,22] Professional socialization and modeling during the medical school years further hardwires a mindset of absolute autonomy, which may then obstruct legitimate changes that are justified by new scientific and client need-driven developments. Therefore, the big challenge for physician leaders is to identify a leadership process by which they can "make" physicians "want" to adopt evidence-based medicine. Because of the lack of a well-established clinical leadership process that delivers results, most healthcare and professional organizations have designed their evidence-based practice guidelines to ignore the issue of physicians' practice behavior. Instead, most guidelines skirt around the physician-practice behavior issue, preferring to focus on the efficiency of care production involving non-physician providers.[23]

Defining Physician Leadership and Its Scope

An appropriate definition of physician leadership is "the ability to motivate a group of peers to achieve particular organizational purposes, and to take physicians where they would otherwise not go, to a delivery system that burdens them with far greater collective accountability for quality and costs."[21] At this point, we need to distinguish between the physician executive who provides clinical leadership for changes in healthcare performance and the executive who happens to be a physician aspiring to organizational executive and leadership positions. A substantial part of the current confusion regarding the leadership skills and competencies required for physicians to become effective leaders can be attributed to this confusion between a physician executive and an executive who happens to be a physician. The former has to pursue competencies to provide clinical leadership, and the latter has to pursue competencies to provide organizational, strategic leadership. Another source of confusion about the physician leader's role arises from confusing leadership for nut-and-bolts management.

Current Status of Physician Leadership Training Programs

As a result, physician executive development programs are often generic management-training programs, often focusing on financial management, strategic management, accounting, and negotiation training, some basic management content, and finally, throwing in some ad hoc leadership concepts. Many programs do not distinguish between the training needs of physicians seeking to acquire clinical leadership competencies and physicians who are looking to train for organizational executive leadership roles. Such programs often lose the beginner physician leader or their organization entirely because the original training objective of the physician leader and/or their sponsoring organization was to seek clinical leadership competencies to achieve quality and cost benchmark goals.

■ FROM CLINICIAN TO LEADER—ESSENTIAL CHANGES IN MINDSET

Physician leadership positions are not for the faint of heart. Healthcare organizations and clinical physicians need to realize the significant changes in mindset needed, and what they need to leave behind in order to prepare for and succeed at leadership roles.[13,14,24,25] Because of the great divergence between physicians' professional socialization and the skills needed to lead in organizational settings, many wrenching psychological adjustments are needed.[14,26] Foremost is a psychological readiness to move from the comfort zone of the clinician's hard-earned autonomy (through the rigorous medical school years) to the discomfort of a dependent role as a manager/leader, because performance and success is no longer measured by their personal clinical expertise but by the (uncertain) performance of other physicians. Other wrenching transitions are from a clinician's identity and pride in their own patients' outcomes to a leader's identity focused on the organization/unit's aggregate performance; from naivety about organizational dynamics to acceptance of organizational realities; from a command and control mindset (in clinical expert versus lay patient relationships) to the persuasion and ambiguity mode in a managerial role; and, finally, from comfortable peer relationships with professional colleagues to accountability-based boss-subordinate relationships with former colleagues.

Leader Sans Attitudinal Change—The Behavioral Consequences
There are several frequently observed ominous behavioral pitfalls, when physicians rising to management positions ignore the behavioral and mindset transitions needed to provide effective clinical leadership. These pitfalls include: insensitivity or downright arrogance and inability to choose staff, over-managing and inability to adapt to organizational hierarchical roles,[27–29] fighting the wrong battles, being seen as untrustworthy, and failing to develop and effectively communicate a strategic vision,[27] dysfunctional responses due to lack of awareness of the organizational imperatives,[27,29] lack of commitment to leading,[27,30] lack of desire to be a manager, lack of management training, insufficient self-knowledge and self-awareness, lack of style flexibility, poor utilization of resources, and inadequate interpersonal skills,[30] lack of dynamism,[30,31] exclusively relying on data sharing and feedback as the tool to realize

outcomes and resolve conflicts,[1,29] and assuming that if one has read every important management text, one is a great manager.[29]

Contextual Factors Hampering the Clinician to Leader Transition

It is important for healthcare managers to understand that most physician executives also have clinical responsibilities, which makes it doubly challenging for him/her to make the mindset transitions. Many complex reasons, including the financial value of their clinical role to the organization, identity of most physicians with the clinical role, and concerns about losing the respect of peers, contribute to this mix of clinical and management responsibility shouldered by most physician leaders.[25,32]

In addition, healthcare organizations need to realize that organizational factors can hamper good physician leaders from being effective. These include poor leadership skills among organizational leaders, poorly defined institutional goals and criteria for judging performance, and inadequacy or lack of control over resources.[30]

How Physicians Reaching Leadership Positions Impact Their Transition

Unlike business leadership, where upward career progression to executive positions is the natural ambition of managers, physicians' move to leadership or managerial positions is a metamorphic transition. There are several pathways from medicine to management that greatly impact how they perform as leaders: management by evolution (sliding into management roles over the years), management by stardom (outstanding clinical accomplishments rewarded with leadership positions), management by default (position defaulting to available physicians due to non-availability of candidates with aptitude and inclination), management by positive choice (consciously chosen as a career path by physicians with a positive attitude toward leadership roles), management by negative choice (motivated by a desire to avoid clinical roles), and management by cultivation (physicians deliberately groomed for management).[27,33,34] Regardless of the default process, unless there is a change in mindset, achieved by a combination of appropriate leadership training and self-development, the result oftentimes is a reluctant physician leader, lapsing into a laissez-faire leader with little goal-driven direction provided to the department or organization.[32,35]

■ LEADERSHIP DEVELOPMENT MODELS

In exploring leadership development models suitable for clinical leadership, it is worth repeating that one has to distinguish between a physician who is in a clinical leadership position and an organizational executive who happens to be a physician. Much of the literature on physician managers/leaders does not make the distinction, and neither do many healthcare organizations. Not distinguishing the two roles and the associated training needs has led to much confusion on the role of formal management education (generally an MBA degree) and whether it is useful to physicians.[32,36,37] Another cause of confusion in training content stems from failing to distinguish between the utility of *strategic versus interpersonal leadership* competencies for effective *clinical* leadership.[38] Strategic leadership concerns competencies in influencing the organization's strategic direction and positioning relative to its environment. Interpersonal leadership deals with influence processes to steer follower performance toward the desired behaviors and goals.

The urgent healthcare reform goals of quality improvement and cost control call for judicious resource use and evidence-based medical practice by practicing physicians in the organization. This requires its physician leaders to have interpersonal leadership competencies, not strategic leadership abilities. The question arises, what interpersonal leadership behaviors and attributes should physician leaders aim for in order to positively influence their physician subordinates and other clinical care providers? In identifying a suitable leadership training model for physicians, healthcare organizations have to bear in mind one significant difference in boss-subordinate dynamics between business organizations and the medical profession: A physician leader (such as medical director, department chair, etc.), regardless of organizational title, will continue to relate to "followers" as a peer (in line with the medical professional code that overrides all other sources of authority). The peers who are "organizational subordinates" have a keen awareness of their professional autonomy and, generally, scant respect for organizational hierarchy. In contrast, in business organizations, regardless of how democratic the organization, it is an unspoken assumption that the boss-subordinate relationship is framed by the organization's goal imperatives and hierarchical accountability.[13,14,39–42]

Lastly, unlike business managers who acquire a natural legitimization of authority when they rise up the management hierarchy, physician managers often face criticism from former peers for having "sold out," abandoning the values of the profession, or being second-class physicians.[13,35,43] Physician executives, during their early management years, face being "ejected from the professional fraternity, with only partial membership in the managers' club."[14,29]

Two professional traditions pose particular challenges in leading physicians.[44] First, physicians generally cherish custom-crafted variation, taking pride in custom-designing care for each patient, which, in dysfunctional form, manifests as resistance to making work easier and more error-proof. Secondly, physicians are trained in "black hat thinking," a style that emphasizes judgment and caution, which beyond a point, may stifle innovation and change. These professionally socialized mindsets that impede the process of leading physicians toward evidence-based optimum medical care are further compounded by physicians' generally high cognitive competence, which can meld into a general resistance to physician leaders' attempts to influence their practice patterns. These widely observed facets of physician behaviors result in an additional dilemma for a transitioning physician leader, "on the path to leadership, they cannot leave the values of physicians behind, but they must leave some of the behaviors behind . . . and they have to learn and practice skills and actions that apply those cherished values to the larger needs and vision of the whole health care enterprise."[14]

Since peers determine professional values, there is no one best answer as to which combination of goals is right. Herein lies a major source of dissipation of a physician leader's effort in contrast to a business executive. The potential multiplicity of directions of followers' inclinations, each equally valid in one or other scheme of values, confronts physician leaders striving to achieve specific organizational goals, which is in sharp contrast to the singular business focus of business leader-follower relationships. The chosen leadership development model should be capable of addressing these dynamics between physician "leaders" and their "followers."

Transformational Leadership—A Leadership Style for Physicians

Transformational leadership appears to be a well-rounded leadership process that is suited to the intricate challenges faced by leading physicians. Bass and Avolio's full range of leadership model[45–47] presents three potential leadership styles that one could engage in when exercising interpersonal leadership: transformational, transactional, and laissez-faire leadership (see Table 18-1). The elements of each of these styles are discussed in the following sections.

Transformational leadership is a constellation of behaviors and attributes that target followers' higher motivations, leading them to become aware of and act upon hitherto latent motivations toward exceptional performance, and ethically motivated goals beyond the call of duty, transcending individual self-interest. Among physicians, exceptional performance translates to healthcare quality improvement, despite the cost-conscious demands of the managed care environment. Transformational leadership components are idealized influence, inspirational motivation, intellectual stimulation, and individualized consideration. Idealized influence results from behaviors and attributes that cause followers to perceive the leader as driven by an overarching vision and mission—a desire to emulate the leader—and instills pride, trust, respect, and optimism among followers. Inspirational motivation involves successful communication and follower identification with the vision, focusing follower efforts, arousing awareness of their own higher goals and motivations, and sustaining a positive emotional arousal and identification with these goals. Intellectual stimulation involves challenging followers to rethink old ways of doing things, arousing awareness of problems, and creating a cognitive-emotional milieu for followers to explore and experiment with their own goals driven by their increasing awareness of their own higher motivations. Intellectual stimulation is particularly relevant for physician leaders, who face the challenge of influencing cognitively autonomous followers toward consensual, value-driven goals. Individualized consideration includes mentoring, coaching, continuous feedback, and linking the individual's current needs to the organization's mission.

Transactional leadership involves successfully establishing an exchange process, rewards for good performance (contingent reward), and negative feedback for deviations from the norm (management-by-exception). Transactional leadership behaviors include contingent reward and management-by-exception, active and passive. Management-by-exception–active refers to a style of active search for non-compliance, followed by corrective actions, while management-by-exception–passive refers to a passive style of no action unless a crisis or negative outcome supervenes. In essence, when the goals of leaders and followers pertain to individual or group self-interest, and the leader essentially engages in an exchange process with followers to achieve their individual or mutual goals, it is a transactional leadership process.[48] When leaders "shape and alter and elevate the motives, values and goals of followers through the vital teaching role of leadership," and, "irrespective of separate interests held by the persons, they are presently or potentially united in the pursuit of "higher goals," the process is transformational leadership.[48]

It is important to note, however, that a transformational leader also has to engage in transactional behaviors, both for achieving short-term goals (which is essential for organizational survival and for the leader to survive in a leadership position!), and for gaining credibility as a transformational leader. Therefore, transformational leadership builds on transactional leadership, and a highly transformational leader is also perceived as highly transactional. Transactional behaviors help the leader to establish trust, when rewards are reliably exchanged for performance as promised. This early "transactional" trust subsequently transfers to trust in the leader's long-term vision and mission, which inspires followers' buy-in and action to actualize the vision.

Laissez-faire is non-leadership, when the leader is perceived as being indifferent to follower actions and organizational outcomes. Each leader manifests a combination of leader behaviors with dominance of one of the three styles.[46] It is important to note that the transformational (or other) style of dominance in a leader is determined by how their followers and supervisors rate the person, not how the person rated him/herself.

Table 18-1 Sample Transformational, Transactional, and Laissez-Faire Leadership Behaviors*

I. Transformational Leadership

Idealized Influence
Proud of him/her
Goes beyond self-interest
Has respect of co-workers
Talks of values
Emphasizes the collective mission

Inspirational Motivation
Talks optimistically
Talks enthusiastically
Clear vision

Intellectual Stimulation
Seeking different views
Re-examines assumptions

Individualized Consideration
Teaches and coaches
Individualizes attention
Helps subordinates develop their strengths

II. Transactional Leadership

Contingent Reward
Assists based on effort
Clarifies rewards
Recognizes achievement

Management by Exception–Active
Concentrates on failures
Tracks your mistakes

Management by Exception–Passive
Puts out fires

III. Laissez-Faire Style
Avoids involvement
Unavailable when needed

---

*Selected items from the MLQ-Form 5X Short (Copyright 1996, 2003 by Bernard M. Bass and Bruce J. Avolio. All rights reserved. Published by Mind Garden, Inc., www.mindgarden.com). Item summaries above are in the permitted format for reproduction by the copyright holder, Mind Garden Inc.

Transformational Leadership Goes beyond Managership

Transformational leadership is one style that goes beyond managership, a distinction highly relevant for physician leaders. An executive is playing a leader's role when he/she innovates, develops, and leads people, trusts subordinates, thinks and acts long-range, asks questions that essentially look at why and what issues, and has their vision fixed on the horizon, originates and challenges the status quo, and does the right things.[49] In contrast, the corresponding *managerial* behaviors are to administer (within existing rules and frameworks), maintain, manage structure, control, think and act short-range, ask questions that essentially look at how and when issues have their eye on the bottom line, use precedents as the guideline for action, work by goals/objectives/status quo already in place, be a good soldier, and do things right. Because clinical work is expert-driven, and care processes are so involved, it is impossible to design rules and procedures exhaustively, to cover every patient diagnosis, treatment plan, or care contingency. The failure to understand this limitation was at the crux of the failure of "micromanaged" care, causing inappropriate care denials to significantly, and sometimes dangerously, erode patient care and patient satisfaction. Transformational leadership allows followers to take their own autonomous course, yet put forth exceptional performance, establish and surpass their own goals, and be self-motivated to establish ever higher goals and standards. Keeping in view the complex web of accountabilities driving clinical practice, professional, scientific, fiduciary, legal, fiscal, as well as personal (self-interest), transformational leadership appears to fit the bill for physicians to exercise clinical leadership.

Empirical Evidence for Transformational Leadership among Physicians

Transformational Clinical Leaders and Organizational Clinical Outcomes
Evidence for the usefulness of transformational leadership behaviors for physician leaders is available from a national study of medical directors of the federally-assisted community health centers (CHCs) in the United States.[50] CEOs of the centers were surveyed, asking them to rate their medical director's leadership behaviors using an adapted Bass and Avolio's Multifactor Leadership Questionnaire (a partial list of summarized items used is included in Appendix 1).[46] The CEOs were also requested to share information on their center's performance in their top-priority clinical programs or aspects. A total of 269 CEOs (41% of the sample population) responded to the survey. From the leadership item ratings, aggregate scores were calculated for each medical director on their manifest transformational, transactional, and laissez-faire leadership styles (how frequently they engaged in the behaviors that add up to each style). For each medical director, scores were also calculated on perceived effectiveness, perceived satisfaction of subordinates, and subordinate extra effort.

The study showed that medical directors with higher transformational leadership scores had superior clinical program achievements that required superior performance of their clinical teams. The priority clinical areas reported were mostly related to improving glycemic control among the diabetic patient population of the center, prenatal care coverage and reduction in low birth weight, hypertensive and asthma patient coverage under evidence-based programs, and functionality scores reflecting clinical outcomes among geriatric and mental health patients. Transformational leadership scores also significantly predicted the CEO's assessments of their effectiveness on all three subjective measures. For both clinical goal achievement and subjective ratings of effectiveness, transactional leaders were also more effective than laissez-faire leaders, although they were less effective than transformational leaders. The medical director's specialty, age, duration of tenure as a medical director, and duration of tenure at the CHC did not alter these relationships.

Does Transformational Leadership Competency Improve with Management Training?

Another significant finding was that medical directors who had significant management training, either a master's degree (in health administration, public health, or business administration), or more than 28 days equivalent of in-service training were rated as significantly more transformational, compared to those without such a degree and less than a week's equivalent of in-service training.[51] The study had some limitations, in being cross-sectional, and in surveying bosses rather than physician subordinates of the medical directors. Yet, its findings suggest that transformational leadership has significant utility for physician leaders to influence clinical practice patterns toward evidence-based practice. Transformational leadership has proven to be an effective tool for improving objective measures of performance in almost every other setting that calls for intellectually and motivationally-driven follower behavior, such as idea generation among computer-mediated group decision-making teams, productivity of industrial research teams, financial unit productivity in financial institutions, military personnel, and nuclear facility safety groups.[52–56]

Ideally, research needs to be more conclusive about a *causal* impact of transformational leadership of physician leaders on influencing their clinical team's patient outcomes. For this, one needs longitudinal studies that show increasing physicians' transformational leadership scores over time results in improved performance of the clinical team. Pending such studies, the dynamics of physician behavior, complex accountabilities in clinical decision making, unique dynamics of physician leader-follower relationships, and historic aloofness of physicians from the hospitals they work for all intuitively point toward transformational leader behaviors as an appropriate tool to influence physician practice patterns toward achieving better quality, cost control, and patient safety in the United States.[44]

■ CHAPTER SUMMARY

- Physician leadership is critical for improving healthcare quality and reducing its cost, the most urgent priorities in the U.S. health system.
- Improving quality and reducing redundancy in healthcare requires a systematic organization-wide process to steer physicians toward evidence-based medicine and value-driven practice behavior.
- Clinical leadership, involving effective interpersonal leadership by adequately prepared physician leaders in healthcare organizations will be the key.
- A complex web of professional, scientific, and other accountabilities and values drives practicing physicians. This is why it takes a physician to lead them, based on a shared understanding of the clinical process.
- Transformational leadership as applied to the interpersonal leadership domain conceptually fits the needs of clinical leadership dynamics.
- A nation-wide empirical study of physician leadership in the context of the federally supported community health centers has found that centers with transformational medical directors have significantly superior population-based clinical outcomes among their patient panels.
- The study also suggests that transformational leadership may be trainable; medical directors with significant management training (either formal degree or in-service training) had clearly higher transformational leadership scores.

Review/Discussion Questions

1. Explain why physicians' practice performance as a group holds the key to achieving sustainable improvements in healthcare quality, cost, and access to care.
2. Explain why clinical leadership is the key to getting physicians on board for achieving hospital/HCO-wide improvements in clinical quality performance.
3. What are the motivations and accountabilities that physicians have to trade-off in their clinical decision making? Are some of these contradictory in the directions they would lead the physician? Why?
4. Outline the challenges faced by physician leaders in their attempts to "lead" physicians toward a common vision of healthcare performance.
5. How should physicians desirous of taking leadership positions prepare themselves to become successful in providing clinical leadership?

6. What are the differences between transformational, transactional, and laissez-faire leadership?
7. Why is transformational leadership likely to be a suitable leadership tool for clinical leaders?

References

1. Berwick DM, Nolan TW. Physicians as leaders in improving health care. *Ann Intern Med*. 1998;128(4):289–292.
2. Leape L. Error in medicine. *JAMA*. 1994;272:1851–1857.
3. IOM (Institute of Medicine). *To Err is Human: Building a Safer Health System*. Edited by LT Kohn, JM Corrigan, MS Donaldson. Washington, DC: National Academic Press; 2000.
4. Starfield, B. Is U.S. health really the best in the world? *JAMA*. 2000;284(4): 483–485.
5. Casalino L, Gillies RR, Shortell SM, Schmittdiel JA, Bodenheirmer T, Robinson JC, Rundall T, Oswald N, Schauffler H, Wang MC. External incentives, information technology, and organized processes to improve health care quality for patients with chronic diseases. *JAMA*. 2003;289(4): 434–441.
6. McGlynn EA, Asch SM, Adams J, Keesey J, Hicks J, DeCristofaro A, Kerr EA. The quality of health care delivered to adults in the United States. *N Engl J Med*. 2003;348(26):2635–2645.
7. Dye CF. Cultivating physician talent: 5 steps for developing successful physician leaders. *Healthc Exec*. 1996;11(3);18–21.
8. Frankford DM, Konrad TR. (1998). Responsive medical professionalism: Integrating education, practice, and community in a market driven era. *Acad Med*. 1998;73(2):138–145.
9. Emanuel EJ, Dubler NN. Preserving the physician-patient relationship in the era of managed care. *JAMA*. 1995;273(4);323-329. (Jan 25)—75% of health care costs driven by physician decisions—maybe sub reference: Baker LC, Cantor JC. Physician satisfaction under managed care. *Health Aff*. 1993;12(Suppl.):258–270.
10. Rosenthal MB, Landon BE, Normand S-LT, Frank RG, Eptstein AM. Pay for Performance in Commercial HMOs. *N Engl J Med*. 2006;355:1895–1902.
11. Lindenauer PK, REmus D, Roman S, et al. Public reporting and pay for performance in hospital quality improvement. N Engl J Med. 2007;356:486–496.
12. Berwick DM. Eleven worthy aims for clinical leadership of health system reform. *JAMA*. 1994;272(10):797–802.
13. McCall MW Jr., Clair JA. In transit from physician to manager—Part I. *Physician Exec*. 1992;18(2):3–9.
14. Guthrie MB. Challenges in developing physician leadership and management. *Front Health Serv Manage*. 1999;15(4):3–26, 45.
15. Lowet PF, Eisenberg JM. Can information on cost improve clinicians' behavior? Lessons from health care trials and management theory. *Int J Technol Assess Health Care*. 1997;13(4):553–561.

16. Davis DA, Thomson MA, Oxman AD, Haynes RB. Changing physician performance—A systematic review of the effect of Continuing Medical Education strategies. *JAMA*. 1995;274(9):700–705.

17. Rosenthal GE, Hammar PJ, Way LE, Shipley SA, Doner D, Wojtala B, Miller J, Harper DL. Using hospital performance data in quality improvement: The Cleveland Health Quality Choice experience. *Jt Comm J Qual Improv*. 1998;24(7):347–360.

18. Lagoe RJ, Aspling DL. Enlisting physician support for practice guidelines in hospitals. *Health Care Manage Rev*. 1996;21(4):61–67.

19. Gamm LD. Dimensions of accountability for not-for-profit hospitals and health systems. *Health Care Manage Rev*. 1996;21(2):74–86.

20. Shortell SM, Waters TM, Clarke KWB, Budetti PP. Physicians as double agents: Maintaining trust in an era of multiple accountabilities. *JAMA*. 1998; 280(12):1102–1108.

21. Merry MD. Physician leadership for the 21st century. *Qual Manag Health Care*. 1993;1(3):31–41.

22. Irvine D. The performance of doctors. I: Professionalism and self-regulation in a changing world. *Br Med J*. 1997;314:1540–1542.

23. Horne M. Involving physicians in clinical pathways: An example for perioperative knee arthroplasty. *Jt Comm J Qual Improv*, 22(2), 115–124.

24. Olson DA, Scott EF, Wright RH. And a doctor shall lead them. . . . *Health Services Review*. 1997;30(50):33–35, 48–49.

25. Kirschman, D. Physician executives share insights. *Physician Exec*. 1996;22(9):27–30.

26. Sullivan, P. MDs aiming for hospital boardroom may face humbling experience, CEO warns. *Can Med Assoc J*. 1998;158(7):918–919.

27. McCall Jr., M.W., Clair, J.A. Why physician managers fail—Part I. *Physician Exec*. 1990;16(3):6–10.

28. McCall MW Jr, Clair JA. Why physician managers fail—Part II. *Physician Exec*. 1990;16(4): 8–12.

29. Kennedy MM, Pickett RB. Seven deadly assumptions for new physician managers. *Physician Exec*. 1995;21(12):47–49.

30. Cummings KC. Why some managers fail. *Physician Exec*. 1988;14(4):6–8.

31. Sterling J. The seven deadly sins of physician management. *Med Group Manage J*. 1998;45(5):17–22.

32. Ottensmeyer DJ, Key MK. Lessons learned hiring HMO medical directors. *Health Care Manage Rev*. 1991;16(20):21–30.

33. Ackerman FK Jr. The role of physicians in executive management. *Med Group Manage J*. 1993;40(5):67–76.

34. Kimmey JR, Haddock CC. Physician executives' characteristics and attitudes. *Physician Exec*. 1992;18(3):3–8.

35. LeTourneau B, Curry W. Physicians as executives: Boon or boondoogle? *Front Health Serv Manage*. 1997;13(3):3–25.

36. Lyons, M.F. Transitional leaders for transitional times. *Front Health Serv Manage*. 1999;15(4):36–41.

37. Kindig, D.A. Do physician executives make a difference? *Front Health Serv Manage*. 1997;13(3):38–42.

38. Pawar BS, Eastman KK. The nature and implications of contextual influences on transformational leadership: a conceptual examination. *Acad Manage Rev.* 1997;22(1):80–109.

39. Heifetz R. Leadership without easy answers (interview by J Flower). *Healthc Forum J.* 1995;July-August:30–36.

40. Greer AL. The shape of resistance . . . the shapers of change. *Jt Comm J Qual Improv.* 1995;21(7):328–332.

41. Kendall ER. When a physician leads quality improvement: An interview with Keith Wilson. *Jt Comm J Qual Improv.* 1994;20(6):344–350.

42. Goldsmith J. Hospital—physician relationships: A constraint to health reform. *Health Aff.* 1993;Fall:160–169.

43. Johnson RL. Physicians as executives: Barriers to success. *Front Health Serv Manage.* 1997;13(3):28–32.

44. Reinertsen JL. Physicians as leaders in the improvement of health care systems. *Ann Intern Med.* 1998;128(10):833–838.

45. Bass BM, Avolio BJ. *Transformational leadership: Manual for the Multifactor Leadership Questionnaire.* Palo Alto, CA: Consulting Psychologists Press; 1990.

46. Bass BM, Avolio BJ. *MLQ Multifactor Leadership Questionnaire, Sampler Set, Technical report, Leader form, Rater form, and Scoring Key for MLQ Form 5x-Short.* Binghamton University, NY: Center for Leadership Studies. (Distributed by Mind Garden, Redwood City, CA); 1995.

47. Bass BM, Avolio BJ. *Full Range Leadership Development—Manual for the Multifactor Leadership Questionnaire.* Palo Alto, CA: Mind Garden; 1997.

48. Burns JM. *Leadership.* NY: Harper & Row; 1978.

49. Bennis W. *On Becoming a Leader.* Reading, MA: Addison-Wesley; 1989.

50. Xirasagar S, Samuels ME, Stoskopf CH. Physician Leadership Styles and Effectiveness: An Empirical Study. *Med Care Res Rev.* 2005;62(6):720–740.

51. Xirasagar S, Samuels ME, Curtin TF. Management Training of Physician Executives, Leadership Style and Disease Management Performance: An Empirical Study. *Am J Manag Care.* 2006;12(2):765–772.

52. Sosik JJ. Effects of transformational leadership and anonymity on idea generation in computer-mediated work groups. *Group & Organization Management.* 1997;22(4):260–287.

53. Keller RT. Transformational leadership and the performance of research and development project groups. *Journal of Management.* 1992;18(3):489–501.

54. Howell JM, Avolio BJ. Transformational leadership, transactional leadership, locus of control and support for innovation. *J Appl Psychol.* 1993;78(6):891–902.

55. Yammarino FJ, Bass BM. Long-Term Forecasting of Transformational Leadership and its Effects Among Naval Officers. Some preliminary findings in Clark KE, Clark MB. *Measures of Leadership.* West Orange, NJ: Leadership Library of America, Inc., 151–170; 1990.

56. Bettin PJ, Hunt PS, Macaulay JL, Murphy SE. Shido: Effective leadership in Japan. In Clark KE, Clark MB, Campbell DE. *Impact of Leadership.* Greensboro, NC: Center for Creative Leadership, 81–94; 1992.

19

Governance and Board Development

Dennis G. Erwin and Andrew N. Garman

Learning Objectives

- Understand the principal roles and responsibilities that governing boards hold in the oversight of healthcare organizations.
- Understand the relationship between the board and the senior leadership of healthcare organizations.
- Identify common committee structures used by boards, and the typical functions of those committees.
- Identify recent trends in the changing nature of board responsibilities, and their implications for governance in healthcare organizations.
- Evaluate the effectiveness of a governing board and its members' contributions.
- Define current and future board membership needs, and develop approaches to meeting those needs.

■ INTRODUCTION

In this chapter, we will discuss governing boards and their roles and responsibilities, how they are structured, and how they operate to fulfill their responsibilities. As you will see, there is wide variety in current practice, and while there are some generally accepted principles of effective practice, these principles provide for considerable flexibility. Hospital and non-profit organizations have many nuances in their governance activities; accordingly, we have attempted to reflect examples of these throughout the chapter.

As background, most healthcare organizations in the United States are organized as non-profit corporations. The secretaries of state authorize the formation of non-profit corporations and the attorneys general regulate their operations in each of the 50 states. Because non-profit corporations are formed to benefit the public for charitable purposes, they are granted exemption from most federal, state, and local taxes. Responsibility to oversee these non-profit healthcare organizations is delegated to governing boards, which are also referred to as boards of trustees or boards of directors. The individual members of governing boards are known as trustees or directors.

Effective oversight, or governance, of healthcare organizations involves ensuring that the organization fulfills its charitable mission and public responsibilities. Such responsibilities are fulfilled by providing appropriate leadership and strategic direction as well as ensuring financial integrity and the delivery of quality and safe patient care in ways that meet the healthcare needs of community members.

■ BOARD ORGANIZATION

An organization's articles of incorporation and bylaws serve as guidelines for the structure and operation of its governing board. These guidelines will typically address the frequency of board elections, the election process for board members and officers, board member terms of office, the powers and duties of board members, the types of decisions requiring board approval, the frequency of board meetings, and even who will preside at board meetings.

Boards vary greatly in how they are organized and how they operate. A recent survey of 616 hospital governing boards reflected this diversity of practices.[1] Respondents to the survey indicated that:

- Although the average membership of their boards was 15–16, smaller boards of less than seven members and larger boards with more than 31 members were not uncommon.
- A number of committees typically support the work of the board. The most common board committees included finance, governance/nominating, quality, and strategic planning, as well as an executive committee.
- The average board met ten times per year. Most boards met monthly but some met as infrequently as quarterly.

- Typical board meeting agendas usually included addressing reports from management and board committees, discussing strategy, setting organization policy, and educating board members.
- Most boards defined board member terms of 3 years, with limitations of three consecutive terms. Although not directly related to governance, fund-raising and solicitation of charitable gifts is an important activity of non-profit governing boards. In fact, many non-profit organizations expect contributions from their board members as part of their services.

■ BOARD OFFICERS

An organization's bylaws will also identify and define the roles and responsibilities of the board members. The board will typically be led by a chairperson (or president), who presides over meetings of the governing board and the executive committee, serves as spokesperson for the board and the organization, appoints committee chairs, establishes the agenda for board meetings and board priorities, and works closely with the chief executive officer and leadership team of the organization.

Other than the chairperson, board officers include a vice chairperson (or vice president), a treasurer, and a secretary. The vice chairperson assumes the responsibilities of the chairperson in the chairperson's absence and serves on the executive committee. The treasurer serves on the executive committee and chairs the finance/audit committee, and the secretary serves on the executive committee and is responsible for the maintenance and accuracy of board minutes. Board minutes are the official record of the activities of the board and document the approval of corporate policy decisions at board meetings.

■ BOARD COMMITTEES

Although most governing boards have the committees mentioned above (executive, finance, governance/nominating, quality, and strategic planning), boards may have additional committees specific to their organizations. For example, non-profit organizations typically have a charitable giving committee, or hospitals often have separate foundation boards to support charitable giving activities.

How a committee operates and its activities vary greatly from organization to organization. Accordingly, each board committee should have a written description of its role, responsibilities, and policies to provide guidance and clarity of expectations. The activities described next are typically associated with each of the major committees.

Executive Committee

Members of the executive committee support the board chairperson in establishing the priorities and key goals and objectives of the board. Members of this committee generally include the board officers and/or the chairs of the various committees, and as such represent a leadership group within the board. Often, members of the executive committee meet in "executive session." The purpose of "executive session" is to handle sensitive issues including the compensation and evaluation of the chief executive officer's performance, or when it is impractical for the entire board to meet.

Finance Committee

The finance committee supports the board in its responsibility to ensure the financial integrity and financial oversight of the organization. As part of this activity, many boards also have an audit committee with responsibility for oversight of the audit function and the independent auditors. This typically includes recommending and selecting the independent auditors and oversight of financial reporting and internal controls. Other functions of the finance committee include working with the chief financial officer to establish appropriate financial and operating information to be reported to the board, and recommending financial policy to the board.

Governance/Nominating Committee

The governance/nominating committee supports the board in establishing and defining the duties and responsibilities of the board and its members, evaluating board structure, nominating and recruiting members of the board, and facilitating board continuing education. Often this committee also has responsibility for overseeing a board assessment process, described in more depth later in this chapter.

Quality Committee

The quality committee supports the board in ensuring that the organization is providing high-quality patient care and meeting the healthcare needs of community members. The quality committee works with the leadership team and, in the case of hospitals, the medical staff to establish appropriate quality measurements reported to the board as well as to the community in meeting public reporting requirements. In hospitals, often the medical affairs committee reports to this quality committee. The hospital's medical affairs committee is typically responsible for evaluating the professional competence and credentials of the medical staff and making recommendations to the board for appointing physicians to the medical staff and granting clinical privileges.

Strategic Planning Committee

The strategic planning committee supports the board in meeting its responsibilities for overseeing the organization's strategic management activities. The strategic planning committee works with the organization's executive team to ensure that the organization is monitoring and adapting to changing community needs within the constraints of the organization's mission, capabilities, and resources.

Charitable Giving Committee and Foundation Board

Charitable giving committees and foundation boards support non-profit boards and their organizations in developing public awareness of the charitable benefits the organization provides. A charitable giving committee's activities may include involvement in soliciting contributions and gifts as well as oversight of board/foundation investments. These activities are coordinated with the organization's director of development or chief executive officer. A foundation board typically operates as a separate board that reports to the governing board. Often, governing boards elect to retain responsibility for managing investments made from charitable gifts received by the foundation boards.

■ BOARD MEETING FORMAT

The formats of board meetings vary widely—a sample agenda follows. The organization's bylaws indicate the necessary notice that must be provided to the members in announcing a meeting, and the proper method of announcement. To have an official meeting, there must be a quorum, which is also defined in the corporate bylaws. To have a quorum, the bylaws generally indicate those who must attend (e.g., the chairperson or vice chairperson) and the minimum number of board members who must be present (e.g., a majority of members).

After calling the meeting to order and ascertaining there is a quorum, some boards request approval of the agenda to ensure all are in agreement with the priorities of the board meeting. Then, the minutes of the prior meeting are usually approved in order for the meeting to be official. The main agenda items are started next. Although meeting structure and content varies, it will often include presentations from the chief executive officer, the chief financial officer, and members of management concerning operations, finance, strategy, and quality, and the chairs of each standing committee will typically present reports outlining key issues from their respective committee meetings. Additionally, outstanding issues from prior meetings may be addressed, while new proposals might be presented or discussed including elections, approval of budgets, capital expenditures, and strategic plans. Discussions are generally involved with each agenda item, and, at any point, motions and/or votes on issues may be requested and discussed. Once all of the agenda items before the board have been addressed, a member moves for the meeting to be adjourned, and a vote is taken to approve adjournment of the meeting.[2]

MEETING OF THE BOARD OF DIRECTORS

Thursday, January 2
ABC Hospital and Health Centers

SAMPLE AGENDA

Call to Order	D. Howard, Chairperson
Invocation	T. Johnson, President
Minutes (for review and acceptance)	
Discussion of Old Business	
New Business Items	
Annual Corporate Compliance Report	L. Soto, Director of Compliance
Annual Board Assessment	Complete and return to Secretary
President's Report	T. Johnson, President
Operations Report	S. Shah, Chief Operating Officer (COO)
Financial Report	A. Viernes, Chief Financial Officer (CFO)
Quality Report	M. Kwasny
Community/Foundation Report	M. Odwazny
Professional Affairs/Medical Staff	L. Aponte, M.D.
Appointments Report	
Marketing/Business Development	T. Jones

Board Member Education: Implications of Sarbanes-Oxley for Non-profit Boards
Adjournment

ATTACHMENTS:
Minutes from Prior Meeting
Compliance Report
Board Assessment
Financial Statements
Balanced Scorecard Report
Charitable Care Report
Credentialing Report
Quality Improvement Plan
Resource Management Plan
Marketing Plan

■ THE RELATIONSHIP BETWEEN SENIOR MANAGEMENT AND THE BOARD

The governing board is ultimately responsible for hiring the chief executive officer, or president, as well as determining his/her ongoing fitness for the role. Based upon the board's understanding of the chief executive's strategies and operating plans, the board and chief executive agree on which decisions should be brought to the board, which the board should "advise and consent," and which should be delegated to the chief executive.[2] Despite delegating certain responsibilities to the chief executive, the board's role is to continually monitor and evaluate the organization's performance in achieving its goals and objectives. In addition, determining how the board will hold management accountable and intervene in the event performance goals and objectives are not met is fundamental to the board's role.

Officially, the chief executive is the only member of management who reports to the board. However, based upon the information and analysis needed by board members and the board committees to make meaningful recommendations and appropriate decisions and policy, board members will typically need to interact somewhat regularly with other members of the senior leadership team, including, at a minimum, the chief financial officer, the chief operating officer, the chief nursing executive, and the chief medical officer.

In addition to organizational goals and objectives, the board is responsible for working with the chief executive in establishing expected personal performance goals and objectives. Monitoring, evaluating, and providing meaningful feedback about the chief executive's performance is an important board responsibility.

■ FIDUCIARY DUTIES

In meeting their responsibilities, members of a governing board are required, both individually and collectively, to carry out their duties using standards of *care, obedience,* and *loyalty.* The *duty of care* requires members to act in good faith, with at least the degree of diligence, care, and skill ordinarily exercised under similar circumstances. The *duty of obedience* requires members to ensure that the leadership of the organization complies with laws, acts within the guidelines established in the articles of incorporation and bylaws, and is faithful to the charitable mission and purposes of the organization. The *duty of loyalty* requires board members to prioritize the interests of the organization and the public above their own self-interests.

In practical terms, these duties require board members to have a commitment to regularly attend board meetings and to familiarize themselves with organizational strategic, operating, quality, and financial matters. In addition, to ensure adherence to activities within the constraints of the organization's charitable and tax-exempt purposes, a periodic board committee review of articles of incorporation, bylaws, due diligence reports from licensing and accrediting authorities, and insurance companies may help to surface noncompliant activities.

To avoid potential conflicts of interest, board members should generally avoid transacting business with the organization they are serving. Any transaction between a board member and the organization they are serving requires full disclosure and evaluation to ensure that the transaction is in the best interests of the organization. Further, any opportunities related to the purposes of the organization that come to the attention of a board member must be presented to the organization before being taken advantage of by a board member.

■ FINANCIAL OVERSIGHT

In connection with the fiduciary responsibilities described above, governing boards are responsible for ensuring financial integrity, developing financial policy, and providing oversight of financial and operating performance. Because virtually all irregularities involve the finances of an organization, the roles of the finance and/or audit committees are fundamental to board governance.

As part of financial oversight, board members generally review an organization's monthly and annual financial statements. Review of the financial statements includes obtaining an understanding the composition of and any changes in the organization's revenue, expenses, and operating margins as well as its assets and liabilities. In addition, governing boards are responsible for understanding and approving the organization's annual operating and capital budgets as well as any significant financings, transactions, and contractual agreements.

The finance/audit committee is also responsible for selection of the organization's independent audit firm and arranging periodic meetings with the auditors to review issues related to the financial statements and weaknesses in financial and accounting controls. Financial oversight might also include meetings with the organization's attorneys to discuss significant legal issues that might have an impact on the organization.

■ OPERATING OVERSIGHT

It is becoming clear that this limited view of the fiduciary role of financial oversight by boards is not adequate. For instance, a view of hospital boards as "stewards of assets" has been promoted.[3,4] Such a perspective requires more than ensuring adequate financial integrity and internal controls; it also

THE SARBANES-OXLEY ACT

In recent years, high-profile business failures such as Enron, Arthur Andersen, WorldCom, and Tyco International along with non-profit problems at United Way; the American Red Cross; and the Allegheny Health, Education and Research Foundation have created considerable popular interest in strengthening the role and oversight of board governance. In 2002, Congress responded to concerns about governance of publicly traded companies by passing the Sarbanes-Oxley Act, also known as the Public Company Accounting Reform and Investor Protection Act. Several policy-makers and scholars (e.g., Orlikoff) have suggested that non-profits should consider adopting relevant elements of the Act, which could include:[5]

- Required review of the appropriateness and effectiveness of internal controls
- Required certification of the financial statements by both the chief executive and chief financial officers
- Assurance of auditor independence and approval of the auditors by an audit committee consisting of board members independent of management
- Bans on personal loans to officers or board members
- Adoption of policies that protect whistleblowers

includes an evaluation of financial and operating performance.[6] Monitoring financial and operating performance is no longer viewed as micromanagement on the part of the board, but increasingly as essential to the board's legal responsibility for oversight. As stewards, understanding the goals and objectives of the organization, ensuring their alignment with the strategies of the organization, and monitoring that they are being achieved in an effective and efficient manner are becoming viewed as fundamental responsibilities. These activities include comparisons of actual outcomes to budgets and plans as well as analyses of trends and activities.

In reviewing the operations of the organization, the board looks for trends and explanations for changes in operating performance. For hospitals, operating information often reviewed by boards includes patient admissions and average daily census, average revenue and expenses per patient day, and average patient length of stay. Other information of interest might include trends between outpatient and inpatient services provided, payer mix, and the case mix index (CMI), a measure of acuity or level of sickness of patients. Hospital board members might also monitor the performance of key departments and service lines (e.g., emergency department, surgery, outpatient imaging, heart and vascular, oncology, and obstetrics/gynecology) to be aware of changes in activity, revenue, expenses, and levels of profitability. Other issues with financial implications that might be appropriate for board-level review include malpractice insurance premiums, write-offs of bad debt, and the costs and reporting of charity care.

HOSPITALS AS COMMUNITY ASSETS: PUBLIC ACCOUNTABILITY AND THE REPORTING OF CHARITY CARE

In reaction to substantial, recent pressure from Congress to ensure that non-profit hospitals are using their tax-exempt status to support the public good, several organizations have provided guidance about how non-profit hospitals should manage and report their community relationships. Influential reports include The Catholic Health Association's "Guide for Planning and Reporting Community Benefit"and PricewaterhouseCoopers' "My Brother's Keeper: Growing Expectations Confront Hospitals on Community Benefits and Charity Care."[7,8] Best practices described in these reports include:

- Establishing board-level community benefits committees with external community members to assure alignment of organizational missions and community benefits.
- Developing stakeholder analyses to assure community needs are met and not duplicated by other hospitals.
- Identifying community benefit programs and their positive impacts in their communities
- Developing and distributing community benefit reports throughout the community.
- Reporting charity care (service for which the hospital does not expect to receive payment due to a patient's inability to pay) at cost.
- Offering discounts to uninsured patients based on managed care rates and their ability to pay.
- Providing patients with financial assistance information and assistance from qualified financial counselors

Taken together, these numerous public reporting requirements strongly support the perspective that hospitals are community assets, and their board members and leaders are publicly accountable for their mindful stewardship.

■ STRATEGIC OVERSIGHT

Another key role of healthcare governing boards is ensuring that the organization is responding and adapting to changing forces in its environment. Such environmental or external forces include changing economics, community demographics, technological advancements, epidemiological changes, regulatory and political changes, and competitor challenges. Each of these forces can substantially affect the viability of healthcare organizations, and they are therefore affecting the way board members and management teams must think about their organizations.

For example, many hospital boards and their senior management teams have tended to be internal in their focus, primarily concerned with operations and not how their organizations may need to adapt and change in response to forces external to their organizations. However, there is an increasing recognition by governing boards of the need to focus on strategic issues and ensure their organizations are responding appropriately to changes to the external environment. Often, to obtain market information about strategic changes and trends, management uses outside services, such as local healthcare associations or consulting firms that monitor and provide some analysis of relevant data.

Strategic management involves several key components including: monitoring elements of the environment external to the organization; evaluating how environmental changes impact the organization; determining how these changes fit with the mission, resources, and capabilities of the organization; and developing action plans to implement necessary and appropriate change and adaptation. All of these activities are crucial responsibilities for senior management. However, because the board is ultimately responsible for determining the mission of the organization as well as approving decisions and policy about the direction and allocation of resources, it typically makes sense for boards to be integrally involved in the strategic planning process. In other words, management has the responsibility to provide the board with relevant information and analysis that is meaningful and helpful to the board in ultimately making strategic and policy decisions.

Senior management and governing boards continue to wrestle with numerous strategic trends and the associated questions of how these trends will impact their organizations, and how their organization might respond in light of its mission, resources, and capabilities.

For instance, a governing board might need to address the implications of an aging and ethnically changing population along with a growing number of uninsured and financially disadvantaged patients in relation to the current services the organization provides, the diversity of the organization's existing workforce, the organization's available resources, and the feasibility of the organization's desired mission.

Another example of strategic challenges a hospital governing board might need to evaluate is the declining access to capital for improving the facility's infrastructure and investing in information technology, medical technology, and electronic medical records in relation to the continuing demand by patients, physicians, and regulators for the most modern facilities and technologies. Finally, a governing board might need to address how the organization will respond to growing competition from other service providers and changing demands for services (e.g., cardiac services, women services, cancer services, pediatrics, neurosciences, surgical services, diagnostic services, ambulatory surgery centers, and end-of-life care).

These strategic conversations provide a governing board and its senior management with the framework to identify the challenges and opportunities for providing improved value and services to its patients, customers, and other constituencies. The resultant development of meaningful strategies and the implementation of appropriate change are probably the most crucial for ensuring the long-term sustainability of organizations.

■ OVERSIGHT OF PATIENT CARE AND RESOURCE UTILIZATION

A key component of any healthcare organization's mission statement is for its staff to provide high-quality care to its patients in an efficient manner with the resources it has available. Accordingly, monitoring and evaluating the quality of patient care and efficiency of resource utilization are pivotal roles of governing boards. Historically, in hospital organizations, the medical staff was viewed as primarily responsible for the quality of patient care. More recently, however, responsibility for the quality of care of patients has become as important as ensuring financial integrity and operating performance.[9]

Working Relationship with Medical Staff

Typically, in hospital organizations, the responsibility for patient care oversight is assigned to the quality committee, which works closely with the medical staff to promote quality patient care. The medical staff works independently from the hospital's senior management, who may not have the appropriate background to inform clinical decision making. To manage this relationship between hospital management and the medical staff, hospitals have medical staff bylaws, which identify the rules and regulations for physicians and other professionals who have been granted clinical privileges at hospitals. Those bylaws are prepared by the medical staff and submitted to the governing board for approval. The medical affairs committee, a committee of medical staff, is typically responsible for evaluating the professional competence and credentials of the medical staff and making recommendations to the board for appointments to the medical staff and granting clinical privileges.

Quality Improvement

In addition to managing medical staff appointments and granting clinical privileges, the governing board monitors and evaluates quality improvement and resource management plans. Numerous types of quality improvement programs exist. For instance, a clinically focused program might establish priorities that concentrate on high-risk, high-volume, or problem-prone clinical practice areas that consider the incidence, prevalence, and severity of patient problems. Many organizations have adopted quality programs with customer-first orientations focused on allowing patients and customers to drive quality goals. Other programs focus on pursuing continuous improvement and best practices or the continuing education and training of staff.

PUBLIC ACCOUNTABILITY AND REPORTING FOR QUALITY PATIENT CARE AND SAFETY

To enhance public disclosure of individual hospital performance and to encourage continuous quality improvement, the U.S. Department of Health & Human Services publicly discloses information reported by hospitals about the treatment of certain medical conditions. Performance by individual hospitals can be compared for 21 quality measurements reported to the Centers for Medicare and Medicaid Services. Those measurements are available at http://www.hospitalcompare.hhs.gov/hospital.[10] The reporting includes measurements of treatments for heart attacks, pneumonia, and surgery patients.

Soon, in addition to reporting the above quality measurements, the results of the Hospital Consumer Assessment of Healthcare Providers and Systems (HCAHPS) Hospital Survey will also be reported. The survey is used by hospitals to collect information about patient satisfaction. The goals of the survey include producing comparable data about hospital care from the patient's perspective, to create incentives for hospitals to improve their quality of care, and to enhance public accountability and transparency of the quality of care (www.hcahpsonline.org).[11]

Although the implications of expanded reporting are difficult to predict, the greater transparency of hospital operations and performance most certainly demand greater accountability by governing boards and senior management to the communities and constituencies they serve.

Efficient Resource Utilization

Promoting quality improvement also requires the board to ensure effective and efficient use of organizational resources. In delivering high-quality care, organizations must work within the constraints of balancing quality against the costs of providing care. In a hospital, for example, resource management plans might include identifying patterns of resource utilization such as overutilization, underutilization, and the scheduling of resources. Elements of such a plan might include: evaluating the medical necessity of admission, continued stay, and the costs of drugs and treatments; discharge practices and case management policies and procedures; the accuracy, timeliness, and completion of medical records; and medical staff policies and rules.

■ CHANGING BOARD MODELS

As indicated in the previous discussions of each of the areas of board responsibilities, many facets of the governance role and process are continually evolving. The traditional governance model of only meeting the most basic fiduciary responsibilities and serving as a "rubber stamp" of management recommendations is clearly obsolete. In most instances, that model has evolved to a level in which the board provides assurance that the chief executive and the management team are meeting the board's expectations and in which the board is remaining informed about significant strategic, operating, and patient care improvement plans and issues. Even this model of providing basic assurance and remaining informed, however, is now being challenged.

The model of governance that seems to be emerging involves board members becoming more engaged in the leadership of organizations. In a more engaged board model, the talents for which board members are recruited are utilized in providing value and supporting the management team in creating high-performing boards and organizations. In this model of governance, board members are expected to provide meaningful advice and insightful thinking to leadership, including contributing to the development of organizational plans and making key decisions.[12]

■ EFFECTIVE GOVERNANCE: CULTURES AND ACTIVITIES

The most effective boards have been described as "robust, effective social systems."[13] They are distinguished by cultures that allow them to candidly and openly discuss difficult information, challenge one another's thinking and beliefs, and conduct meaningful reviews of board-level and individual board member performance.

A study of both effective and ineffective boards identified numerous activities associated with effective board governance.[14] These activities included: board members ensuring that they understood the organization, its cultures, and values; the board's responsibilities; the complexities of issues from multiple perspectives; the board's accepting their responsibilities for stakeholder relationships; and their ensuring a strategic approach.

Using these activities as a basis for evaluating board performance, a study of 64 non-profit hospitals found that boards conducting more of these activities were associated with better organizational performance.[6] Findings such as these make a strong case for ongoing board assessment and development to enhance board performance.

■ BOARD ASSESSMENT

Many boards engage in periodic assessments concerning their overall performance and opportunities for improvement. Such assessments may include questions such as: Are we addressing the right issues and giving them the appropriate time and attention? Are we evaluating the right information? Do we have the right membership? Are board members exhibiting appropriate behaviors and providing value? By compiling open and honest responses to questions of these types, boards are in a better position to make appropriate changes and enhancements to improve performance. Below are some areas that are frequently helpful for boards to self-assess.

Establishing Board Priorities and Setting the Agenda

Identifying and prioritizing the areas that are most important to the board and then determining the amount of time and attention the board will allocate to those areas is an important assessment exercise. It may be useful to identify the areas where board members are currently focusing their time and energies (e.g., financial oversight 20%, capital budgets 20%, administrative duties 30%, etc.) and where the board members feel they *should* be spending their time (e.g., strategy 40%, physician relations 25%, operational improvement 25%, etc.). Comparing and contrasting the results can provide a basis for discussing how the board may wish to refocus its priorities and efforts. For example, a board meeting may be overloaded with management presentations with little discussion or serious questioning or input from board members. Negotiating or managing the board agenda such that the priorities of the board and the organization receive the appropriate time and attention can improve the board's focus on issues of greater priority and areas in which the board contributes the most value. Controlling the agenda in this way can also allow more time to educate board members concerning the nuances of complex issues, as well as to engage in productive discussion.

Additionally, having senior management conduct the same analysis of the board could provide useful information in helping the board and management negotiate their respective roles and initiate a meaningful discussion of priorities.

Determining Information to Be Monitored and Evaluated

Board members are often given a substantial amount of information to monitor and evaluate. The quality of the information the board receives, including when and in what format they receive it, is critically important to the board's ability to conduct its work effectively.[12] Too little information or missing information will create "blind spots" in the board's judgment; conversely, too much information (e.g., lengthy presentations and reports without meaningful analysis) can overwhelm a board member's capacity for processing this information.

Member Skills and Experience Assessment

Boards that are clear about the issues that will be most important to them are also in the best position to identify the skills and experiences that will be most helpful for future board members to have. Assessing the skills and experience of existing board members and comparing those to the future needs of the organization can help boards make better decisions about changes in the composition of board membership. For example, if the board views changing demographics in the community and the movement of a competitor into the organization's market as significant issues, which may require the organization to adapt and respond, it may consider focusing on recruiting new members who have a deeper understanding of the healthcare industry, the changing needs of the community, and/or experience with strategic planning and change management.

Member Performance Assessment

In addition to evaluating board member skills and experience, assessing board member performance provides an opportunity to support members in making more meaningful contributions to the board. Some boards have their members self-assess as frequently as every board meeting on the quality of their contributions (e.g., whether they read the packet and came to the meeting adequately prepared, contributed to the discussions, and spoke with appropriate candor). Boards may also ask members to complete a set of peer feedback surveys, which will then be aggregated and the results reported back to individual board members. Areas in which members might be evaluated include: their knowledge of the organization and the healthcare industry; their knowledge of areas such strategy, finance, patient care, technology, or marketing; their ability to understand specific technical issues, provide quality input, and ask thoughtful questions; and their ability to understand their roles as board members and to interact effectively with management and other board members.

Diversity

As representatives of community assets serving the needs of multicultural communities, board members who can interface and speak on behalf of these communities can help ensure the organization is keeping their interests in mind. Research also suggests that board and senior leadership roles have not been keeping pace with the diversification of the U.S. population.[15] It is therefore important for hospital boards to also assess their ability to hear, respond to, and include those they serve in the workforce and in decision and policy-making.

■ BOARD MEMBER EDUCATION

Healthcare delivery is influenced by a highly complex set of factors; even if board members have considerable expertise in their own fields, they often need additional grounding in healthcare. Accordingly, board member education is important for ensuring board effectiveness and productivity. Many boards will sponsor initial and ongoing educational programs for board members, which can include orientations, annual retreats, and regular items on the board's meeting agenda. Subjects that are particularly useful for board member orientation include:

- A general overview of the healthcare industry, to provide board members with an understanding of the framework within which healthcare organizations operate (e.g., the healthcare delivery system, major payers, regulators, and accrediting agencies).
- The mission, vision, philosophy, and values of the organization, as well as its history.
- The structure of the organization, including bylaws; an organization chart; and a summary of departments and their functions, policies, and relationship with constituencies (e.g., the medical staff).
- The organization's strategy including: market description; significant competitors; market share; community demographics; and current strengths, weaknesses, opportunities, and threats.
- An overview of financial, operating, and quality programs and reports.
- A review of board minutes for the prior year to understand the activities and major issues recently addressed by the board.

Board education activities can also provide a forum for exposing members of the organization's management team to the board. This can serve the dual purpose of providing board members with multiple perspectives of the organization, as well as familiarizing them with key leaders responsible for running it on a day-to-day basis.

CONSENT AGENDAS

To provide more time during board meetings for board member education and the discussion of strategic and substantive issues, many boards have adopted consent agendas. Consent agendas include non-controversial administrative and financial items requiring board approval but not requiring board discussion before the board votes. Such items might include approval of board minutes and routine minor expenditures or contracts needing board approval but already reviewed by committees. All information and supporting documentation along with motions or policy resolutions about such matters should be provided to board members in advance of the board meeting and then simply voted on as one item.

Important items that would not be appropriate for a consent agenda include adoption of the organization's mission; strategic, operating, and quality plans; annual operating and capital budgets; executive compensation arrangements; or any matters that might be controversial.

■ CURRENT ISSUES AND CONTROVERSIES

Currently, there are a number of questions regarding optimal board structure and process being debated. Several of these are described below.

Board Member Independence

Independent board members are not employees and do not conduct business with the organization. Some authors (e.g., Orlikoff) have argued that a majority of members of a board should be independent.[5] The recommendation comes from the concern that board members who are part of management may not have the appropriate objectivity to make decisions in the best interests of the communities they serve. On the other side of the discussion, independent board members, who serve part-time and on a volunteer basis, certainly do not have the ability to make the same time commitment, nor do they have the same knowledge of the organization as will the organization's leaders; thus a critical mass of board members from senior management may be essential to effective board operations.

Separation of the Board Chairperson and the Chief Executive Officer

There is increasing convergence of opinion that the chairperson and the chief executive officer should not be the same person. In circumstances in which an organization has a dominating chairman/chief executive, the chief executive lacks accountability. Division of the roles gives the board chairperson responsibility for leading the board, controlling the board agenda, establishing appropriate committees, and managing the nomination and selection of board members.

Paid vs. Unpaid Board Members

Although few board members of non-profit organizations are currently compensated, some have argued that board members should be paid, given the increasing challenges and responsibilities of boards, as well as the expectations for more active contributions from board members. Doing so might entice board members to be more engaged in meeting preparation and attendance, and payment might enhance the ability to recruit the most competent and qualified board members. The counter-argument is that payment undermines the very essence of a non-profit organization, and if a person is unwilling to serve in this role without pay, then they may not have the ideal personality "fit" for the role.

■ CHAPTER SUMMARY

- Governing boards assume responsibility for oversight of non-profit organizations and refer to members as trustees or directors.

- There are wide varieties of ways in which boards are structured (e.g., number of members) and in which they function (e.g., frequency of meetings).

- Most boards have a number of subcommittees, including an executive committee as well as finance, governance/nominating, quality, and strategic planning committees.

- The role of the board has been changing in recent years. The general trend has been toward greater expectations for involvement and accountability; some are recommending that boards require larger proportions of independent members and even consider payment for service.

Review/Discussion Questions

1. What are the three "duties" the board is responsible for upholding? What is an example of a circumstance in which each might serve as a guiding principle?

2. This chapter has described several important trends in the nature of board member responsibilities. What are some important general themes you noticed in these trends? What do you think their implications may be for future board members?

3. Given the increasing challenges and responsibilities of boards, as well as the expectations for more active contributions from board members, some have suggested that board members should be paid for their time and trouble. Discuss the pros and cons for paying board members.

Learning Activity

Case Study: What Not to Do

The failure of Allegheny Health, Education, and Research Foundation (AHERF) has become a case study in how "not" to govern an organization. The study of AHERF's rise and fall tells a story about a senior management team that manipulated the governing board and the financial community, intimidated staff and employees, and operated without any constraints. This failure in governance challenges governing boards to examine their practices and their obligations as stewards of community assets and the public trust. Below is brief information about AHERF along with a few of its board's practices.

Break into groups, and have each group select one or two of the board practices. Discuss the problems with the board's practice, and then discuss how to improve them.

THE BANKRUPTCY OF ALLEGHENY HEALTH, EDUCATION, AND RESEARCH FOUNDATION (AHERF)[16]

In July 1998, AHERF filed for bankruptcy, thus becoming the largest non-profit health-care bankruptcy in history with over $1.3 billion in debt and 65,000 creditors. Further, in June 1999, the AHERF's officers and directors were sued for $1 billion in damages for breech of fiduciary duty, gross negligence, and management and corporate waste.

As background, AHERF was formed as a non-profit corporation in 1983 with a single, prosperous hospital, Allegheny General Hospital. In 1986, AHERF had $274 million in assets, revenues of $195 million, and 4000 employees. By 1997, the organization had grown (almost exclusively by acquisition) to $2.20 billion in assets, $2.05 billion in revenues, and 31,000 employees.

Sherif Abdelhak, hired as chief executive officer in 1906, orchestrated the organization's aggressive acquisition program, growth, and ultimate demise. Ultimately, the AHERF board of directors fired Abdelhak in June 1998 for hiding cash transfers used to cover up the financial problems of AHERF.

Below are several descriptions of AHERF's board practices:

1. AHERF's business and acquisition strategy appears to have been based on a flawed vision, one that the board should have challenged but did not. Board members were discouraged from asking "tough questions;" those who did question AHERF's plans were either pressured to conform, or found themselves subject to term limitations and removed from the board.

2. The board was dominated by an alliance between the chief executive officer and the board chairperson. Board meetings were "scripted affairs, intentionally staged to limit oversight and participation."[16] Board members received large stacks of reports and information of up to 1000 pages, with minimal time to review them, and often the information was not reviewed.

3. Acquisitions were completed without proper due diligence, and sometimes even without the approval of the board. In numerous instances, failing organizations were acquired with no turnaround plan or subsequent monitoring to evaluate improvement in operating performance.

4. The organization had a network of ten different boards responsible for its various operations and a large parent board varying in size from 25 to 35 members. No one seemed to have access to a complete overview of the organization, or specific accountabilities for it. Moreover, until 1998 AHERF did not prepare a consolidated financial statement reporting a complete picture of the entire operation.

5. Board membership was viewed as a "social activity or community service" rather than as a fiduciary duty.

6. Board members consisted of leaders in the community with numerous apparent conflicts of interest. For example, five AHERF board members were from the organization's lender, which completed transactions without board approval.

Failures of accountability and oversight extended even beyond these listed items, to include relationships with external auditors and bond-rating agencies and bond insurers, as well as a lack of oversight by the state attorney general's office.

References

1. Lockee C. *Raising the Bar: Increasing Accountability, Transparency, and Board Performance.* The Governance Institute's 2005 Biennial Survey of Hospitals and Healthcare Systems; 2005.

2. Colley J, Doyle J, Logan G, Stettinius W. *What is Governance?* New York: McGraw-Hill; 2006.

3. Chait R, Holland T, Taylor B. *Improving the Performance of Governing Boards.* Phoenix, AZ: Oryx Press; 1996.

4. Taylor B, Chait R, Holland T. (1996). The New Work of the Nonprofit Board. *Harvard Business Review,* 74:5, September-October 36–46.

5. Orlikoff J. Building Better Boards in the New Era of Accountability. *Front Health Serv Manage.* 2005;21(3):3–12.

6. McDonagh K. Hospital Governing Boards: A Study of their Effectiveness in Relation to Organizational Performance. *Journal of Healthcare Management.* 2006;51 November/December:377–391.

7. Catholic Health Care. *Guide for Planning and Reporting Community Benefit.* 2007. Accessed March 24, 2007, from http://www.chausa.org/Pub/MainNav/ourcommitments/ CommunityBenefits.

8. PricewaterhouseCoopers. *My Brother's Keeper: Growing Expectations Confront Hospitals on Community Benefits and Charity Care.* 2007. Accessed March 24, 2007, from http://www.pwc.com/extweb/pwcpublications.nsf/docid/38BE1BA9F194D10F85257308005936AB.

9. Biggs E. *The Governance Factor: 33 Keys to Success in Healthcare.* Chicago, IL: Health Administration Press; 2003.

10. US Department of Health & Human Services. *Hospital Compare.* 2007. Accessed on March 24, 2007, from http://www.hospitalcompare.hhs.gov/Hospital/Search.

11. CAHPS Hospital Survey. *Hospital Care Quality Information from the Consumer Perspective.* Accessed on March 24, 2007, from http://www.hcahpsonline.org.

12. Nadler DA. Building Better Boards. *Harv Bus Rev.* 2004;82(5):102–111.

13. Sonnenfeld JA. What Makes Boards Great? *Harv Bus Rev.* 2002;80(9): 106–113, September. 109.

14. Jackson D, Holland T. Measuring the Effectiveness of Nonprofit Boards. *Nonprofit and Voluntary Sector Quarterly.* 1998;27:159–182.

15. Health Research & Educational Trust. *Hospital Governance: Initial Summary Report of 2005 Survey of CEOs and Board Chairs.* Accessed March 24, 2007, from http://www.hret.org/hret/programs/leadergovern.html.

16. Based on Burns L, Cacciamani J, Clement J, Aquino W. The Fall of the House of AHERF: The Allegheny Bankruptcy. *Health Aff.* 2000;19(1):7–41.

20

Organization Development for Terrorism and Natural Disasters

Ahmed Adu-Oppong, Gerald R. Ledlow, Mark Cwiek,
James A. Johnson, and M. Nicholas Coppola

Learning Objectives

- Why it is important to incorporate the organizational contingency plan into the overarching goals of the organization's strategic planning initiative.

- Why the form that the threat of terrorism could take should include chemical, biological, radiological, nuclear, and explosive, with special emphasis on bioterrorism.

- How to prepare the organizational workforce for disaster management.

- What the organizational needs are for disasters and how to be able to undertake threat evaluation for the organization.

- What the different kinds of threats faced in society are today, and how to prepare for them.

- How to communicate the organizational contingency plan to the employees of the organization.

- Why it is important to establish a disaster control command center. Also tips on how to manage it.

■ INTRODUCTION

Since the publication of the 9/11 commission, the government has issued guidance for securing our homeland. The Department of Homeland Security, born out of the 9/11 commission report, was given the mission of building a foundation for the future direction in homeland security. Healthcare organizations have been significantly affected by this act, and will continue to be in the upcoming decade.

Furthermore, in 2002, the Department of Homeland Security (DHS) published the National Strategy for Homeland Security, which outlined six critical mission areas necessary to defend the United States. These include: intelligence and warning, border and transportation security, domestic counterterrorism, protecting critical infrastructures and key assets, protecting against catastrophic threats, and emergency preparedness and response. Foundations necessary to address these critical areas were also identified. They are law, science and technology, information sharing and systems, and international cooperation. The National Strategy was formulated based on the content and provisions of the Homeland Security Act of 2002. Since 2002, the Department of Homeland Security has expounded upon these areas—and constructed corresponding departments.

It is a long-term goal of the DHS to assist universities, organizations, and federal government agencies in creating sanctioned degrees and certificate programs in Homeland Security as a method to better protect our nation. In fact, the Hart-Rudman Commission Report suggested an increasing need for homeland security education to protect against threats to United States' soil. The report suggests that the strategy to defend the country is up to the educated, that is, those with the knowledge and education to prevent the disaster. As a result, it is incumbent on future healthcare leaders to be aware of these opportunities and receive education and training as appropriate to their organization's mission.[1]

■ SIGNIFICANCE TO HEALTHCARE LEADERS

Disaster comes in many forms. Whatever the form disaster may take, the organization has a responsibility to plan proactively and to protect its employees, its stakeholders, its local community, and its assets. It is therefore important that the organization have a contingency plan that addresses the spectrum of known risks, from natural disasters (such as hurricanes) to terrorism risks (such as bio-terrorism). Terrorists can use weapons made from chemical, biological, radiological, nuclear and explosive agents, pathogens, and elements. Of particular note, there are different kinds of biological terrorism/biological weapons that can be used in a terrorist attack that the organization needs to be aware of such as anthrax, plague, Q fever, tularemia, and influenza. The threat should be understood relative to one's own industry and the goods or services that the industry produces. Some of the potentially high-risk industries include shipping, communications, media, utilities, **healthcare delivery**, finance, travel, defense suppliers, mass producers, distributors of food, and any business operating in global markets.

Strategic planning is an organization's process of defining its corporate strategy and direction, and making decisions on allocation of resources (including people and financial capital) to pursue that strategy. The work product normally is represented as a formal strategic plan. The strategic plan is used as a guide to define functional areas such as technology, marketing, and so forth. The strategic plan is used also as a guide to define the operations of sub-units of the organization, such as divisions, departments, and so forth.

It is important for the strategic plan of the organization to include the organization's business contingency plan (BCP) for natural disasters and terrorism, because protecting the workforce makes excellent business sense. Keeping the BCP high on the strategic priorities list is more about "how it is done" and not "what is done." It is the job of the senior leadership to establish BCP methodology and then guide the company through the processes in an efficient and thoughtful manner. By combining the company's resources, risk mitigation efforts can become more effective and efficient, and BCP can become a stronger discipline within the company. Key business issues can be identified and prioritized proactively within the company. Risk mitigation goals should be valued as part of the business decision-making process and as based on a holistic view of the issues at hand. The more integrated the process for identifying and assessing potential risks to the business within the strategic plan, the easier the decisions can be made by the BCP management team.

A company typically is made up of many departments, strategic business units, business processes and of course its overall workforce. Ideally, all of these components align around the company's strategic plan and support of the company's mission, vision, and objectives. Healthcare organizations likewise are comprised of many different business units that work together to produce healthcare services for the communities they serve. The basic responsibility of the management team is to assure the continuation of the company by providing cost-effective products to their consumers and keeping an eye on the bottom line and making a profit. For the company to survive, it has to be innovative and flexible, and it needs to provide services and/or products that are valued by their customers. BCP must follow the same philosophy. For BCP to be successful within the company, executive leadership and the BCP planners must have agreement on what disasters could disrupt the business, and then strategically align the business operations around acceptable contingency plans for minimizing business disruptions. Every business should develop a business contingency plan as part of its strategic plan, as a principal means of protecting its future.

Companies have many departments that seek to evaluate and mitigate risks. However, these departments seldom communicate effectively with each other. Each department has its own agenda, and often risk mitigation is not centrally planned within the company. Too often, companies do not require their departments to look at the same risks at the same time. This decentralized approach is too often ineffective and redundant. The integration of BCP into the company's strategic plan, on the other hand, can add value by aligning critical business units and key individuals around company issues associated with BCP.

In most business endeavors, people (human resources) constitute a significant and valuable asset, responsible for production and ultimately profit or net margin. Protecting the workforce and their families, customers, suppliers, and other stakeholders should be an essential and moral core value of the organization. Bioterrorism and infectious diseases potentially threaten business operations at the heart of its productivity, by attacking the people, their families, and the communities where the business thrives. One only has to look at the recent anthrax "attack" in the U.S. Capitol to realize how disruptive bioterrorism agents can be. The postal service was paralyzed for a time. If this had been a non-government business enterprise, it would be a rather straightforward exercise for the company to calculate impact in terms of lost revenue and increased costs.

Just as the world seemed to have turned the corner from the arms race among superpowers, another threat, perhaps more ominous, is upon the world: biological warfare. Biological agents and pathogens increasingly are becoming a concern to business entities throughout the world.[2] Companies now need to integrate business contingency planning into the strategic planning process so the organization can quickly return to a functional state as rapidly as possible in the aftermath of a disaster. This integration needs to be endorsed and led by the senior management team, so that all members of the organization can see the value put on these efforts.

■ THE THREAT

"Black biology, the research on bacteria, viruses, and toxins for the purpose of creating weapons of mass destruction, is the nightmare of security experts in western countries and is also beginning to capture the attention of scientists and politicians. . . . Bio-weapons have become the 'poor man's nuke'."[3] Religious extremists, state-sponsored terrorist groups, criminals, and the mentally unstable are the most probable candidates to employ biological terrorism. The rapid increase in present knowledge of biotechnology and the global biotechnology business, including information available on the Internet, seems to contribute to the widespread possibility of biological agents to be used as weapons.[4] There exists real concern about rogue nations, undefined stockpiles of weapons, global terrorist networks, and financial resources available to deranged and fanatical individuals. In addition, advances in genetic engineering and molecular biology have empowered microbiologists to engineer new organisms that are not only more lethal than endemic pathogens but are also resistant to antibiotics and other prophylaxis.[5]

Today, up to 18 countries are suspected, if not confirmed, to have biological weapons research and development programs in place, and of the seven countries listed by the U.S. State Department as sponsors of international terrorism, at least five are known or suspected to have bioweapons programs.[6] Some estimates suggest that at least 20 nations are developing biological agents for use as mass casualty producing weapons.[7]

The most worrisome threats, according to researchers, are biological terrorism agents such as smallpox, anthrax, and plague.[7] It is important to reiterate that terrorists can use various means to achieve their evil goals, including agents that are chemical, biological, radiological, nuclear and/or explosive. A 1969 United Nations expert panel determined that the cost to produce mass casualties over one square kilometer was $600 for a chemical weapon, $800 for a nuclear weapon, $2000 for a conventional weapon, and only $1 for a biological weapon.[8] Also very worrisome, small nihilist teams are operating in different parts of the world.[7] "Experts believe that the ability to respond to acts of terrorism in the future will depend on our ability to recognize and react to a highly infectious, invisible agent promptly and appropriately—without panic and with a high degree of organization. Emergency personnel will also have to recognize new weapons: deadly bacteria and viruses may be easily disseminated from a bursting light bulb, an aerosol can, or a spray bottle."[9]

Countries that have attempted to acquire nuclear weapons are also suspected of developing biological weapons; North Korea, Libya, and Iraq are topping the list of most threatening nations. Biological weapons are easy to manufacture when compared to other weapons of mass destruction.[8] Biological weapons can be made by using the same fermentation technology that produces antibiotics, vaccines, wine, and beer. Many agents such as those that produce anthrax and the plague can be collected around the globe from the soil or from diseased animals.[6] The Working Group on Civilian Bio-Defense has identified the variola virus (smallpox) and bacillus anthracis (anthrax) to be the greatest threat from terrorists.[6] Bioterrorism and infectious disease experts seem to agree that it is just a matter of time before a biological agent will be used as a weapon of terrorism.[9] Biological agents reportedly are attractive to terrorists because these agents can be released and the perpetrators long out of the country before signs and symptoms begin to appear in the population.[10]

"Preparedness for mass casualties, whatever their cause, is an established and legitimate mandate of public health."[11] The lack of integration of public health, healthcare, law enforcement, education systems, and mass media to deter and counter bioterrorism is a primary obstacle that must be overcome.[12] Most county and city public health agencies have not dedicated serious resources into bioterrorism preparedness.[13] Effective communication is the most critical first step (and ongoing process) between key stakeholders, businesses, healthcare facilities, medical personnel, public health, medical laboratories, veterinary systems, and law enforcement. Only with effective communication can there be hope to deter and to respond to biological terrorism and infectious diseases in general.

Preparedness

The most critical step in preparing for a large-scale mass destruction attack is organizing and training staff to respond to the potential mass chaos that will occur when a disaster or terrorist event happens to better prepare for chaos situations (in the spirit of "contingency planning"), consider reasonable preparedness measures and put them in effect as soon as possible. Implement detection systems. Place special emphasis on technological innovation, research and development, medical countermeasures, and preparation for handling bioterrorist threat situations. Provide phased and prioritized education to emergency personnel, first responders, individuals in high-threat situations, and the general public.[7] Community preparedness is a critically important issue. The reader is advised to review the series, Community Preparedness and Response to Terrorism, where a community preparedness model[2] and structure are discussed.[14,15]

When developing the business contingency plan, roles and responsibilities must be clearly communicated and understood by the people developing the plan. Senior management of the company should be responsible for strategic decisions and the development of overarching principles. Management teams should be responsible for developing the various parts of the plan and for assuring that the contingency plan meets the expectations of senior management, who approves the business contingency plan and provides oversight.

As stated above, senior management must set clear priorities, goals must be set, and an integrated, organized effort needs to be set into motion to achieve these goals.[12] A system must be put into place to sustain the effort from the international, national, regional, state, and local levels. A top-down strategic plan that allows local flexibility and that is implemented at each level of society is required to strike a blow against bioterrorism and to respond effectively when "black biology" is inflicted. A wide variety of activities need to be taken, from developing vaccines, to building biological agent detectors (such as the mail sniff box), to setting up decontamination systems. These activities may prove in many ways difficult to pursue, but they are of critical importance. Resources must be positioned so that they can be moved quickly from location to location. National and state funding of these efforts, especially in the areas of public health and community preparedness, are paramount. Business political support is necessary to raise the priority of these efforts, and to help ensure that collaboration between all entities is maintained.

Risk mitigation strategies and business contingency plans can be logically thought through when cross-functional teams identify and assess potential business disruptions. It is important to include key suppliers, vendors, and customers in this planning process. A cross-functional team approach allows each area to give their perspective of what they believe are the issues and solutions.

Detection of biological agents is often difficult. Various organizations currently are developing technologies to improve the speed and accuracy of methods for detecting and determining what biological agent is threatening people in a specific location.[6] The first sign of attack would be a number of individuals presenting with signs and symptoms. As such, surveillance systems are being developed that will identify an event rapidly so that medical countermeasures (prophylaxis to treatment) can be started quickly. Response teams are being organized, fielded or planned under the umbrella of the National Disaster Medical System, the Centers for Disease Control and Prevention (CDC). Various public health and advocacy agencies are involved, and the military also has several response teams in the United States. The National Association of County and City Health Officials (NACCHO), representing almost 3000 public health agencies, are active in building a bioterrorism response capacity.[13] The first step in the process is identification. The local hospital laboratories may well be the sentinels that sound the alarm that a bioterrorist event has occurred. It is up to the BCP developers to identify the organized response team within their locality and how to maintain communications when there is an attack.

National, regional, and statewide epidemiological systems are necessary to identify, track, and control resource allocation, and must be fully integrated within the multi-tiered medical laboratory system, the CDC (including the Health Alert Network), and public and community health systems.[8] The CDC received $178 million in fiscal year (FY) 1999 to prepare for bioterrorism and to establish this network of laboratories (the Laboratory Response Network). In addition, the CDC received $52 million to establish a pharmaceutical stockpile of drugs, vaccines, prophylactic medicines, and antidotes for a bioterrorist event response.[4] The integration of the Laboratory Response Network (LRN) in the National Electronic Disease Surveillance System (NEDDS), a system that would replace more than 70 different disease-reporting systems operated by the CDC into a single system, should be a high priority. Improvement in the capability and communication systems of clinical laboratories is critical in supporting counterterrorism efforts. It is imperative that the local healthcare facility's microbiology laboratory integrates into the LRN, where protocols are utilized to either rule out bacterial agents (those that could be from bioterrorism acts) or refer such specimens on to the next level of laboratory within the network.[16] Even if biological pathogens are affecting a community without a bioterrorist event, infectious diseases are the second leading cause of death and leading cause of disability—adjusted life years worldwide—so implementing the appropriate BCP protects the workforce and thus protects business.[17]

With an effective identification and control system, quick response assistance can come to the aid of a business. The CDC has developed a national pharmaceutical stockpile of "push packages" that can be delivered by two aircraft within 12 hours anywhere in the United States. These packages include therapeutic and prophylactic supplies.[18] This system would be supported by national level vendor-managed inventories that would be delivered within 24–36 hours and would be prepared specifically for the biological incident. Critical Incident Stress Management teams from the mental health community can play an important role in controlling and managing a bioterrorist event.[19]

Education is the first level of defense in the war against bioterrorism. Education of medical personnel, police/law enforcement officials, and public health officials in the identification, containment, and control of biological agents is a high priority. Businesses must insist that the healthcare system(s) nearest their operations are aware of the importance of preparing for bioterrorism. "A large proportion of hospitals probably are poorly prepared to handle victims of chemical or biological terrorism. Surveys of hospital emergency departments have found broadly prevalent deficiencies in knowledge, plans, or resources for responding."[20]

Increasingly, biological agents and pathogens are becoming a concern to business entities throughout the world. Consider the following:

- Infectious diseases are the second leading cause of death and disability in the world (and an ill workforce does not produce effectively or efficiently).
- Travel at the international, national, and regional levels facilitates the spread of infectious disease (many times before first signs and symptoms of the disease present).
- Infectious disease prevalence can be reduced and controlled.
- Bioterrorism, using infectious diseases to cause harm in a planned and vicious manner, is an increasing threat to communities and businesses worldwide.
- Knowledge, planning, and preparation can reduce the impact of bioterrorism.

Core Competencies in Homeland Security for Healthcare Leaders

The NCES (2002) defines competency as "the combination of skills, abilities, and knowledge needed to perform a specific task." An individual achieves competency by having the knowledge, skills, and ability required to effectively perform the activities of a given occupation.[21,22] Figure 20-1 depicts the necessity of having a foundation of traits and characteristics relevant to the subsequent learning process. For the health service executive, this could include having experience in emergency management, police activities, information technology, or business management. From this foundation, skills, abilities, and knowledge are added and developed within the learning process. For instance, the health service executive would gain skills in emergency management, strategic planning, terrorism, etc., or build upon existing knowledge by expanding the scope of the foundation.

Without an established professional entity acknowledging standardized core competencies, healthcare professionals may find it difficult to develop appropriate job descriptions, which may impact any competitive advantage held by employing a homeland security executive in the organization.[22]

Currently, two educational consortiums exist with focus on education to support the homeland security/defense mission. Formed first was the Homeland Security and Defense Education Consortium (HSDEC), which established the following tenets:

1. Ensure the Department of Defense (NORAD/NORTHCOM) role in and perspective on homeland security adequately and accurately reflects in educational initiatives.
2. Promote and facilitate homeland security related education program development.

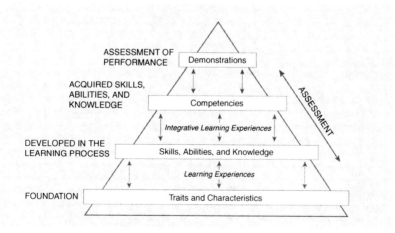

Figure 20-1 A Hierarchy of Postsecondary Outcomes.

3. Focus and facilitate homeland security related research and development.
4. Encourage cooperation between consortium institutions.

The second consortium, the National Academic Consortium for Homeland Security (NACHS) comprises public and private academic institutions engaged in scientific research, technology development and transition, education and training, and service programs concerned with current and future U.S. national security challenges, issues, problems, and solutions at home and around the world. The specific objectives of the NACHS are to help:

1. Improve understanding of national security issues, especially terrorism and strategies for counterterrorism.
2. Promote development of better-informed public policy, strategy, plans, and programs regarding national security issues.
3. Develop new technologies and transition those technologies into effective, practical, and affordable solutions to (current and future) international and homeland security problems.
4. Educate and train the people required by governmental and non-governmental organizations to effectively accomplish international and homeland security roles and responsibilities.

Both the HSDEC and NACHS have furthered the education components of homeland security into proposed standardized curriculum-based programs. To support the need for the components of the curriculum, professional core competencies should be the foundation of any program.

Once specified knowledge, skills, and abilities are acquired, the healthcare executive will be considered competent to perform within their profession. As a result, through assessment of performance competency components, healthcare organizations will be able to continually demonstrate an ability to respond appropriately to threats.[22]

Business Threat Evaluation

Every business entity should develop a sense of how vulnerable it is in the wake of a bioterrorism attack. Table 20-1 is provided as a place for many businesses to begin assessing their relative risk by virtue of their business size, location, dependence on human performance, and the mission/product/service of the entity. After the business entity scores itself on the following table, the authors suggest that a score in the moderate range (5–7 points) or above should be considered a warning for the entity to put serious resources into developing bioterrorism contingency plans.

The authors suggest that communities assess their level of risk for bioterrorism and develop appropriate contingency planning by using Table 20-2.

Table 20-1 Biological Terrorism Threat Evaluation for an Organization

Points	1. Size of Business	2. Dependence on Human Resources to Perform Mission	3. Location of Business	4. Mission/Production of Business
0 ROW 1	Very small (>20 people)	Very low	Rural area	
0.5 (half a point) ROW 2	Small (21–50 people)	Low	Suburban (Small city >100,000)	Businesses and corporations with international direct customers or suppliers, local government, food services, business and corporations with over $100 million in revenue per year
1 ROW 3	Medium (51–100 people)	Moderate	Small city (>100,000)	Minor electrical and fossil fuel interchanges and hubs/network hubs, biomedical equipment, state government, national finance & banking, emergency services organizations (not deployed)
1.5 (one and a half points) ROW 4	Large (101–500 people)	High	Suburban (Large city)	Moderate electrical and fossil fuel interchanges and hubs/network hubs, medical goods supply, international finance & banking, transportation, military weapons or products, food production, law enforcement, emergency services organizations (deployed), biotechnology
2.5 (two and a half points) ROW 5	Very large (more than 501 people per location)	Very high	Large city	Major electrical and fossil fuel interchanges and hubs/network hubs, pharmaceuticals or vaccine production, mass media, food processing or central storage, healthcare, dental, veterinarian facilities and medical laboratories, mail or delivery services, national level government, armed services

(continues)

Table 20-1 Biological Terrorism Threat Evaluation for an Organization (continued)

Note: For each area (1–4) use the highest point level that approximates your business situation.

Step 1. Determine the size of your organization under #1 and write down corresponding point level;

Step 2. Determine human resource dependency level under # 2 and write down point level;

Step 3. Determine location of organization under # 3 and write down point level;

Step 4. Determine mission/industry under # 4 and write down point level; and

Step 5. Add all points together where 8–10 = high threat, 5–7 = moderate threat, 2–4 = low threat, and <2 = negligible threat; of course more preparation moderates the threat level downward,.

Table 20-3 is prepared for communities and businesses located in those communities as an indicator of approximate threat level related to bioterrorism, and the concomitant need to develop a community-wide Bioterrorism and Infectious Disease Preparedness Plan, a Community Collaboration Plan, an Infection Control Plan, a Post-Exposure Management Plan, a Workforce Education Program, and an Off-site Contingency Plan.

Table 20-2 Bioterrorism Threat Evaluation for a Community—Composite

Points	1. Population of a Defined Geographic Area	2. Industrial–Production Composition of Area	3. Traveler Traffic per Year
0	>50,000	>5% of ROW 4 or 5 in Table 2	>50,000
.34	50,000–99,999	6–9% of ROW 4 or 5 in Table 2	50,000–99,999
1.34	100,000–499,999	10–19% of ROW 4 or 5 in Table 2	100,000–999,999
2.34	500,000–999,999	20–29% of ROW 4 or 5 in Table 2	1,000,000–2,499,999
3.34	<1,000,000	<30% of ROW 4 or 5 in Table 2	<2,500,000

Note: For each area (1–3) use the highest point level that approximates your location's situation.

Step 1. Determine the size of your population under #1 and write down corresponding point level;

Step 2. Determine industrial-production composition level under # 2 and write down point level;

Step 3. Determine traveler traffic in and out of your location under # 3 and write down point level;

Step 4. Add all points together where 8–10 = high threat, 5–7 = moderate threat, 2–4 = low threat, and <2 = negligible threat; of course more preparation moderates the threat level downward.

Table 20-3 Business and Community Preparation Guidance Based on Threat Level			
Business and/or Community- Composite Threat Level Measure	Bioterrorism and Infectious Disease Preparedness Plan (Priority Level)	Community Collaboration Plan with Action Steps and Establishment of Command and Control Authority	Infection Control Plan, Post-Exposure Management Plan, Workforce Education Program, and Off-site Contingency Plan
>2 points	Low	Moderate to low	Moderate to low
2–4 points	Moderate	Moderate to high	Moderate
5–7 points	High	Urgent	High
8–10 points	Urgent	Urgent	Urgent

■ BUSINESS INVOLVEMENT: WHAT SHOULD BE DONE

Business leaders need to take responsibility for addressing concerns about the possibility of bioterrorist activity. Awareness is the key. Leaders should inform all their key stakeholders, from the Board of Directors to the employees, that preventive as well as response policies/programs are under way. This may take place in the form of briefings, in-service workshops, simulations and mock exercises, security enhancements, and coordination with local health facilities. Many businesses will want to develop disaster plans that help victims and their families remain in the information loop or in some cases to evacuate the workplace. If the threat level is high for the organization, a security audit by an outside firm might be in order. Additionally, the human resources department and the business center will need to have business contingency plans and backup systems to deal with business downtime. Some type of communication to the public and customers will also be essential. Additionally, work with your local community, utilizing an assessment system, such as the community preparedness scorecard.[23] There are several "critical success factors" for an organization to consider, and these should include the following:[24]

1. Workforce training (i.e., a well informed workforce)
2. Mitigation of confusion
3. Time management (time is critical)
4. Building a response capacity
5. Economic constraints
6. Coordination with local health agencies
7. Mitigation of fear and panic

Training

Training is essential for all personnel. This could be in the form of aware-ness enhancement or, for businesses at greater risk, actual training in dis-ease detection and early intervention. Additionally, the training of at least one "disaster coordinator" or "health coordinator" would be important. This individual can serve as a resource person, advisor, counselor, and or-ganizer. They also could have the responsibility for staying informed and maintaining contact networks with local health agencies. Ideally, this co-ordinator would receive continuing education through CDC, WHO, ACHE, or some other organization that provides periodic updates on skills and knowledge needed to be effective in this role.

Mitigation of Confusion

Mitigation of confusion is a critical success factor in managing any crisis. The natural tendency of humans in a state of confusion is to panic. If this occurs, more harm can result. Training, preparedness, and prior discus-sion of the range of possibilities and response scenarios all help to miti-gate confusion. Fast, clear communications to all personnel is essential. No one should be left in the dark on these matters. Some organized pro-tocols for testing and prophylaxis will help provide much needed reas-surance that the business cares for its people and is taking appropriate steps. Finally, a key to avoiding confusion is the development of roles and responsibilities that are clearly understood and communicated widely.

Time Management

Time is critical in all matters pertaining to infectious disease. Early signs, early diagnosis, early warning to the non-infected, and early interven-tion all have positive implications for the decreased spread and eventual decreased impact of the disease.

Response Capacity

Response capacity may be in the form of trained personnel, along with needed equipment and proper training. It also includes working with lo-cal health agencies to develop a quick response to a crisis. There are fi-nancial considerations such as cost of training, supplies, equipment, and down time that should be part of the capacity building within the busi-ness. Some might even consider a "bioterrorism crisis reserve" for con-tingency planning.

Mitigation of Fear and Panic

There is no better way to decrease stress and anxiety in anticipation of a possible bioterrorism attack, and likewise no better way to control for panic after an attack, than putting in the requisite time and resources to properly train the workforce and larger community. This should include the design of a disaster-control command center where all communications originate. When there are but a few people directing the response, it tends to minimize panic and maximize effective distribution of information.

■ A PREPAREDNESS PLAN

Address the following areas in the BCP:

- A collaboration plan including area healthcare; public health; veterinary, physician, and medical group practices; and law enforcement with specific preparation action steps (stockpiling appropriate levels of material, training, etc. . . .) and with the local hospital(s) addressing the planning necessities presented in Aimee Stern's "Bioterrorism" in *Hospital & Health Networks* pages 58–60.[25]
- Reporting of incidents and possible incidents and how it will be done.
- Infection control practices and procedures and decontamination procedures.
- A post-exposure management plan for employees (prophylactics and vaccines and a plan to prevent secondary infections).
- An off-site contingency operation plan.
- An education plan (prospective and concurrent to an attack) and a public relations plan.[4]

Components of an Effective Response to Bioterrorism[10]

- Establish protocols for suspicious packages (protocols are at http://fbi.gov).
- Establish a response command and control structure where critical decisions can be made (should be community based).
- Develop and implement a training and awareness program for the workforce and with local healthcare, public health, and law enforcement officials.
- Ensure surveillance systems are in place (LRN, etc. . . . .).
- Implement the business contingency plan.

Cost of Business Involvement

Consider the following when preparing a budget for preparation of a bioterrorism attack, the response sequence, and the recovery phase in the BCP:

- Cost of detection devices
- Cost of personal protection devices such as masks and body covering

- Cost of vaccines and prophylaxis (Cipro, etc. . . .)
- Cost of training: training professionals, resources, and personnel hours
- Cost of constructing evacuation avenues, decontamination sites, and "safe rooms"
- Cost of temporary or permanent loss of business function
- Cost of securing substitute personnel in case of temporary or permanent loss of regular personnel
- Cost of insurance coverage: general liability, health, life, and workers compensation

It is imperative that the business entity's risk manager understands the insurance and coverage implications of each carrier's policies related to bioterrorism. Are there "Acts of War" exclusions, or any other exclusions/ modifiers that proscribe or limit coverage? Will the health and life insurers cover the cost of vaccines or personal protection devices based on the business' level of threat? Planning the insurance aspects of bioterrorism should be taken as seriously as every other phase of disaster preparation.

Sample Forms for Organizational Contingency Planning for Disasters and Terrorism

The following forms (Figures 20-2–20-6) are from www.ready.gov and provide a simple, "get started" approach to thinking in terms of readiness, preparedness, and contingencies.

Open for Business Worksheet

Computer Hardware Inventory

Use this form to:

- Log your computer hardware serial and model numbers. Attach a copy of your vendor documentation to this document.

- Records the name of the company from which you purchased or leased this equipment and the contact name to notify for your computer repairs.

- Record the name of the company that provides repair and support for your computer hardware.

Make additional copies as needed.

Keep one copy of this list in a secure place on your premises and another in an off-site location.

HARDWARE INVENTORY LIST

Hardware (CPU, Monitor, Printer, Keyboard, Mouse)	Hardware Size, RAM & CPU Capacity	Model Purchased	Serial Number	Date Purchased	Cost

Figure 20-2 Open for Business Worksheet.

Emergency Supplies
Talk to your co-workers about what emergency supplies the company can feasibly
provide, if any, and which ones individuals should consider keeping on hand.
Recommended emergency supplies include the following:

Water: amounts for portable kits will vary. Individuals should determine what amount they are able to both store comfortably and to transport to other locations. If it is feasible, store one gallon of water per person per day, for drinking and sanitation.
Food: at least a three-day supply of non-perishable food
Battery-powered radio and **extra batteries**
Flashlight and **extra batteries**
First Aid kit
Whistle to signal for help
Dust or filter masks, readily available in hardware stores, which are rated based on how small a particle they filter
Moist towelettes for sanitation
Wrench or **pliers** to turn off utilities
Can opener for food (if kit contains canned food)
Plastic sheeting and **duct tape** to "seal the room"
Garbage bags and **plastic ties** for personal sanitation

Figure 20-3 Emergency Supplies.

The following will give you an idea of what it may cost to develop a disaster protection and business continuity plan. Some of what is recommended can be done at little or no cost. Use this list to get started and then consider what else can be done to protect your people and prepare your business.

No Cost

- Meet with your insurance provider to review current coverage.
- Create procedures to quickly evacuate and shelter-in-place. Practice the plans.
- Talk to your people about the compan's disaster plans. Two-way communication is central before, during and after a disaster.
- Create an emergency contact list, include employee emergency contact information.
- Create a list of critical business contractors and others whom you will use in an emergency.
- Know what kinds of emergencies might affect your company both internally and externally.
- Decide in advance what you will do if your building is unusable.
- Create a list of inventory and equipment, including computer hardware, software peripherals, for insurance purposes.
- Talk to utility service providers about potential alternatives and identify backup options.
- Promote family and individual preparedness among your co-workers. Include emergency preparedness information during staff meetings, in newsletters, on company intranet, periodic employee emails and other internal communications tools.

Under $500

- Buy a fire extinguisher and smoke alarm.
- Decide which emergency supplies the company can feasibly provide, if any, and talk to your co-workers about what supplies individuals might want to consider keeping in a personal and portable supply kit.
- Set up a telephone call tree, password-protected page on the company website, an email alert or a call-in voice recording to communicate with employees in an emergency.
- Provide first aid and CPR training to key co-workers.
- Use and keep up-to-date computer anti-virus software and firewalls.
- Attach equipment and cabinets to walls or other stable equipment. Place heavy or breakable objects on low shelves.
- Elevat valuable inventory and electric machinery off the floor in case of flooding.
- If applicable, make sure your building's HVAC system is working properly and well-maintained.
- Back up your records and critical data. Keep a copy offsite.

More than $500

- Consider additional insurance such as business interruption, flood or earthquake.
- Purchase, install and pre-wire a generator to the building's essential electrical circuits. Provide for other utility alternatives and backup options.
- Install automatic sprinkler systems, fire hoses and fire-resistant doors and walls.
- Make sure your building meets standards and codes. Consider a professional engineer to evaluate the wind, fire or seismic resistance of your building.
- Consider a security professional to evaluate and/or creae your disaster preparedness and business continuity plan.
- Upgrade your building's HVAC system to secure outdoor air intakes and increase filter efficiency.
- Send safety and key emergency response employees to trainings or conferences.
- Provide a large group of employees with first aid and CPR training.

Figure 20-4 Cost of Developing a Disaster Protection and Business Continuity Plan.

Open for Business Worksheet

Insurance Coverage Discussion Form

Use this form to discuss your insurance coverage with your agent. Having adequate coverage now will help you recover more rapidly from a catastrophe.

Insurance Agent: _____

Address: _____

Phone: _____ Fax: _____ Email: _____

INSURANCE POLICY INFORMATION

Types of Insurance	Policy No.	Deductibles	Policy Limits	Coverage (General Description)

Do you need Flood Insurance?   Yes _____ No _____

Do you need Earthquake Insurance?   Yes _____ No _____

Do you need Business Income and Extra Expense Insurance?   Yes _____ No _____

Other disaster-related insurance questions:

_____

_____

_____

_____

Figure 20-5 Open for Business Worksheet.

Sample Business Continuity and Disaster Preparedness Plan

❏ PLAN TO STAY IN BUSINESS	If this location is not accessible we will operate from the location below:
Business Name	
Address	Business Name
City, State	Address
Telephone Number	City, State
The following person is our primary crisis manager and will serve as the company sokesperson in an emergency.	Telephone Number
	If the person is unable to manage the crisis, the person below will succeed in management:
Primary Emergency Contact	
Telephone Number	Secondary Emergency Contact
Alternative Number	Telephone Number
Email	Alternative Number
❏ EMERGENCY CONTACT INFORMATION	Email
Dial 9-1-1 in an Emergency	
Non-Emergency Police/Fire	
Insurance Provider	

Figure 20-6   Sample Business Continuity and Disaster Preparedness Plan.

■ CHAPTER SUMMARY

The threat of natural or terrorism disasters having a negative impact on business is perhaps greater today than ever before. The integration of the BCP into the strategic plan of the company can add real value by aligning all the key departments and staff around company issues associated with disaster preparedness. The threat of biological weapons is more real in today's society due to the limited cost of their production, the availability of the production knowledge through the Internet and other sources, and their ease of dissemination once produced. All businesses should evaluate their threat level based on the nature of their business, their size, and the community in which they are located.

For prompt and better response to disasters of such nature, the BCP has to identify collaboration with the local, county, state, and/or federal agencies and healthcare providers in the business area to understand what their capabilities are in handling such attacks. For the organization's BCP to be successful, it should include workforce training, mitigation of confusion, timely identification of the event, building a response capacity, coordination with local health agencies, and mitigation of panic using the command control center where all communications are coordinated.

References

1. Homeland Security Act of 2002.
2. Ledlow G, Johnson J, Cwiek M. Bioterrorism and business: Think globally, act locally. In Delener N, Chao C. (eds.) *Global Business and Technology Association International Conference; Beyond Boundaries: Challenges of Leadership, Innovation, Integration and Technology.* 683–693; 2002.
3. Breithaupt H. Toxins for terrorists: Do scientists act illegally when sending out potentially dangerous material? *EMBO Reports.* 2000;1(4):298–301.
4. Leach DL, Ryman DG. Biological weapons: Preparing for the worst. *MLO Med Lab Obs.* 2000;32(9):26.
5. Dennis C. The bugs of war. *Nature.* 2001; 411(6835):232–235.
6. Kortepeter MG, Cieslak TJ, Eitzen EM. Bioterrorism. *J Environ Health.* 2001;63(6):21.
7. Sandström G. A Swedish/European view of bioterrorism. *Ann N Y Acad Sci.* 2000;916(1):112–116.
8. Henderson DA. (2000). Bioterrorism. *Int J Clin Pract.* 2000;115 Supplement 115:32–36.
9. Hagstad D, Kearney K. Bioterrorism: Reacting promptly and appropriately to a highly infectious, invisible agent. *Am J Nurs.* 2000;100(12);33.
10. Canada Communicable Disease Report (IM). General Collection. 2001;27(4), February 15, 2001-02- 28 10:19:14, ISSN: 1188-4169.
11. Geiger HJ. Terrorism, biological weapons, and bonanzas: Assessing the real threat to public health. *Am J Public Health.* 2001;91(5):708.
12. Lawler A. The unthinkable becomes real for a horrified world. *Science.* 2001;293 Sept 21:2182–2185.

13. Fraser MR, Brown DL. Bioterrorism preparedness and local public health agencies: Building response capacity. *Public Health Rep.* 2000;115(4):326–330.

14. Johnson J, Ledlow G, Cwiek M. *Community Preparedness and Response to Terrorism* (A three volume series). Westport, CT: Praeger/Greenwood Publishers; 2005.

15. Ledlow G, Jones W, Johnson J. *Community Preparedness and Response to Terrorism: Governmental Collaboration and the Community Model.* Westport, CT: Praeger/Greenwood Publishers. Vol 1; 2005.

16. Jortani SA, Snyder JW, Valdes R Jr. The role of the clinical laboratory in managing chemical or biological terrorism. *Clin Chem.* 2000;46(12):1883–1893.

17. Fauci AS. Infectious diseases: Considerations for the 21st Century. *Clin Infect Dis.* 2001;32(5):675.

18. McLaughlin S. Thinking about the unthinkable: Where to start planning for terrorism incidents. *Health Facil Manage.* 2001;14(7):26–30.

19. Simon JD. Nuclear, biological and chemical terrorism: Understanding the threat and designing responses. *Int J Emerg Ment Health.* 1999;1(2):81–89.

20. Wetter DC, Daniell WE, Treser CD. Hospital preparedness for victims of chemical or biological terrorism. *Am J Public Health.* 2001;91(5):710–716.

21. Chyung SY, Strepich D, Cox D. Building a competency-based curriculum architecture to educate 21st-centruy business practitioners. *Journal of Education of Business.* 2006;81(6):307.

22. Gauthier G, Palacios C, Kitchens J, Coppola MN. *Executive Companies in Health Education*, Army-Baylor Program, Fort Sam Houston, TX (unpublished); 2007.

23. Contact Dr. Gerald R. Ledlow at gledlow@georgiasouthern.edu for more information.

24. Friesen M, Johnson J. *The Success Paradigm.* London: Quorum Books; 1995.

25. Harner A. Will you be ready when your patients need you most? *MGMA Connexion.* 2001;1(3):40–41.

CHAPTER

21

Organization Development and the Future

James A. Johnson

Learning Objectives

- To better understand the theory and practice of organization development.
- To better value the philosophy of organization development in a changing world.
- To identify critical foci for organization development in the future.

■ INTRODUCTION

We are imbedded in an era of major social and cultural change with many challenges compelling us to manage health organizations with greater efficiency, effectiveness, and value.[1,2] Many believe we are engaged in the refinement of the best healthcare system in the world and others foresee that we are on the verge of a major reinvention that leads to universal care for all. If this is so, then we will need new knowledge, tools, skills, technology, policies, and particularly new perspectives. With exponential increases in information, interconnectivity, technological breakthroughs, and scientific discovery, there must be an unwavering commitment to life-long learning and a healthy embrace of change.

Healthcare organizations are fundamentally dependent upon people and require an extensive range of roles to accomplish their tasks and goals.[2] The process of leading and managing complex organizations, considering the scope and scale of healthcare delivery, can be daunting. In the leading and managing of healthcare organizations, organizational development, closely tied to organizational purpose, mission, vision, culture, and strategy, becomes a "critical success factor."[2,3,4]

■ DEVELOPMENT PRACTICE AND PHILOSOPHY

Organizational development involves assessment of the culture, training and learning needs, and human dynamics across the organization. Thus, health organizations need to manage knowledge appropriately and create a culture that enables the organization to learn continuously. Organizational purpose, mission, vision, culture, and strategies inform organizational development plans, and those drive group and individual learning and change opportunities. Managing organizational knowledge and fostering organizational learning are a necessity in the fast-paced information and bio-information world of healthcare.[2]

Organization development (OD) is a preferred approach in a growing number of organizations to dealing with change.[1] The processes of OD are designed to improve the ability of an organization to deal with changes in its environment as well as internal changes in an effective way that also meets the needs of its members. Organization development, more than most approaches, has demonstrated considerable success in working through the natural resistance to change we see in organizations. This is in part due to the way OD empowers participants in the change process with understanding and a commitment to the desired change. It embraces a philosophy of participation, mutuality, and the value of knowledge at all levels of the organization. At the core of any OD effort will be the involvement of employees in developing a commitment to change. This occurs for the following reasons:

- They are intimately familiar with the current system and can make valuable contributions to the change effort, increasing its chances of success.
- They become knowledgeable about what will happen as a result of the change, reducing fear of the unknown.
- They are acting in a way that is supportive of the change by being a part of the process and their beliefs about the change become more positive.

An excellent resource for further information on OD is the Organization Development Institute with its international network of practitioners and information dissemination.[5]

■ DEVELOPMENT IN A CHANGING WORLD

Change is inevitable and development really is not an option but a necessity. Planned change and the managing of change are critical to organizational survival and success.

There are key foci, or what Johnson and others have called "critical success factors" that will gain increasing attention in the coming decades.[3,6]

Values Renewal

As futurist Ian Morrison asserts, "Health care is in need of renewal, reinvigoration, and leadership."[7] We desperately need creativity and innovation, on the one hand, and pragmatic long-overdue execution of well-established ideas, on the other. All healthcare systems are the products of the culture and thus an organizational embodiment of societal values. Morrison identifies these core values in U.S. society as pluralism and choice, individual accountability, ambivalence toward government, innovation, volunteerism, anti-monopoly, and competition. The manager is often faced with difficult decisions that are opposed to or consistent with these values. Some organizations even conduct a values audit to ascertain their own core values. Others establish a "values statement" that is co-equal to their mission statement. There is also an emerging trend toward values alignment for organizations to assure they are doing what they say they are and the initiatives and programs are aligned with all stakeholders.

Creating Sustainable Organizations

Health organizations have been slower than other organizations in the business sector to adopt principles and practices of sustainability. This approach embraces the "triple bottom line," which means a co-equal focus on: (1) financial viability, (2) social responsiveness, and (3) environmental responsibility. Healthcare organizations have become increasingly adept at managing finances and their missions tend to be socially responsible in their communities, yet when it comes to environmental practices they are quite dismal. There are few examples of "green hospitals" trying to reduce their environmental impact through energy conservation. This will have to change as society expects more and as we begin to see the value of operating from the triple bottom line.

Managing Workforce Complexity and Globalization

With advances in transportation and international commerce, we see an ever-shrinking world. In fact, the term "global village" is widely used, as we perceive the interconnectedness of today's diverse societies and organizations. With globalization, new challenges emerge. Recent examples include infectious diseases like the HIV pandemic and emerging threats such as the Avian Flu and West Nile Virus. Also, there continues to be the threat of terrorism and the possibility of economic upheaval.

Globalization also brings with it more immigration and thus a changing workforce. There is increasing workforce complexity. U.S. demographics have dramatically shifted with the increased number of Hispanics and Asians entering the labor pool. Many bring education and skills that can be useful in health organizations. Additionally, healthcare delivery must be culturally sensitive to be effective in reaching these various populations.

In addition to a more globalized workforce and patient population there is an increasing intergenerational demographic. For the first time in history, there are four generations in the workforce. Although this is an exciting time, it is not without challenges. Working with the generations requires patience and understanding. Each generation brings a new perspective, but we need to learn to value the new ideas, and embrace the change that each new generation brings. Thus, the healthcare manager must help the organization adapt to a more diverse workforce as well as more diversity in the populations being served.

Disaster Preparedness and Crisis Management

With the possibility of natural disaster always present and man-made ones such as terrorism looming in our collective psyche, it is imperative for all organizations to focus on community and organizational preparedness. Additionally, organization development, education, and training are necessary, as are inter-organizational exercises and partnerships.

A successful, comprehensive emergency management program of preparedness, response, and recovery will help the organization through what could be its most difficult challenge. The manager will be center stage during these trying times and can expect to be pulled in many directions by board members, clients, employees, and their own families. If ever there is a time for multi-tasking, this will be it. However, those managers who have an organization-specific plan will do much better. As we all know, a plan is only as good as its implementation. There will be a need to modify decisions on the ground and to adjust accordingly. This is a kind of organizational improvisation that will call upon all the skills and knowledge addressed in the previous chapters.[9]

■ CHAPTER SUMMARY

The world is changing so fast that organizations and individuals who do not change quickly will become less and less effective. Managers and leaders of health organizations in the 21st century will have to anticipate change and create change. They will need to be grounded in organization theory, must be keen observers of organization behavior, and must have the skills and values needed to engage effectively in organization development.

Review/Discussion Questions

1. Identify the core reasons for involving employees in any change process. What happens when you do not?
2. Is organization development a philosophy or a practice process? Is it both?
3. Discuss each of the four future foci (values, sustainability, globalization, and preparedness). What current events in the world portend the necessity for addressing these in health organizations?

Learning Activities

1. Watch the film "An Inconvenient Truth" and discuss in class the many implications for health, health organizations, and planned change.
2. Visit the website of the World Health Organization, http://www.who.int, and identify four global health challenges. Discuss how health organizations might address these global health challenges.
3. Visit the website of the Sustainability Institute (http://www.sustain abilityinstitute.org), and discuss ways in which hospitals and other health organizations can adopt sustainability practices and values.

References

1. Kilpatrick AO, Johnson JA. *Handbook of Health Administration and Policy.* New York: Marcel-Dekker; 1999.
2. Johnson JA, Ledlow GR, Kerr BJ. Organizational development, training, and knowledge management. In Fried B, Johnson JA, Fottler M. *Human Resources in Healthcare: Managing for Success* (2nd ed.). Chicago, IL: Health Administration Press; 2005.
3. Friesen M, Johnson JA. *The Success Paradigm.* Westport, CT: Quorum; 1995.
4. McIlwain T, Johnson JA. Strategy: planning, management, and critical success factors. In Kilpatrick AO, Johnson JA. *Handbook of Health Administration and Policy.* New York: Marcel-Dekker; 1999.
5. Cole D. *Organization Development Institute.* 2007. Accessed May 6, 2007, from http://www.odinstitute.org
6. Johnson JA, Breckon DJ. *Managing Health Education and Promotion Programs: Leadership Skills for the 21st Century.* Sudbury, MA: Jones and Bartlett; 2006.
7. Morrison I. *Health Care in the New Millennium: Vision, Values, and Leadership.* San Francisco, CA: Jossey-Bass; 2000.
8. Johnson JA, Kennedy M, Delener N. *Community Preparedness and Response to Terrorism: The Role of Community Organizations and Business.* Westport, CT: Praeger; 2005.
9. Johnson JA. Johnson JA. Community preparedness and response: The Katrina experience. *Social Science Perspectives Journal.* 2006;33(1):20–27.

INDEX